Corrective Exercise Solutions to Common Hip and Shoulder Dysfunction

Evan Osar

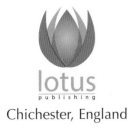

lotus
publishing

Chichester, England

First published in 2012 and reprinted with corrections in 2014 by
Lotus Publishing
Apple Tree Cottage, Inlands Road, Nutbourne, Chichester, PO18 8RJ

Illustrations Amanda Williams
Photographs John Eatinger
Text Design Simon Hempsell
Cover Design Paula Morrison
Printed and Bound in the UK by Bell and Bain Ltd

Disclaimer
The information contained herein is not intended to be a substitute for professional medical advice, diagnosis, or treatment in any manner. Always seek the advice of your physician or other qualified health provider with any questions you may have regarding any medical condition or before engaging in any physical fitness plan.

British Library Cataloguing-in-Publication Data
A CIP record for this book is available from the British Library
ISBN 978 1 905367 26 9

Library of Congress Cataloguing-in-Publication Data
Osar, Evan, 1969-
The integrated movement system : a corrective exercise approach to common hip and shoulder dysfunctions / Evan Osar.
    p. ; cm.
Includes index.
ISBN 978 1 905367 26 9
I. Title.
[DNLM: 1. Shoulder Joint--physiopathology. 2. Exercise Therapy--methods. 3. Hip Joint--physiopathology. 4. Joint Diseases--therapy. 5. Movement. WE 810]

617.5'8106--dc23
2011042904

CONTENTS

ACKNOWLEDGEMENTS

Anyone who has undertaken the task of writing a book or performing any activity that takes several intense months of dedicated effort understands the challenges, mental gymnastics, frustrations, and elations that are part of the inevitable journey towards the task's completion. And they also understand the special individuals behind the scenes, who often remain anonymous yet are instrumental in the successful completion of the task.

First, I would like to thank Jonathan Hutchings and Lotus Publishing for giving me the opportunity and the creative freedom to produce something that I hope will benefit the industry. An author could not ask for an easier individual and publishing company to work with.

A special thanks also goes out to my friend and colleague Laree Draper. I appreciate all the support from her and her husband, Dave.

To the multitudes of mentors and industry giants who have taught, inspired, and motivated me to continue to learn and grow, I am forever grateful. Although too many to mention, several stand out for the particular role they played in my evolution as a movement specialist.

Linda-Joy Lee is one of the kindest and brightest minds in the field of rehabilitation. Her passion for learning, teaching, and sharing her corrective treatment and exercise strategies have helped me understand the importance and intricacies of cuing and kinesthetic awareness in changing an individual's motor control system. My techniques and observation skills have been improved by studying extensively over the years with LJ.

Dr. Pavel Kolar has contributed greatly to our understanding of stabilization, and his techniques and strategies for developing dynamic neuromuscular stabilization are on the cutting edge of rehabilitative and movement re-education. Dr. Kolar, and his assistants Alena Kobesova, MD, PhD, Martina Jezkova, PT, and Zuzana Suzan, PT, are some of the humblest individuals in this field; I would like to thank each of them for their contribution to my knowledge. Dr. Kolar's work on dynamic neuromuscular stabilization has been a great influence in the development of the corrective exercise strategies contained in this book.

The late Vladimir Janda has possibly contributed more to our understanding of muscle inhibition, muscle imbalances, and the role of the nervous system in the development of movement patterns than perhaps any other individual. While he is missed, his work will live on in all of us who continue to be the beneficiaries of his contributions.

Shirley Sahrmann is one of the pioneers of utilizing corrective exercise as a means of improving movement patterns. Her work inspired me from the beginning of my career and her influences can be seen throughout this book.

The late Drs. George Goodheart and Alan Beardall completely changed the face of the chiropractic profession with their contributions to understanding muscle inhibition and detection through precision muscle testing. The collective contribution of Dr. Goodheart's *Applied Kinesiology* and Dr. Beardall's

Clinical Kinesiology has forever changed the way clients with muscle inhibition and movement dysfunctions are evaluated and treated.

Robert Lardner and Ed Flaherty are two of the finest physical therapists I have had the pleasure of working with and are equally great individuals. Both men selflessly share their passion and knowledge, and my patients are the beneficiaries of their collective knowledge. I am fortunate to know these men both as professional colleagues and as friends.

To *Integrative Movement Specialists™* Teams I, II and III: each of you has made a decision and dedicated the time and energy to advance your training to better serve your clients. Thank you for letting me be part of your journey. Keep empowering and educating the world to the importance of proper movement. Together, we can change the world.

When it comes to corrective exercise and improving movement patterns, Gray Cook is at the top of the industry. It has been said that genius is the process of making complex topics simple to understand and Gray has a knack for doing just that. Mike Boyle is one of the greatest strength and conditioning coaches in the industry. He continues to learn and grow, which demonstrates his passion and dedication to his craft. He is one of the few individuals within the health and fitness industry who is humble enough to admit when he makes mistakes and does not let his ego get in the way of being open to new ideas. These two men motivate and inspire the fitness industry by selflessly sharing both their wisdom and their experience.

I would like to extend a special note of gratitude to the following individuals:

Models: Steven Schmoldt, ACE-CPT, IMS, and Melissa Posh – thank you for your friendship and support on this project.

Facility: Core Fitness Chicago – thank you for the use of the facility during the photo shoot.

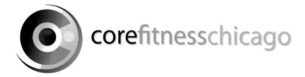

Finally, a special thank you to my beautiful wife, Jenice. You allow me the space, provide the encouragement, and challenge me to be the best that I can be. I thank you for empowering me everyday to be the change I want to see in the world.

DEDICATION

This book is dedicated to all my clients and patients who allow me the privilege and honor to serve them and learn from our experiences together.

INTRODUCTION

This book has not been written to make you agree with the concepts contained within. It has not been written to say that this is the gospel way of doing things. And it most certainly is not written to say that this is the way it will always be. It also is in no way saying that this approach works one hundred percent of the time for one hundred percent of the individuals you will interact with in your profession. This book was written for one and only one purpose: to make you think. If reading this book makes you stop and think, if it raises questions, or if it challenges your thought process, then I have done my job.

With the plethora of great resources that are available to the fitness and health care professional, what makes this book so different from others of a similar topic? This simple but profound quote by James Dyson, the founder of the vacuum manufacturer Dyson, sums it up nicely – "We fix the obvious problems others seem to ignore." This powerful statement resonates because as a movement specialist I am constantly working to find the absolute best solution for the movement dysfunctions of my clients and patients, by addressing the obvious movement faults that other therapists and trainers have ignored.

What are the obvious things that our colleagues tend to ignore?

1. **Breathing:** Too many of our colleagues assume that, just because a client or patient presents to us and is breathing, they are using a correct strategy. Studies on individuals with chronic pain, anxiety disorders, and respiratory challenges including asthma, allergies, and chronic obstructive pulmonary disease (COPD) demonstrate that these individuals often experience alterations in their breathing strategies. How many of our clients fit into one of these categories? At a rough estimation, I would guess 75% of them, and they represent the clients and patients who have the most difficult time adopting proper breathing habits, because they underestimate, as I once did, the global improvements in health that result from achieving more ideal respiratory patterns.

2. **Appropriate progressions:** In our haste to get clients to perform the 'sexy' exercises that we (and they) think they need to accomplish their goals of playing sport, losing weight, or performing their job, we allow them to perform exercises that are too demanding for their current level of conditioning. Why? With the explosion of the Internet and mass media (DVDs, cable programming, and infomercials), our clients and patients have never had more access to information and so many 'experts' who seem to have the magic cure for weight loss, solutions to solving pain, and strategies for making them look and perform like a professional athlete. They come in with their expectations and reality television success stories, expecting us to deliver similar results. Unfortunately, they only see the success stories (through no fault of their own as the 'experts' like to keep their failures hidden from the general public) and don't hear about the many individuals who were unable to complete the program due to pain, fatigue, or functional limitations, or who were not helped by the magic cure. Individuals in the last groups are the ones who generally seek the services of a chiropractic physician, physical therapist, or fitness professional.

3. **Education, empathy and empowerment:** I used to think my job as a chiropractic physician was to solve every patient's problems and get them out of pain – if I failed to do this, then I had failed them. As a conditioning specialist I thought my job was to help my clients get into the best shape of their lives, achieve the body of their dreams, and enable them to do any recreational activity

of their choice – and if I failed to do this, then I was a failure. So, while I was able to help quite a few patients and clients in my early years, I never felt like it was enough and that I was actually failing as a practitioner. Seeking solutions, I attended innumerous conferences and observed my colleagues for countless hours, only to become more discouraged as many of them expounded on all their success stories. However, it slowly became evident to me that a lot of these 'experts' would only speak of their successes, while, as I observed many of them, I would witness faulty movement patterns in their clients and patients. Over the years, as I made my way around the lecture circuit, both as an observer and as a presenter, I realized that the majority of top presenters, in the fitness industry especially, worked with high level athletes – those rare individuals who succeed at the college and professional level. It became shockingly apparent to me, albeit over the course of several years, that while relatively few coaches and trainers work with high level athletes they are the ones setting the parameters for training and conditioning. That is not necessarily problematic except when you consider that most of us in the fitness industry fields of rehabilitation don't work with athletes. In fact, although many of our clients may participate in recreational activities, our clients are anything but athletic, yet, much to their detriment, we have been encouraging them to adopt the training programs and strategies of the higher level athletes. They don't have the genetics, the motor control, the training habits, the mental aptitude, or the recuperative habits of the professional athlete – just some of the training habits. It is not hard to guess what happened and is happening to the general population at an alarming rate – increasing cases of repetitive injuries, a rise in the number of pain and anti-inflammatory medication prescriptions, and more and more cases of degeneration, chronic pain, and fatigue.

As our society moves further from ideal health and well-being, overwhelmed by physical, emotional, and financial stressors, I can now clearly see what our role is in this industry, as well as what our role is for our patients and clients. Our responsibilities are threefold:

i. **Educate:** to help clients and patients understand what constitutes health and what is and is not appropriate for them in terms of exercise, movement, and adjunctive therapy (medications, surgery, other therapies), based solely upon their individual needs and wants.

ii. **Empathy:** to meet clients and patients where they are at, without judgment or ego and let them know we are here to help.

iii. **Empower:** to make a difference in their lives by being a positive influence, by listening, by encouraging them, and by providing solutions through working either with us with someone else who is better suited to meet their needs and wants.

In no way am I suggesting that clients should spend 60 minutes lying on a table, breathing and meditating themselves into shape or out of pain (although this approach may also hold some validity), in lieu of resistance training. What I am saying is that if we as fitness and health care professionals are to accept the liberty of working with clients and patients, then we must also assume the responsibilities that come with the job: the responsibility of assessing and marrying their needs and wants; the responsibility of empowering them every time we interact with them; and the responsibility of being the solution to the health care crisis that our clients and patients need and want.

IT'S ALL ABOUT THE PRINCIPLES

"As to methods there may be a million and then some, but principles are few. The man who grasps principles can successfully select his own methods. The man who tries methods, ignoring principles, is sure to have trouble." (Ralph Waldo Emerson)

As previously stated above, if we want to become the solution to the health care crisis, then we have to become the change we want to see. How we create that change begins by understanding the principles of human movement. While there are many methods, there are only three simple principles that apply to the rehabilitation, training, and/or conditioning of the human movement system.

The principles are: improve respiration, achieve optimal joint centration, and integrate these activities into fundamental movement patterns. What does this mean? Simply that:

1. Respiration must be optimized, and this activity must be coordinated with activation of the deep stabilizers.

2. There must be optimal joint centration.

3. Respiration and centration must be integrated and incorporated into fundamental movement patterns.

While these principles may seem overly simplistic, as B.J. Palmer, son of the founder of the field of chiropractic D.D. Palmer, used to say, "Great principles like great men are simple." These principles are paramount to function of the human movement system, and the lack of or deficiency in any one of the three principles will lead to movement dysfunction.

Did you notice that nothing was said about any particular method of achieving the three principles? There was no mention of Pilates, although Pilates incorporates all three principles. There was no mention of yoga, although each of the three principles can easily be seen in the practice of yoga. And there was no mention of functional training, CrossFit, sport-specific training, the Barre Method, the Dailey Method, kettlebells, or any of the over one hundred different types of exercise methods that have come and will undoubtedly keep coming over the next few years. Why is this? Simple – they are all methods – nothing more than different methods of getting the individual to accomplish their functional goals.

One question is sure to arise as you read this, because it always does whenever I present this concept at my internships and workshops. Which is the best method for me to use with my clients to accomplish these principles? To that I answer simply – "It depends." While this answer always frustrates the questioner, it does need some clarification. It depends largely upon what the functional goals of your client are, what level your client is currently at, what their health history is, and most importantly, how effective the trainer or therapist is at adapting and using their method while applying the principles. I think all of us can agree that Pilates and CrossFit are at far different ends of the training spectrum. And there are very few similarities between the Barre Method and kettlebell training. However, don't people get better from performing Pilates, CrossFit, and functional training (by better I am referring to the client's definition of better, which includes feelings of increased strength, improved body aesthetics, and/or overall sense of feeling better)? The answer is resoundingly – yes. So which is the best method for your client? I will answer it this way. The value and effectiveness of your method is only proportional to the ability of that method to accomplish the three principles while simultaneously reducing the client's risk of injuring themselves. If your method does this, then it is the best method to use with the client. Please note that I did not say injury prevention, as it is impossible to prevent all injuries. However, the goal is always to reduce the client's risk by teaching them how to breathe better, improve their ability to centrate, and perform fundamental movement patterns.

This book is not about my method or anyone else's methods. It is all about integrating the concepts and principles into your current routine to enable your patients and clients to accomplish their functional goals while reducing their risk of injury. If you accomplish these goals, then your method works and you have succeeded as a true testament of the word 'professional'. I hope that this book can serve you well in your education in the understanding and application of improving and/or enhancing functional movement.

I only have one small request as you read this book and that is you keep an open mind. As Malcolm Forbes once stated, "Education's purpose is to replace an empty mind with an open one." And so it is with this thought in mind that I offer this book as a resource to you.

THE PROBLEM

"Nothing is more revealing than movement." (Martha Graham)

The prime focus of this book is to present strategies and techniques that can be utilized to improve human movement. Why the focus on movement? Let's consider some statistics:

- The United States spends approximately $2.1 trillion on health care each year or 16% of its gross domestic product. This is, by far, greater than any of the other developed countries, yet the United States ranks 50th out of 224 countries in life expectancy.

- Americans spend approximately $216 billion on prescription medications every year – a large majority of this cost is related to treating musculoskeletal symptoms.

- Arthritis and other musculoskeletal conditions are cited as the most common causes of chronic disabilities in working age adults. While there are only approximately 18 cases out of every 1,000 persons between the ages of 18 and 44, the number of individuals experiencing these conditions rises remarkably to 56 between the ages of 45 and 54, and to 99 for those between the ages of 55 and 64.

- There are nearly 157 million visits to doctor's offices for musculoskeletal conditions at a cost of $215 billion per year.

- The obesity rate for individuals between 18 and 64 years of age has more than doubled in the period 1971 to 2005.

And if you think this epidemic is limited to just adults, check out these statistics on the state of the health of our children:

- Nearly half of all injuries in children participating in sports are the direct result of overuse, and the majority of these occurred not while they were playing their sport but rather while they were at practice.

- According to the National Electronic Injury Surveillance System for the year 2001, there were approximately 14,000 injuries related to football. While this makes sense because of the aggressive and contact-nature of the sport, there were almost 700,000 injuries in basketball.

- There has been a 150% increase in physical education class injuries between the years of 1997 and 2007, with most of these being sprain/strain-type injuries.

- Nearly one-third of children are obese.

It is rather safe to conclude that there is something fundamentally wrong with our movement system and these statistics just begin to tell the story of our current state of dysfunction. Our society is moving from production and manufacturing that was representative of the United States economy at the turn of the 20th century, to a predominantly service-driven economy in the 21st century that is characterized by more time sitting in front of a computer, in meetings, or on the phone. Coupled with increasing technology and automation that further limits how much we need to move, together with a nutrient-depleted, overly processed, and genetically-modified diet, this creates a human architecture that is far from capable of handling any increases in demands that may be imposed upon it. An example of this is the approximately 200,000 non-contact anterior cruciate ligament injuries that occur every year in the United States. Many of these are in non-athletic individuals and occur as a result of stepping off a curb, across an uneven surface while playing their weekend sport, or while walking and suddenly changing directions. A client who sits on their way to work, sits at work, sits on their way home from work, and then sits once they get home will be ill-equipped to deal with any changes in their center of gravity or momentum, or with situations that demand them to react dynamically, like their weekend golf or softball games. They are also likely not to have consumed a well-rounded, nutrient-dense diet that would provide them the ground substance to develop, regenerate, and optimize the function of the connective tissues of their body, making them more susceptible to decreases in performance and to increases in the likelihood of developing illness or injury. And these individuals in all likelihood will not have sleep patterns that are conducive to proper recuperation and will have a stress level that is out of alignment with their ability to manage their stress, adding further stresses to an already overwhelmed system. It is not hard to see why this individual will suffer from non-contact injuries as well as any of the common overuse injuries that plague modern society.

These are the individuals who most often present to the fitness professional for their services. Unfortunately, rather than being the solution that these clients need in order to effectively and appropriately deal with common musculoskeletal issues, the fitness industry often becomes a part of the problem. Individuals are told by their health care professionals to just go and exercise, to strengthen their 'weak' back or knees, or to simply move and that will make them better. They are further encouraged by commercials that urge them to just 'do it' and train harder, and operate under the premise of 'if there is no pain, there is no gain.'

As mentioned in the introduction, training the general population the same way as professional athletes and/or military personnel presents several challenges. Remember, the individuals who the professional conditioning coach works with are a rather homogenous population. They are between the ages of 18 and 35 – recall that the rate of arthritis and musculoskeletal pain increases three to five times between the ages of 44 and 65. They have made it to a high or professional level of performance and represent the 1% of the population with the genetics, skill set, recuperation, and training that enables them to perform at that level. They have above-average recuperative rates, meaning that they can take more stress than the average person before breaking down. And they have greater access to health professionals such as chiropractic physicians, massage therapists, and athletic trainers, as well as therapeutic modalities such as whirlpools, ice baths, ultrasound, and electronic muscle stimulation. They often receive treatments every single day and more often than that if they are injured.

Our clients receive treatment once or twice a week at best and possibly do some self-care, hardly equating to the amount that the athlete receives. Sleeping habits are likely different as our clients and patients rarely report receiving 7–8 hours of quality sleep per night. If an individual has the ability to make it to a high level in dance, athletics, or military service, they are in the select minority of motor skill proficiency, notwithstanding the amount of training and coaching that went into the effort. They often have access to better coaches and spend more collective time working on their skills. Many general population clients just assume their body will function the way they want. Very few athletes get to the highest levels without dedicating significant time, energy, and attention on their craft. This leaves us with a very significant challenge as we work with the general population clientele.

THE CHALLENGE

In his book *How the Mighty Fall*, author Jim Collins discusses cancer and how it is harder to detect in the early stages but easier to treat, and how it reverses in the advanced stages, where it is easier to detect but much harder to treat. A similar analogy can be made about movement patterns – it is much harder to detect the subtleties of compensatory movement in the early stages although easier to correct them, and much easier to detect errors in chronic movement dysfunction however they are much more difficult to change.

What makes movement patterns so challenging to correct in the later stages than in the earlier stages? And what makes our clients' movement so dysfunctional in the first place? It is important to ask these questions as they are at the beginning of the journey to understand the marvels and complexities of the human body as well as provide a framework for both the correction and education processes that will help a client return to function. Too often clients are told that there is nothing that can be done outside of medication or surgery, or worse that the pain and/or limitations in movement are all in their head. Unfortunately, for all the advances in medical technology, there are no fewer incidences of movement dysfunction; however, there has been a greater confidence in syndrome and conditional diagnoses because they are now proven by advancements in imaging techniques.

Part of the issue with this disconnect is the fact that there are no medical machines or blood tests that 'test' to prove movement dysfunction. The best that these tests can prove is either there is or there is not pathology within the given region, meaning muscle inhibition cannot be seen in any test based on medical standards. Poor stabilization in a single leg stand does not register in any standardized equipment. However, the manifestations of these poor movement and stabilization strategies can be graphically visualized on a radiograph or MRI image. Osteoarthritis, more accurately described as degenerative joint disease, is just one manifestation of poor movement strategies and is not simply a process of getting older. Non-traumatic labral tears within the shoulder or hip are not the result of poor genetics or hereditary weakness, but rather the result of poor stabilization of the humeral and femoral heads within their respective articulations. Disc bulges and herniations are the result of poor stabilization strategies, leading to either overcompression or instability at or around the area of the disc pathology.

So what's the point of all this? The point is not to discount genetics or hereditary causation – father, mother, grandmother, sister, or anyone else the client would care to mention – but rather suggest that individuals are way more responsible for what happens to their musculoskeletal system than the intangible hereditary factors. We have to educate clients and patients that while they do not have control over hereditary factors they do have control over how they move, how they eat, how they recuperate, and how they manage their stress. Give them back their power and then empower them to make changes.

Why do we lose function, particularly stability, range of motion, and movement efficiency? While there are multiple causes of these issues, they essentially fall into one of three primary categories: poor neurodevelopment, injuries, and learned behaviors.

- **Lack of optimal neurodevelopment:** Dr. Vaclav Vojta, a Czechoslovakian neurologist focusing on the challenges of motor rehabilitation in children, suggested that one-third of children never develop optimal central nervous system function. This often manifests in poor patterning and many of the postural/movement dysfunctions we see in our adolescent and adult populations.

- **Trauma including surgeries, injuries (chronic and acute), and emotions:** These factors affect how an individual is able to both stabilize and create efficient movement. Surgery will always lead to muscle inhibition and alterations in motor control throughout the system. Trauma generally results in a reflexive stiffening of the injured region and subsequent compensatory alterations in the stabilization and movement systems.

- **Learned behaviors:** These are patterns that we adopt, based not necessarily on engrained neurological patterns, but rather on things we learn throughout our life. Everything from lifestyle (occupation, sports, and exercise choices) to adapted postures and movement habits learned in childhood, from mimicking what we see to adopting a 'gripping' pattern to appear slimmer, has a dramatic effect on our movement patterns. Unfortunately, the very thing we use to improve our movement dysfunction – exercise – is an often-overlooked contributor to altered movement patterns. For example, many of the exercises we perform are in direct opposition to the functional patterns engrained in our nervous system. Consider the crawling child where the spine is moved around the fixed limbs. Many of the exercises we perform in the gym, such as barbell squats, barbell rows, biceps curls, and bench presses, utilize the trunk and limbs in the exact opposite way they were intended: the trunk is fixed and the limbs move around the fixed trunk.

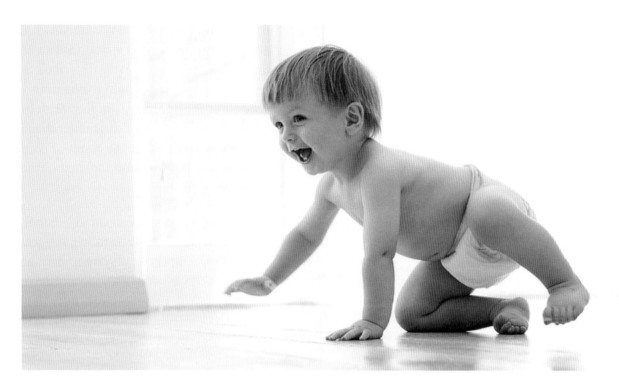

Notice how the developing child in the image above moves his spine around stable extremities (right hip and left shoulder). This develops simultaneous limb stability (right side hip and left side shoulder) and spinal mobility. The majority of the exercises we perform with our clients do the exact opposite – they move the extremities around a fixed spine. Often these patterns are performed in a bilateral fashion which fixates and locks the thorax, creating compensatory hypermobility in the extremities. This is not to suggest that these exercises are bad but rather point out the long-term effects these exercises have on the mobility of the thorax and stability of the shoulder and hip complexes.

What about exercise cues that we often use when instructing our clients? Generally, we cue our clients to 'tighten the core' or 'squeeze the glutes' or 'pull the shoulder blades down and back.' These cues often get the intended response of increased activation of the abdominal wall, glutes, and scapular retractors respectively. However, the biggest problem clients have is not in activating prime movers but rather activating the stabilizers as well as coordinating the timing and efficiency of using these muscles. The result of these exercise cues is increased problems such as compression syndromes at the spine and hips, as well as stabilization issues of the scapulothoracic region.

Additionally, whether we like to admit it or not, most of us have been influenced by learned behavior. As young children we watch and adopt the postures, mannerisms, and movement patterns of our parents, peers, and social influences. Models who are taught to hang off their hips and overly extend through their thoracolumbar junction influence many young girls. Moreover, we are influenced by our fashion, including things such as wearing high-heeled shoes, overly supportive athletic shoes, use of orthotics, etc. – each of which affects an individual's stabilization and movement patterns.

Ultimately, these learned behaviors can lead to stiffness and rigidity of the spine and thorax, which in turn leads to common movement impairments including:

- compensatory hypermobility patterns at the scapulothoracic, thoracolumbar, and lumbopelvic regions;

- reflexive tightness of the glenohumeral (shoulder) and femoroacetabular (hip) joints;

- altered respiratory mechanics necessitating the increased utilization of the accessory respiratory muscles and further perpetuation of these patterns.

While the medical field is quick to blame genetics and old age, the resultant poor stabilization and movement patterns that result from improper neurological development, trauma, and learned behaviors are the most common reasons for the majority of our client's degenerative conditions, chronic pain, and decreases in overall performance.

(The previous section has been modified and adapted from the original article 'Assessing the Fundamentals: The Thoracic Connection' – Part 1 of a 2-part series written by Evan Osar and published on www.ptonthenet.com).

THE SOLUTION

Our job, as well as our challenge as fitness and health care professionals, is to help clients and patients recognize the intimate relationship between how they move and what happens to their body as a direct result of how they move. Regardless of genetics, trauma, disease, past experiences, thoughts, beliefs, and previous learned patterns, we can help our patients and clients create positive changes. This is not to suggest that someone with multiple sclerosis or just having suffered a stroke will ever return to a high level function they had prior to the disease. But it is not up to us to place restrictions or limitations upon them. Our job is to teach and empower them to regain their strength, stability, movement awareness, and confidence so that they can achieve the highest level of function they are able to, given their current state. Empower them to challenge their current level with the faith that the nervous system is capable of so much more than it is often given credit for.

Improving movement should not demand the same investment as the professional athlete requires to make it to an elite level; however, it deserves no less attention. The days of 'just doing it' are over. Technology rules and for that we have paid dearly – the cost being dysfunction of our movement system. No longer can we simply recommend exercise and hope that everything is going to work correctly. We need a strategy that improves the individual's tolerance to stress and uses the most effective techniques to achieve this goal. While there are a lot of tools available to the fitness professional, this book presents a powerful approach based upon the principles of human function.

Because so many patients and clients present to medical doctors, chiropractic physicians, physical therapists, and fitness professionals, with movement dysfunction of the extremities, this book will focus on the hip and shoulder. The focus will be on the functional anatomy and kinesiology, as well as the common movement dysfunctions and corrective strategies for improving function. However, it is difficult, if not impossible, to discuss the hip and shoulder without giving attention to the thoracopelvic core. The thoracopelvic core will be discussed briefly throughout the book as this region is an overlooked cause of, as well as a solution to, many common hip and shoulder conditions. It is with the hope that, by improving the fitness and health care professional's awareness of common dysfunctions and straightforward solutions, they can become advocates for their patients and clients in taking control of their own health. Through this approach, we can team with mainstream medicine and effectively become the solution to the health care crisis.

HOW THIS BOOK IS ORGANIZED

This book is designed in three parts to help you make the most of the information presented within. The first part is an introduction to movement and the components of the movement paradigm, including muscles, joints, proprioceptors, and fundamental movement patterns. It also addresses some of the underlying problems that are recognized as keys to the development and prevalence of movement dysfunctions. The second part discusses functional anatomy and kinesiology of the shoulder and hip complexes, including some of the common dysfunctions as well as several concepts that are necessary for improving function of these regions. An assessment of the trunk, hip, and shoulders is also included in this section. The third part will demonstrate the corrective exercise and movement progression, based on the principles that were set up in the first two sections of the book. Included in this book are tables that contain both descriptions of the exercises, including setup, alignment, activation strategies, and what your client should be feeling. Additional tables are designed to supply you with clinical keys. All these are designed to provide you with clinically applicable techniques, strategies, and/or 'aha' moments to help make the information connect and add even more relevance for you and your patient/client.

This information has been developed from the collective contributions of innumerous great minds within the health, fitness, and rehabilitation industries, many of whom were discussed in the acknowledgement section. To reiterate one key concept that was presented in the first few lines of the preface: this information is not meant to replace things you are doing that currently work, or to say that this is the only way to do things, or to imply this is the way things will always be done. As Ralph Waldo Emerson said, "I wish to say what I think and feel today, with the proviso that tomorrow perhaps I shall contradict it all." It is likely that in the near future, as research and methodology improves and continues to grow, we will likely find ways that are even more effective and enable us to make even greater changes in the way our patients and clients move. Until then, we will keep true to the principles and take full advantage of the opportunities that are presented to us in each patient and client we interact with.

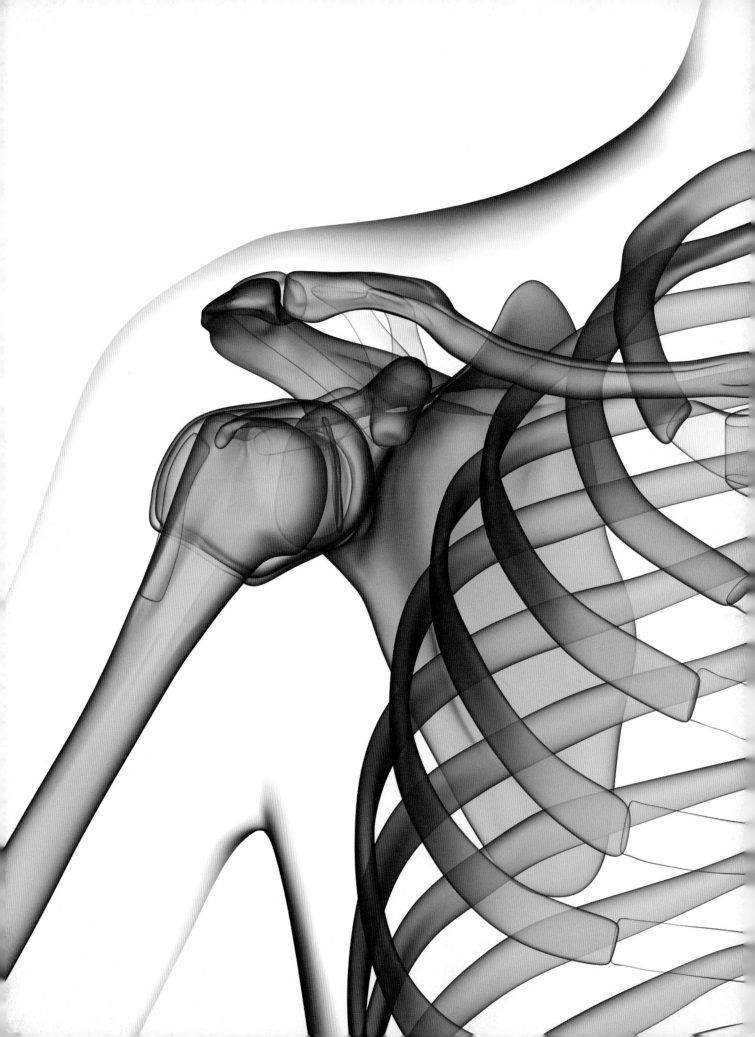

part I

Introduction to Movement:
The Functional Elements

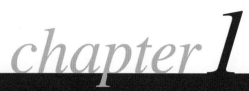

The Functional Movement System

CHAPTER OBJECTIVES

To identify and understand the functional components of movement

To explain and identify the key functions of muscles

BIOMECHANICS

Understanding movement requires a brief introduction to biomechanics. Biomechanics is the study of motion and the internal and external forces that act upon the body. This study is largely based upon looking at joint mechanics, internal forces, and external forces and loads as well as the effects of gravity, momentum, and ground reaction forces.

Kinesiology is the study of motion based on the activity of the muscle system. It is important to have a basic understanding of the biomechanics involved with motion to enable a better appreciation of the kinesiological activity of the muscle system.

Looking at the human gait cycle provides a rather unique look into the biomechanics of the lower extremity. The human gait cycle, like many movements in life, is a series of loading and unloading events that occur in an orchestrated fashion through the kinetic chain. To help demonstrate the biomechanics, as well as provide an example of why muscles act in a particular way, a rather basic evaluation of the gait cycle will be provided below.

As the body moves from the initial contact phase through the midstance phase, the lower extremity is considered to be loading or going through pronation. These phases are designed to decelerate the forward momentum of the body as well as provide shock absorption both from the body weight moving over the lower leg and from the ground reaction forces that travel from the foot back up the kinetic chain. It is important to note that during this phase most of the muscles of the lower kinetic chain are being eccentrically loaded, which will help the body take advantage of both the elastic and contractile properties of the myofascial system, helping to conserve energy and make the push-off phases of the cycle more physiologically efficient. During this loading phase, the hip is moving through relative flexion, adduction, and internal rotation; the knee is moving into flexion, abduction, and internal rotation; and the ankle-foot complex is moving through dorsiflexion, abduction, and eversion.

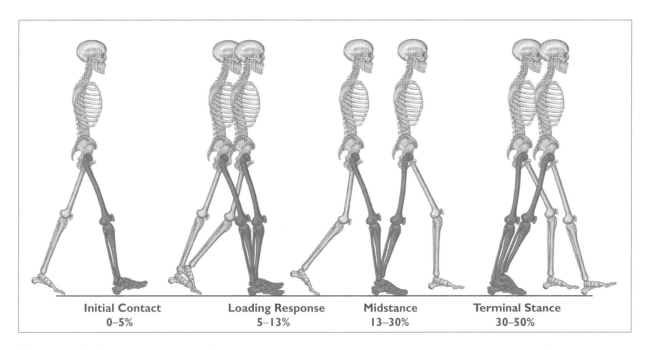

The gait cycle: initial contact through terminal stance.

As the body moves over the stationary leg from the end of the midstance phase through the terminal stance, the lower kinetic chain transitions to an unloading or acceleration phase. This motion takes advantage of the elastic components of the myofascial system as well as concentric muscle contractions to help propel the body forward. During this supination phase, the hip is extending, abducting, and externally rotating; the knee is extending, adducting, and externally rotating; and the ankle-foot complex is plantar flexing, adducting, and inverting.

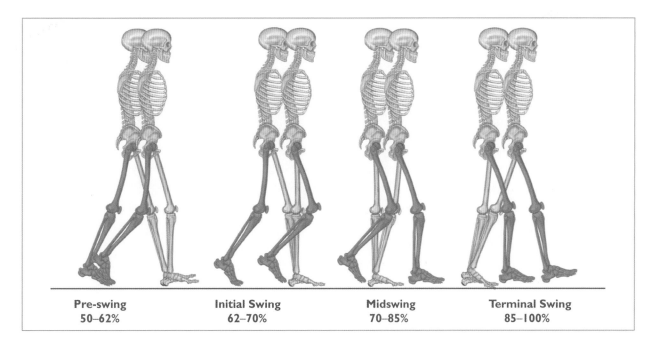

The gait cycle: pre-swing through terminal swing.

The tri-planar motions of the hip, knee, and ankle-foot complex are summarized in the table below.

Movement	Sagittal Plane	Frontal Plane	Transverse Plane
Hip			
Pronation	Flexion	Adduction	Internal rotation
Supination	Extension	Abduction	External rotation
Knee			
Pronation	Flexion	Abduction	Internal rotation
Supination	Extension	Adduction	External rotation
Ankle-Foot			
Pronation	Dorsiflexion (ankle)	Abduction (foot)	Eversion (foot)
Supination	Plantar flexion (ankle)	Adduction (foot)	Inversion (foot)

This section took a brief look at the biomechanics and the role of gravity, external forces, internal forces, and ground reaction in the development of motion. A brief understanding of biomechanics helps to develop an awareness and appreciation of the functional role of the muscular system, which will be the next area of focus.

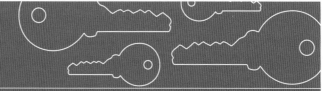

Key To Success
Is Motion Ever Given for Free?

Functional training gurus often look at lower extremity pronation or the loading phase of gait and claim that these motions are 'given for free.' In other words, because gravity is pulling the body towards the ground and the fact that the lower extremity remains relatively fixed as the body moves over the leg, they make the incorrect assumption that the body does not have to actively participate in these motions. However, just because gravity is pulling the body into these motions, it does not mean they are just naturally going to happen. For example, clients often lack internal hip rotation on the side of low back instability. When they walk, they are not instantly given this motion because of the pull of gravity or surrounding biomechanics. Often they will compensate for this lack of motion by increasing motion at another joint, such as the knee or foot. They will overly abduct the knee and/or over-pronate the foot in the absence of internal rotation of the hip. Another example can be seen during the squat pattern and the action of the tibialis anterior. During the squat pattern, while the motion of the knee moving over the foot creates a relative dorsiflexion of the ankle, this does not suggest that the tibialis anterior is sitting idly by and not participating in the motion. The tibialis anterior assists knee flexion by pulling the knee towards the foot. The toes rising from the floor during the descending phase of the squat is often indicative of overactivity of the extensor digitorum longus, substituting for an inhibition of the tibialis anterior. Inhibition of the tibialis anterior is often a cause of improper squat mechanics and must be evaluated in the presence of knee pain or limitations in ankle dorsiflexion during this pattern.

KEY: It is important to realize that no motion is given for free and any muscle that is connected to a moving joint should be taken into account when assessing and correcting movement patterns. Also consider that just because gravity assists a motion, it does not mean the muscle system does not have to work in that direction. As Vojta suggested, muscles work in two directions, both proximally and distally. Therefore, it is vital that all muscles be functionally considered and evaluated in the presence of movement dysfunction.

KINESIOLOGY

Kinesiology is the study of motion based on the activity of the muscle system. The muscle system, including the proprioceptive and fascial systems, is integral to the development of coordinated and efficient movement. This section will take a deeper look at the components of the muscle system and look at the interplay between these systems in developing optimal movement. Additionally, this section will provide a view of functional anatomy that is not often considered, which will, however, be key in the development of the corrective exercise and training paradigm presented later in this book.

PROPRIOCEPTION

Performance of complex movement patterns – such as returning a volley in tennis, controlling the body and center of gravity while riding a bicycle over a pothole, or initiating a fine motor pattern when, for example, playing a song on a piano – all require a highly tuned proprioceptive system. Proprioception is essentially the awareness of our body in space, based on information received by specialized systems and receptors within the body. This includes information that is received from the eyes and within the vestibular system located in the inner ear. The eyes are important for the anticipation and navigation of the external environment. The righting reflexes help maintain the eyes level with the horizon and can be a cause for the development of postural alterations in the presence of a long leg, flat foot, or intra-pelvic torsion. The vestibular apparatus located within the inner ear provides information about posture and balance as well as the position and movement of the head.

There are several types of receptors that are responsible for providing the central nervous system with information regarding the position, tension, rate of change, and pressure within the body. These specialized receptors are known as 'mechanoreceptors' and help detect the conscious sensation of movement within the body, also referred to as kinesthesia. Several of these are discussed below.

THE THREE KEY REGIONS OF MECHANORECEPTORS

How do muscles know what to do? Muscles always act under guidance from the nervous system, based upon the information it receives from the proprioceptive system. Continuous feedback from each muscle to the nervous system is carried out by mechanoreceptors, including information about what the body is doing at each instantaneous moment as well as the rate and length of change that is occurring. There are three main regions of proprioception: the muscle spindles located within the muscle belly, the golgi tendon organ located within the musculotendinous junction, and the joint structure. Muscle spindles are located within the muscle belly near the musculotendinous junctions (see overleaf).

They contain several intrafusal muscle fibers that keep the muscle spindle taut as the muscle changes length. If the muscle is stretched too far or too fast, the muscle spindle sends a reflexive signal back to the central nervous system, initiating a stretch reflex and contraction of the affected muscle. This helps to maintain the muscle length and joint position and minimize the effects of a potential injury. The muscle spindle is most responsible for the reciprocal inhibition response, whereby it inhibits the functional antagonists during a muscle contraction. When a muscle is reciprocally inhibited secondary to injury, trauma, or overuse, it can be activated by tapping, electrical stimulus, sustained stretch pressure, brisk manual pressure, and/or vibration to increase activation of the muscle spindles. These techniques will be discussed further in the corrective exercise section of the book.

Muscle spindle activity can set off a reaction that is referred to as the 'muscle stretch reflex', otherwise known as the 'myotatic reflex'. This reflex causes a contraction around excited spindles, causing a reflexive contraction of the muscle. The muscle spindle reflex 'servo-assists' (serves and assists muscle contraction), as it potentially a) enables the brain to cause a muscle contraction with less nervous energy, b) allows a muscle contraction independent of the level of the loads, and c) counteracts muscle fatigue or additional muscle dysfunction (Guyton 1991).

Golgi tendon organs (GTOs) are located within the musculotendinous junction. These fibers also contain sensory fibers and respond to an increase in tension within the muscle. They respond by creating inhibition of the muscle, thereby protecting the muscle attachments from potential injury. The GTO monitors the internal tension and force of a muscle and responds to increases in muscle tensions. It can create an inhibitory response, known as 'autogenic inhibition', which at times can be so strong that it can lead to relaxation of the entire muscle. This reaction, also known as the 'lengthening reaction', has been suggested but not proven to keep the muscle from rupturing or avulsing at its bony attachment

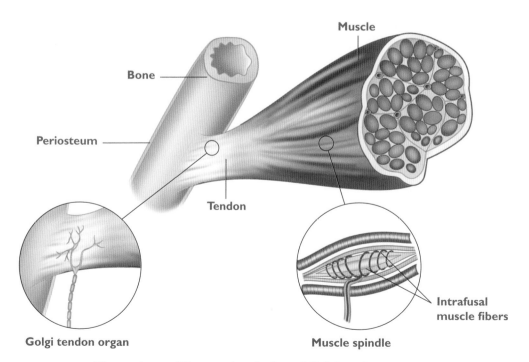

The anatomy of the muscle spindle and Golgi tendon organ.

site. The GTO is also likely to inhibit overactive fibers so there is overall better recruitment of all the individual muscle fibers of a muscle, thereby minimizing potential muscle damage (Guyton 1991).

The joint capsule and ligaments surrounding the joint contain several types of receptors that are responsible for monitoring joint position and movement. While they don't send information regarding joint tension, they are important in relaying information on movement, position, compression, traction, and palpation and have a strong influence on motor feedback and resultant muscle function (Umphred 2007).

One additional source of sensory feedback comes from the cutaneous receptors located within the skin. They are particularly dense in the palms of the hands and soles of the feet. These receptors detect pressure and touch, and play an important role in the kinesthetic portion of the learning process as well as in developing optimal movement strategies.

TYPES OF MUSCLE FIBERS

There are essentially three types of muscle fibers that are present within skeletal muscles – type I, type IIa, and type IIb – and all muscles contain varying percentages of these fibers (Guyton 1991). Type I muscle fibers are regarded as slow twitch because their rate of contraction is generally slower than type II, which are the fast twitch fibers. Type I fibers are generally more aerobic in nature and considered fatigue resistant. Type II fibers are able to generate higher levels of force than type I and are easily fatigued. Type II fibers are further subdivided into type IIa fibers, which tend to have characteristics of both type I and type II fibers, and type IIb, which tend to be more characteristic of type II fibers (Baechle and Earle 2000). Type I muscle fibers are usually found in greater concentrations in the postural muscles and likely have a greater concentration of proprioceptors. The deeper spinal muscles, for example the rotators and intertransversarii, have been shown to contain a four to seven times greater concentration of muscle spindles than the more superficial multifidus, and thus seemingly function as length transducers and position sensors (McGill 2007). In all likelihood the local joint stabilizers of the shoulders and hips similarly contain a higher level of proprioceptors than the corresponding global muscles of the regions. The functions of the muscle fibers are summarized in the table below.

Characteristics	Type I	Type IIa and IIb
Energy system	Aerobic	Aerobic and anaerobic
Force production	Low	Intermediate to high
Color	Red	Intermediate to white
Fatigability	Low	Intermediate to high
Fiber size	Small	Intermediate to large
Location	Deep	Intermediate to superficial
Proprioception	High	Intermediate to low
Function	Posture and stabilization	Movement and gross stabilization

TYPES OF MUSCLE CONTRACTIONS

Muscles contract to produce some type of reaction within the joints they control. Concentric contraction, or contractions where the attachments of the muscles are approximating each other, creates movement. This muscle shortening is responsible for overcoming a resistance, resisting gravity, and/or accelerating the position of the body. Eccentric contraction, on the other hand, is where the muscle attachments are moving away from each other to decelerate a movement. These contractions are illustrated in the examples below.

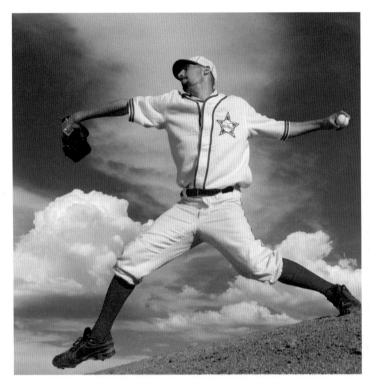 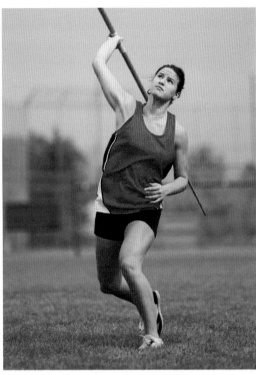

During the early cocking phase of a baseball throw, the athlete has to eccentrically decelerate rotation in his trunk and left shoulder (image to the left). The athlete concentrically contracts to accelerate her trunk and arm through the early phase of the javelin release (image to the right).

Isometric contractions are contractions in which there is no change in the length of the muscle. They serve two important functions in the body:

1. Stabilization: Isometric contractions are important in centrating and stabilizing the joint during movement. Loss of this stabilization function leads to a loss in the optimal axis of rotation, resulting in a decrease in movement efficiency as well as increased wear and tear on the joint (see page 27). The local stabilizers help control the intersegmental position of the vertebrae, while the global mobilizers create gross movement of the spine. In the shoulder, the rotator cuff muscles co-activate in a relatively isometric fashion to stabilize the humeral head in the glenoid fossa. Similarly, the local stabilizers of the hip, including the psoas major and deep external hip rotators, provide joint centration of the femoral head so that the global muscles can produce general movements of the hip joint. This concept will be expanded upon in the hip and shoulder sections.

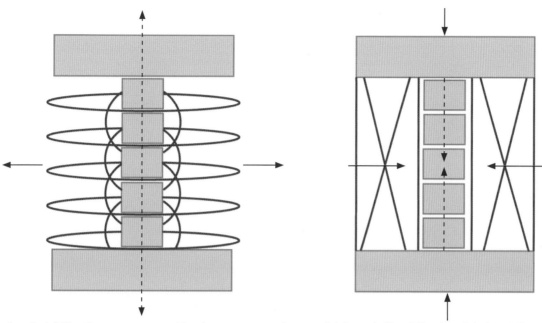

The local stabilization system provides intersegmental control (above left), while the global stabilization system (above right) provides global stabilization of the trunk and spine.

2. The amortization phase of gait or plyometric training: Isometric contractions function as the transition between eccentric and concentric contractions. At the end of the eccentric phase, there is a fraction of time where the muscle is no longer lengthening, yet the muscle hasn't started shortening. This generally occurs around the midstance phase of gait. Alpha motor neurons signal the agonists to contract and use the elastic energy that has been stored from the eccentric phase (Baechle and Earle 2000). If this transition lasts too long, there will be a subsequent decrease in the stretch reflex and amount of resultant concentric force that can be produced (Baechle and Earle 2000). It is possible that the length of the amortization phase determines the difference between first and second places in elite runners, and between getting repetitive running injuries, such as shin splints or plantar fasciitis, and producing an efficient gait pattern. The longer the individual spends in contact with the ground, the more potential they have to overload the soft tissues and joint structures of the lower kinetic chain and, subsequently, the longer it will take to get out of this position.

Eccentric contractions essentially load or pre-stretch the muscle system necessary to help maximize concentric contractions or the unloading phase of movement, while isometric contractions function between these transitions. These functions, along with other common terms, are summarized in the table below.

Eccentric Contractions	Isometric Contractions	Concentric Contractions
Loading phase	Stabilization phase	Unloading phase
Pronation	Stabilization	Supination
Deceleration	Stabilization	Acceleration

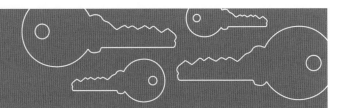

Key To Success
The Relationship Between Muscle Contractions and Repetitive Injuries

A significant number of musculoskeletal injuries are the result of overuse or repetitive movements. Generally these injuries are caused by habitual movement patterns that are perpetuated and engrained during repetitive exercise. Common overuse injuries of the lower extremities — such as iliotibial band syndrome, patellar tendonosis, shin splints, and plantar fasciitis — are the result of the combined effects of poor joint centration and inefficient eccentric control of pronation. Therefore, the corrective exercise approach should focus on improving the client's ability to centrate their joints and then teaching the client how to move out of and back into these controlled positions. Once they have achieved this ability, they can be moved into functional movement patterns and eventually return to sport or functional activity.

KEY: Improving movement patterns and reducing the potential for overuse injuries requires the client to develop better joint stabilization and eccentric control of their body and should be the primary goals during the corrective exercise strategy.

THE LOCAL AND GLOBAL MUSCLE SYSTEMS

While no muscle truly works in isolation, muscles can be differentiated based upon their primary functional activities. Hodges, Lee, Comerford, and others have differentiated between local and global muscle systems based upon characteristics such as their location, time of contraction, effect on the joint, and response to dysfunction. Regardless of this differentiation, the local and global muscle systems must work in harmony to provide smooth and coordinated movement. For example, failure of the local system results in global muscle overactivity, necessitating the muscles of the extremities giving up their movement role in exchange for aiding proximal stabilization (Umphred 2007). Descriptions of the local and global muscle systems are given below.

The local muscle system, otherwise referred to as the 'deep muscle system', is responsible for the segmental stabilization of the trunk and spine in addition to the glenohumeral (shoulder) and femoroacetabular (hip) articulations. The functional role of these muscles lies beyond the strength of their contraction. There are several key factors related to their functional role in stabilization and movement.

1. They are non-direction specific, meaning they contract regardless of the direction of motion. The muscles of the global muscle system, however, are direction specific; referring to certain directions will activate them, while otherdirections of motion do not cause activation. For example, the deep muscles of the shoulder and hip, collectively referred to as the 'rotator cuff' muscles, function to maintain joint centration of the respective glenohumeral and femoroacetabular joints, regardless of position of the joints. In contrast, the global muscles, for example the superficial muscles of the trunk and spine, tend to respond only when the direction of motion requires their specific activity.

2. They have a feed-forward function, meaning they contract just before the global system to provide proximal stability to the joint prior to distal motion. This is an automatic response and this function is often compromised after injury or joint dysfunction.

3. There is general co-activation of these muscles to provide intersegmental stability so the prime movers can perform their role of global movement. This co-activation is required to maintain joint centration and to balance forces across all articular surfaces during global movement.

The global muscle system, also referred to as the 'superficial muscle system', consists of the muscles most responsible for movement. They are also responsible for gross stabilization and are generally the muscles that are involved in clients who demonstrate bracing-type stabilization strategies. Unlike the local muscles, which often become inhibited secondary to joint injury, the global muscles frequently respond to injury by becoming hypertonic and overactive.

The differentiation between local and global muscles of the trunk and spine and the shoulder and hip complexes has been expanded upon in the table overleaf.

Region	Local Muscle System	Global Muscle System
Trunk and spine	Diaphragm	Rectus abdominis
	Transversus abdominis	External and internal obliques
	Multifidi and other short segmental trunk and spinal muscles	Superficial erector spinae
	Psoas major and minor	
	Quadratus lumborum	
	Pelvic floor	
Hip	Psoas major and minor	Superficial fibers of gluteus maximus
	Pelvic floor	Gluteus medius
	Gemelli	Hamstring complex
	Obturators	Quadriceps
	Deep fibers of gluteus maximus	Tensor fasciae latae
		Adductor complex
		Sartorius
		Piriformis
Shoulder	Supraspinatus	Pectoralis major and minor
	Infraspinatus	Latissimus dorsi
	Teres minor	Serratus anterior
	Subscapularis	Trapezius
	Biceps brachii	Rhomboids
		Deltoids
		Coracobrachialis
		Subclavius
		Teres major
		Triceps brachii

While this discussion is not meant to suggest any one muscle is more important than another, understanding this functional muscle relationship will prove helpful when discussing muscle imbalances and the development as well as the perpetuation of dysfunctional movement patterns.

EFFECT OF INJURY AND TRAINING ON LOCAL AND GLOBAL MUSCLES

Reflexive inhibition can be described as muscular inhibition following joint injury. There is evidence that suggests that this inhibition most affects the local (one-joint) stabilizers rather than the global mobilizers. For example, the vastus medialis has shown inhibition and atrophy rather than the rectus femoris in clients who were experimentally induced with knee pain or in those clients with long-standing patellofemoral pain.

Specific training methods have also been shown to change muscle fiber recruitment as well as have an inhibitory effect on the local stabilization system. Ballistic- or plyometric-type training protocols have been shown to positively increase jumping height in participants of a six-week training program. However, there was a subsequent decrease in the strength of the soleus during the program, suggesting that this type of training preferentially recruits the global mobilizers over the local stabilizers – gastrocnemius versus the soleus in this case (Ng 1990). These findings suggest have several implications when rehabilitating or training clients who experience movement dysfunction.

1. Many clients demonstrating movement dysfunctions have local imbalances between the stabilizers and prime movers. Performing high level plyometric, jumping, and/or ballistic exercise is likely to perpetuate this dysfunction as it tends to favor the two-joint, global mobilizers over the local, one-joint stabilizers. This is one of the reasons that slower and controlled movements are favored during the corrective exercise and early in the return-to-activity phases of the movement paradigm.

2. Clients who have experienced an injury/surgery and/or pain or joint swelling are likely to experience reflexive inhibition and exhibit clinical signs of inhibition (weakness and atrophy of the local joint stabilizers). Performing high levels of plyometric, jumping, and/or ballistic exercises will further train the muscles of the global system generally at the expense of the local system, causing further perpetuation of this dysfunction.

3. Performing higher level ballistic exercises will tend to cause greater levels of fatigue and accumulation of metabolic waste products. Fatigue and pain will alter the client's ability to detect mistakes and will impede ideal motor patterning. Again, this will make it easier and easier to facilitate the dysfunctional patterns (Law of Facilitation) while making it harder and harder to program in ideal neuromotor patterns.

AGONISTS, ANTAGONISTS, SYNERGISTS, AND STABILIZERS

Agonists are also known as 'prime movers' or the muscles that are most responsible for a particular movement. Antagonists are the muscles that oppose the agonists. More realistically speaking, there is no muscle that is solely responsible for any particular action – only muscles that are more or less appropriate. Lombard's paradox (1907) suggests that muscles work as functional agonists. For example, during the squat pattern, both the quadriceps and hamstrings contract during the ascent phase of the movement. The quadriceps work to extend the knee, while the hamstrings work to extend the hip and assist knee extension, thereby providing functional antagonism at the knee joint. Most movements in the body, including running, function in this manner (see image below).

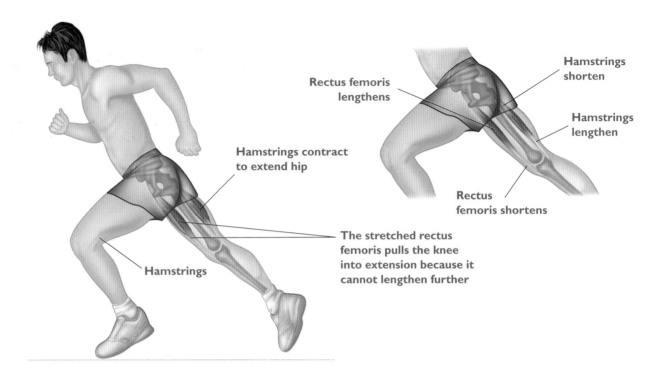

Rectus femoris lengthens

Hamstrings shorten

Hamstrings lengthen

Hamstrings contract to extend hip

Rectus femoris shortens

The stretched rectus femoris pulls the knee into extension because it cannot lengthen further

Hamstrings

With the hip flexed and knee bent, the hamstring can assist knee extension by restraining the lower leg as the body progresses over the support leg.

Synergists are muscles that aid the prime movers. Very few muscles work in an isolated manner and synergists can function to assist the prime mover in the specific action it performs, or it can function as more of a stabilizer of the joint. When the prime mover is inhibited by pain, joint effusion, or improper neurological input, the synergists are called upon to assume the role of prime movers. This is referred to as 'synergist dominance'.

Stabilizers are responsible for maintaining a static joint position against adjacent or distal joint movement. For example, as the right trapezius moves the right arm into abduction, the left trapezius and spinal erectors act to stabilize the spine against movement of the contralateral arm. During flexion of the arm, the scapulothoracic stabilizers must fixate the scapula against the thorax as well as stabilize against the weight of the arm and whatever is being lifted.

When there is optimal co-activation between functional antagonists, there is maintenance of the joint position. In the presence of muscle inhibition, one or more of the functional agonists become dysfunctional and the joint is pulled in the direction of the functioning muscles. This alters the joint position as well as the instantaneous axis of rotation, thereby compromising joint stability.

UNDERSTANDING MUSCLE FUNCTION

"The greatest obstacle to discovering the shape of the earth, the continents, and the ocean was not ignorance but the illusion of knowledge." (Daniel Boorstin)

A common premise within learning environments is that the more that is learned about a certain topic, the more the current and accepted knowledge is challenged. Understanding muscle function is a direct example of this premise. This section will expand upon the discussion of the previous sections and categorize the three primary functions of muscle contractions. Additionally, several of the functional roles that muscles play in the development of ideal movement patterns will both expand upon current knowledge and subtly challenge some long-held beliefs.

FUNCTION #1 – PERFORM MOVEMENT

It is common for students to be taught anatomy based upon the individual muscle's origin and insertion. In other words, the insertion of the muscle is brought towards the origin of the muscle, therefore producing the assigned action of the muscle. For example, the biceps brachii is assigned the primary function of flexion and supination of the elbow, and the secondary function of shoulder flexion. From anatomic position, which was the position from which the early anatomists studied the body, that appears to be a valid interpretation of the biceps brachii's function. If looking at the biceps brachii function in activities of daily living – such as bringing a glass up to one's mouth, lifting dishes out of a dishwasher, or combing one's hair – the assigned functions would seem to be validated.

However, similar to much in the body that is only modestly understood and oft misinterpreted, that is only half the story. In studying children, Vaclav Vojta described muscle function based on reflex locomotion and the child's developmental function. He pointed out that muscles don't simply work in a proximal fashion, as in pulling the insertion towards the origin, but are just as important in their distal function. In fact, he is credited with stating that muscles need to function in two directions – both eccentrically and concentrically (Cohen 2010).

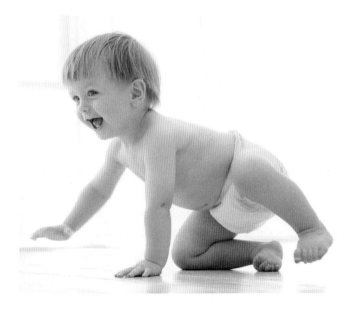

Using the biceps brachii example from above, because of its origin on the superior edge of the glenoid labrum, the biceps brachii functions to pull the scapula over the stable upper extremity as is seen in the crawling child. The open-chain function, or origin-to-insertion-based action of the biceps brachii is to perform elbow flexion. In the developing child, the biceps functions to pull the scapula over the stable arm. This functional action will be trained by using modifications of child developmental patterns to correct movement dysfunction as well as improve performance.

A second example can be seen with the pectoralis major. Traditional muscle anatomy texts list flexion, adduction, and internal rotation of the shoulder as its function. Again, looking at the developing child, the pectoralis major plays an equally important role in crawling. As the child progresses over the stationary arm, the pectoralis major functions to draw the torso towards the stationary arm. This function can also be seen in sport, where baseball pitchers, quarterbacks, and javelin throwers will hold the lead arm stable and use the pectoralis major of the lead arm to help drive rotation of the trunk around that arm.

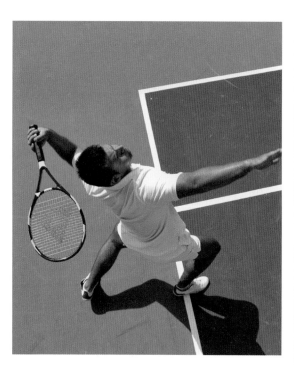
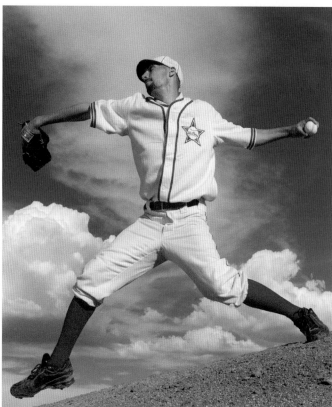

The lead arm in the athlete produces a stable base for trunk rotation. In this way, the athlete will utilize the pectoralis major, along with its synergists – the pectoralis minor, serratus anterior, and anterior deltoids of the lead arm – to assist trunk rotation. Additionally, a reciprocal action of the upper extremities will be utilized as the lead arm is internally rotating as the external arm is externally rotating (see images of athletes above). This serves to both wind up the kinetic chains and stabilize the shoulder complex.

Another example is the piriformis, which is assigned the function of external rotation of the hip. While it performs this function in an open-chain manner, in the crawling child the piriformis works to rotate the pelvis around the stationary lower leg. This action can be seen in activities such as throwing a kick while performing martial arts. The athlete's right piriformis along with the other external hip rotators, function to rotate the pelvis around the stationary lower leg as she performs a roundhouse kick (image opposite left). The child uses his right piriformis to help rotate his pelvis over the femoral head to propel himself forward (image opposite right).

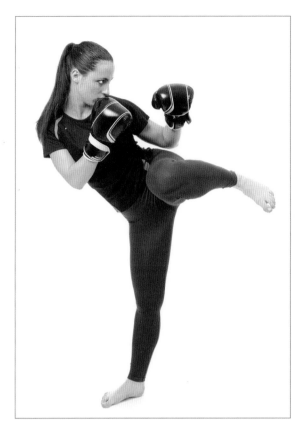

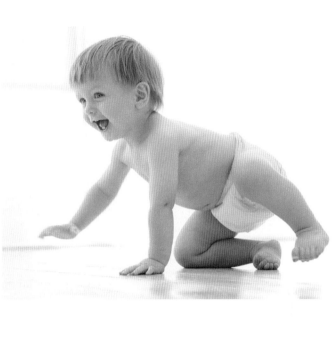

Similarly, muscles can also perform actions based upon how they react to the foot or hand being in contact with the ground. Traditional anatomy looked at the open-chain function of muscles, in other words when the foot is off the ground. However, their function can change rather dramatically when the foot is in contact with the ground. For example, in open-chain function, the hamstring complex will flex the knee and decelerate knee extension. In the closed-chain function, the hamstring complex functions to decelerate anterior pelvic rotation and assist knee extension. As the body is progressing over the fixed foot, the hamstring is assisting hip extension. It is also pulling on the tibia (its distal attachment), which aids knee extension as the body moves over the foot. Likewise, the gastrocnemius has the open-chain function of assisting knee flexion. As it decelerates ankle dorsiflexion during gait, it pulls on its proximal attachment on the femoral condyles to assist knee extension as the body passes over the fixed foot.

One additional concept based on this theory of muscle function, adopted from the child development model, is the idea of using the upper extremities to drive trunk motion. During the crawling pattern, the child uses one arm to stabilize the upper extremity and spine as the opposite arm reaches forward. This patterning helps the child develop stability in the fixed arm and corresponding side of the thorax, while the free arm helps maintain thoracic mobility. There are two key points here to help in making sense of these actions.

1. The majority of scapular stabilizers – including the latissimus dorsi, rhomboids major and minor, as well as all three divisions of the trapezius – have spinal attachments. While these muscles have never been assigned a spinal function, their attachment to the spine suggests they play a role in spine function.

The rhomboids, trapezius, and latissimus dorsi collectively function to rotate the spine towards the fixed upper limb. With elbow support, as in crawling or plank position, the triceps and biceps brachii can draw the scapula towards the fixed elbow (see arrows in below left image, indicating line of muscle pull). This function can be seen in the developing child – the prone elbow support position stabilizes the child's upper extremity. As they reach with the contralateral arm, the scapular stabilizers of the supported arm help rotate the spine.

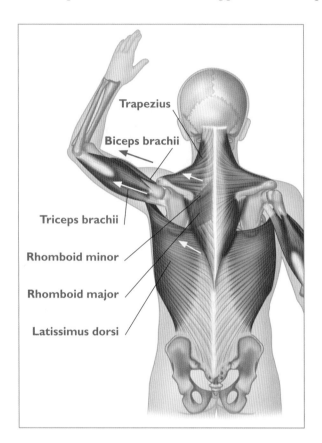

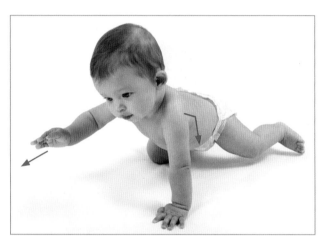

2. As the child stabilizes on his left upper extremity and reaches with his right arm, the left scapular stabilizers aid rotation of the spine. The child stabilizes his trunk with his left arm, while the motion of the free arm helps mobilize the right side of their spine and thorax. This is an important consideration in exercise, as traditional resistance exercise can often create rigidity of the thorax. The main reason for this is that bilateral patterns require the arms be moved over a fixed thorax. In the developing child this pattern rarely occurs and when it does, it is usually not performed with significant resistance or in a repetitive fashion.

Bilateral patterns such as chest presses, upright rows, and curls require the thorax to be used as the stable point, as the loaded extremities are moved around the thorax. Additionally, patterns such as barbell squats, deadlifts, and farmer's walks can also drive thoracic stiffness because the thorax is used as a stable point for lifting. While the thorax should be fixed during these types of patterns, perpetual use of these patterns can drive rigidity and stiffness of the thorax. Although this type of rigidity may be useful for muscle hypertrophy and certain athletic activities, hypertrophy of the muscles of the thorax can lead to stiffness of these muscles, and the resultant hypomobility is

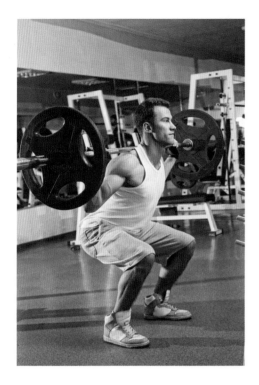 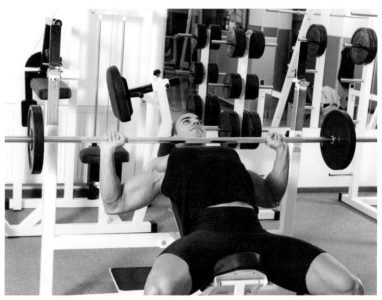

Examples of barbell patterns that can create trunk rigidity: barbell squat (left) and barbell chest press (above).

often responsible for the onset of several of the more common dysfunctions of the movement system. Two examples are:

i. Rigidity of the thorax results in decreased motion and compensatory hypermobility of the cervical and lumbar regions of the spine. This is a common cause of spinal instability in these regions and resultant pathologies of the disc and tissue structures of the spine.

ii. Rigidity of the thorax decreases the client's ability to achieve three-dimensional expansion of the thorax during respiration. This leads to increased activity of the accessory muscles of respiration – mainly the scalenes, sternocleidomastoid, and pectoralis minor – to assist elevation of the thorax during breathing. This causes global reactions in the body, including driving the forward head and shoulder positions, contributing to headaches and anxiety, poor overall levels of oxygenation, and rises in blood pressure.

If bilateral patterns will be performed or have to be performed as part of an athletic training program, they should be followed with patterns that help mobilize the thorax. Unilateral and alternating patterns can help restore thoracic mobility by using the free arm to drive rotation of the thorax while the free arm stabilizes the shoulder complex and ipsilateral of the thorax.

This concept of limb function may seem to contradict Gracovetsky's theory of the spinal engine and that spine motion drives motion of the extremities (Gracovetsky 2008). However, this theory presented here is not to dismiss his notion but rather to add to it by suggesting that the extremities can be used to assist both stabilization and mobility of the spine, helping to create a more functional expression of traditional exercise patterns. These two functions will be incorporated into the corrective exercise and training strategy that follows later in the book.

FUNCTION #2 – TRANSFER OF ACTION

Another concept that traditional anatomy books do not discuss is that muscles can create motion across a joint that they don't cross. For example, the vastus lateralis and medialis do not cross the hip joint; however, each contributes to internal and external rotation of the hip respectively. With the foot fixed on the ground, contraction of the obliquely oriented fibers of the vastus lateralis pulls the thigh towards its distal attachment on the patella, creating internal rotation of the hip. Similarly, the vastus medialis helps contribute to external rotation of the hip as the oblique nature of the fibers pulls the thigh over the fixed lower leg (image right).

With the distal aspect of the kinetic chain stabilized by the ground, the co-contraction of the vastus lateralis and medialis extends the knee and helps to pull the thigh and pelvis over the tibia.

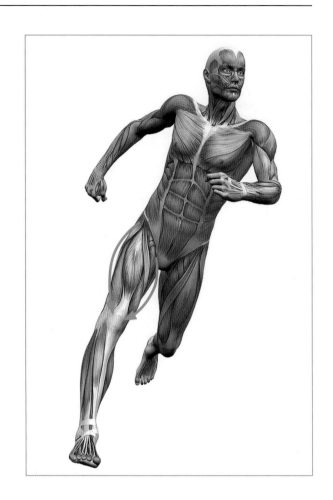

FUNCTION #3 – ACT AS THEIR OWN ANTAGONISTS

Muscles can act as their own antagonists, depending on the joint angle they cross. Several examples are given below.

1. The upper fibers of the pectoralis major assist shoulder flexion, while the lower fibers assist shoulder extension.

2. The upper fibers of the trapezius elevate the scapula, while the lower fibers depress the scapula.

3. The anterior fibers of the deltoid flex and horizontally adduct the humerus, while the posterior fibers extend and horizontally abduct the humerus.

4. The anterior fibers of the gluteus medius flex and internally rotate the hip, while the posterior fibers assist extension and external rotation of the hip.

5. The medial head of the gastrocnemius internally rotates the tibia, while the lateral head assists external rotation of the tibia.

These antagonistic roles enable muscles to function more efficiently and produce more fluid motion in virtually an infinite variety of joint positions and functional activities.

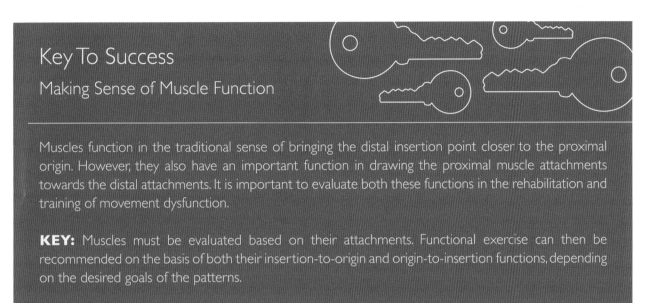

Key To Success
Making Sense of Muscle Function

Muscles function in the traditional sense of bringing the distal insertion point closer to the proximal origin. However, they also have an important function in drawing the proximal muscle attachments towards the distal attachments. It is important to evaluate both these functions in the rehabilitation and training of movement dysfunction.

KEY: Muscles must be evaluated based on their attachments. Functional exercise can then be recommended on the basis of both their insertion-to-origin and origin-to-insertion functions, depending on the desired goals of the patterns.

FASCIA

Fascia, a sheet or band of dense, irregular connective tissue, can be found throughout the human body, essentially invested within all its structures. The joint capsules of diarthrodial joints, aponeuroses (for example the abdominal aponeurosis and thoracolumbar fascia) as well as ligaments and muscles are essentially well-organized arrangements of fascia (Schleip et al 2005). Fascia, not unlike ligaments, was once thought to be an inert connective tissue functioning as a simple connection between muscles and organs. Recent research has indicated that fascia is much more than a simple connective tissue structure and that it indeed contains contractile fibers that are responsive to mechanical stimulation (Schleip and Klingler 2005). In fact, these myofibroblasts have been found not only in fascia but also in the other, often thought of as passive, structure of ligaments (Schleip and Klingler 2005).

These contractile fibers have been found to be more concentrated in tonic muscle tissues than in phasic muscles and thereby add increased stiffness to these muscles (Schleip and Klingler 2005). This evidence suggests that increased stiffness in the tonic musculature may play an important role in joint stabilization and postural support. Activation of these fibers may have the short-term benefit of improving reflexive muscle action and therefore improving joint stiffness (Schleip et al 2005).

Dysfunction of the contractile elements of the musculofascial system has been suggested as one of the contributors of chronic pain. Inhibition of the ligamentous mechanoreceptors has been shown to decrease muscle activation responses. While this response has only been tested in cats, it is postulated that a similar response is present in humans and may explain muscle inhibition following injuries to soft tissue structures of joints. Individuals with chronic low back pain demonstrate decreased concentrations of mechanoreceptors, which can alter proprioception and ideal coordination of muscle activation. Decreases in both ligamentous and fascial tissue concentrations of these mechanoreceptors affect both the ability to generate appropriate levels of tissue and therefore joint stiffness, as well as diminish the proprioceptive feedback from these tissues to the central nervous system.

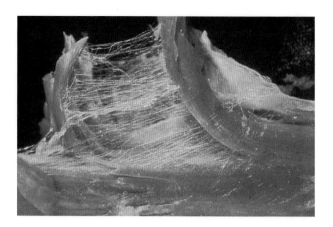

A magnification of myofascial tissue – individual muscle fibers within the cotton floss of the endomysial fascia. Photograph courtesy of Ron Thompson.

FUNCTIONS OF FASCIA

Fascia provides an interconnection between all components of the human body, including connections from muscle to muscle (forming continuous chains of muscles), tendon to bone, tendon to ligament or joint capsule (thereby improving dynamic joint support), bone to bone, viscera to bone, and viscera to viscera. Collectively, these relationships form an interdependent system responsible for supporting, resisting, and moving the body. This interdependence aids in the development and control of tensegrity within the human body.

Coined by Buckminster Fuller (architect and author) in 1961, 'tensegrity' describes the ability of the musculofascial system to develop tension and maintain the integrity of the system. The tensegrity model is based on an architectural design that features a continuous tension-resistant connective system and non-continuous compression-resistant rods or beams (bones). For example, the guy wires of a tent function as the non-contractile tension regulators, while the central and supportive beams of the tent act as the compression-resistant beams. In the human body, the myofascial-ligamentous system functions as the tension regulators, while the bones oppose the compressive forces of gravity, body weight, and

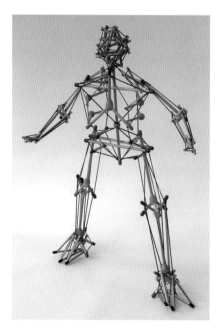
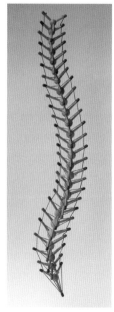

Tensegrity structures, when stressed, tend to distribute rather than concentrate strain. The body does the same, with the result that local injuries soon become global strain patterns. Photograph courtesy of Tom Flemons.

external loads as well as those from muscular contraction. Tensegrity enables the musculoskeletal system the ability to provide significant but yielding support, without, however, succumbing to either externally or internally generated forces. The loss of this tensegrity function as a result of acute trauma (surgery or motor vehicle accident) or repetitive trauma (habitual movement patterns) disrupts this tensegrity function and leads the client to adopt compensatory stabilization and movement strategies. Because of the interconnected nature of the tensegrity system, alterations in fascial tension anywhere along the kinetic chain will render effects across the system.

TYPES OF FASCIA

Fascia can be found both superficially, such as in the thoracolumbar and plantar fascia, and at a deeper level. The superficial layer helps support the skin, numerous muscle attachments, and the fat pads as in the feet. It has also been suggested that fascial thickenings, known as 'retinaculum', over the hands and feet help keep the tendons from bowing during finger and toe flexion. Similarly, the thoracolumbar fascia functions to restrict the contraction of the lumbar erector spinae to help 'stiffen' the trunk. The deeper fascial layers support the muscles and viscera as well as provide a pathway for blood vessels and nerves.

While dispersed among all the tissues of the body, areas that exhibit increased activity and require extra support – such as the low back, hip, and foot – demonstrate an increased thickness of fascia. Additionally, these areas have been shown to contain an increased concentration of myofibroblasts (Schleip et al 2006).

While fascial thickenings are evident throughout the body, there are four distinct thickenings of these myofascial networks that directly aid support of the low back, hip, and foot. These include the thoracolumbar fascia of the back, the abdominal aponeurosis, the fascia lata of the leg, and the plantar fascia of the foot and will be discussed briefly below.

THE THORACOLUMBAR FASCIA

There are three layers of the thoracolumbar fascia (TLF), which function to maintain integrity of the thoracopelvic canister (TPC). The anterior layer connects the quadratus lumborum and intertransverse ligaments. The diaphragm and psoas major have extensive fascial connections to this layer, which functions to co-activate and stabilize the thoracolumbar junction of the TPC. The middle layer blends with the anterior layer and provides attachments for the transversus abdominis muscle. The posterior layer blends with the other two layers and envelops the erector spinae musculature. It also connects the contralateral latissimus dorsi and gluteus maximus, forming the posterior oblique chain. The TLF is important in stabilizing the TPC and sacroiliac joints, as well as adding support to the shoulder and hip complexes. It is also important in rotational control of the trunk and spine. Therefore, alterations in the position and/or control of the extremities can affect stability of the TPC and vice versa.

THE ABDOMINAL FASCIA

The abdominal fascia, also referred to as the 'abdominal aponeurosis', comprises several alternating layers that provide attachment sites for the abdominal muscles. The abdominal muscles and their invested fascia form several decussating layers (cross at angles that form an 'X' pattern) that are integral to the stability of the TPC and therefore stabilization of the hip and shoulder complexes.

The deepest of the abdominal muscles, the transversus abdominis, has attachments to both the abdominal fascia and the TLF. Its fibers are the only pure horizontally oriented fibers in the body, suggesting its important role in stabilization and maintaining integrity of the TPC. The external oblique, the largest of the abdominal muscles, interdigitates with the serratus anterior muscle at the anterolateral costal margins and inserts into the anterior abdominal fascia. It fascially blends with the contralateral internal oblique muscle to form a muscular chain around the anterior aspect of the thorax and abdomen. The rectus abdominis fascially blends distally with the transversus abdominis, internal oblique, pyramidalis, and adductor longus muscles at the pubic symphysis and thus helps to stabilize this joint. Interestingly, the pyramidalis, an often forgotten abdominal muscle, is also responsible for tensing the linea alba, which may help create a better fascial pull on the linea alba from the other abdominal muscles. Clinically speaking, this muscle will commonly demonstrate inhibition in clients who have lost internal hip rotation, necessitating a specific corrective intervention of the pyramidalis when attempting to restore hip range of motion.

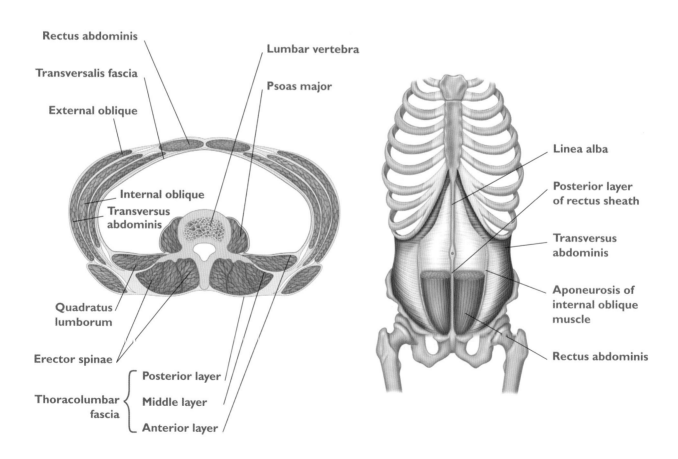

THE FASCIA LATA

The fascia lata, also referred to as the 'iliotibial tract', is one of the thickest expansions of fascia within the body and provides proximal attachments for both the gluteus maximus and the tensor fasciae latae, which takes its name from its insertion point. The iliotibial tract lies superficial to the vastus lateralis and inserts distally into Gerdy's tubercle at the lateral tibial condyle. Contraction of the vastus lateralis causes it to push laterally into the iliotibial fascia, developing a hydraulic amplifier effect upon the iliotibial tract. Along with co-contraction of the gluteus maximus and tensor fasciae latae, this activation helps convert the lower extremity into a rigid lever for supporting body weight during closed-chain lower extremity movements.

THE PLANTAR FASCIA

The plantar fascia, essentially a continuation of the Achilles tendon, attaches from the base of the calcaneus, covers the bottom of the foot, and inserts into all five digits of the foot. This band acts as both a support of the underlying muscles, thereby assisting stabilization of the foot, and a shock absorber for the body. It has been referred to as a prime stabilizer in that it helps prevent collapsing of the mid-foot during the midstance phase of gait as the person's body weight passes over the supporting structure of the foot. Through its connections to the Achilles tendon, gastrocnemius, hamstring complex, sacrotuberous ligaments, erector spinae, and epicranial fascia, the plantar fascia has essentially direct communication with the entire body. Inhibition of the intrinsic foot musculature can often lead to losses of structural integrity within the plantar fascia, which contributes to increased pronatory stresses at the hip, knee, and ankle/foot complexes, and resultant stabilization issues of the lumbopelvic region. Likewise, poor proximal control of the TPC and/or lower extremity pronation tends to overload the plantar fascia, creating many of the common lower extremity compartment and overuse syndromes.

FASCIAL RESPONSE TO TRAUMA AND INJURY

Trauma and injury have been shown to decrease the concentration of intrafascial substances such as type I collagen and hyaluronic acid. This causes alterations in fascial tissue that favors the initiation of inflammation and scar formation, while hindering muscle recovery (Lindsay 2008). This is another cause and perpetuator of movement dysfunctions of the hip and shoulder complexes.

FASCIA AND HYDRATION

The myofascial system is sensitive to hydration levels in the body. Early signs of dehydration are cramping and fatigue, while joint and muscle pain can be indicative of more advanced stages of dehydration (Meyerowitz 2001, Batmanghelidj 1995). Improper hydration levels from exogenous sources (not consuming enough hydrating fluids and/or overconsumption of dehydrating fluids), as well as immobilization (either post-injury or as a result of chronic limitations in range of motion), can lead to decreased tissue mobility, creating adhesions, and promote scar tissue formation within the fascia (Lindsay 2008). Beyond the obvious benefits of maintaining proper intracellular and blood fluid volumes, adequate hydration has been suggested as a means of improving tissue mobility within the fascia (Lindsay 2008, Chek 2004, Meyerowitz 2001, Batmanghelidj 1995). The loss of tissue mobility within the fascia is one significant contributor to loss of movement efficiency and the reason for instituting specific soft-tissue techniques such as myofascial release, origin-insertion techniques, and/or foam rolling prior to the initiation of corrective exercise.

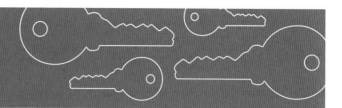

Key To Success

Can Improving Hydration Levels Aid Movement?

As noted, hydration levels within the body can affect tissue mobility. But can improving hydration levels maintain and/or improve the development of ideal movement patterns? Unfortunately, this is a challenging question to answer because there is little evidence to suggest that this is even possible. There is evidence of muscle cramping and decreased performance with lack of proper hydration, and inadequate hydration has been shown to create specific changes, such as the development of adhesions within the myofascial system, that will undoubtedly affect movement patterns. There is, however, anecdotal evidence from alternative health practitioners suggesting the beneficial relationship between proper hydration and health. For example, Goodheart noted that patients who were dehydrated would demonstrate multiple muscle weaknesses during muscle testing, and that drinking a glass of water would restore generalized strength (cited in Walther 2000).

So how much water or fluid should an individual consume for optimal health and muscle function? Unfortunately, this is almost a rhetorical question based upon who is questioned as there are so many varied opinions on the topic. And often the research only adds to the confusion. For example, one study looking at the effects of caffeinated and non-caffeinated beverages showed that there were no significant changes to the hydration levels of healthy men with the consumption of hydration carbonated, caffeinated caloric and non-caloric colas, and coffee. However, an interesting note is that this study was funded by a grant from The Coca-Cola Company (Grandkean et al 2000). Similar studies found no difference in hydration levels between consuming plain water versus other beverages.

So what about the 6–8 glasses of water per day rule? While 8 glasses per day has unscientifically stood the test of time as the gold standard, this would equate to about 64 ounces per day (8 glasses at 8 oz per glass). It is unlikely that most of the population drinks this much water and is often contradicted by researchers who suggest there is no proof of needing to consume this amount (Valtin 2002). It is interesting to note, however, that 64 ounces of fluid intake was not enough to replace the fluid weight lost in the research subjects in the study conducted by Grandkean and colleagues. In fact, the authors suggest that perhaps the 64 ounces fluid recommendation is not a sufficient quantity for maintaining adequate hydration levels and also make note of research that supports the inverse relationship between fluid consumption and cancer risks (Grandkean et al 2000).

KEY: So just how much water should be consumed on a daily basis for optimal health? The consensus among health experts, in other words those who look to optimize health and not merely look at the absence of disease as a sign of health, is that there is a chronic dehydration epidemic. Paul Chek and Steve Meyerowitz recommend one-half of an individual's body weight in ounces (90 oz of water for someone weighing 180 lb), while Mark Lindsay recommends 0.6 ounces times body weight in pounds (106 oz for someone weighing 180 lb) for achieving optimal health and tissue mobility. Even greater fluid intake has been recommended for those individuals who are exercising and sweating profusely. While there seems to be no agreement between the researchers and the health experts, there is enough anecdotal clinical evidence to suggest that increased water consumption is warranted for achieving and maintaining tissue mobility and overall health for most individuals.

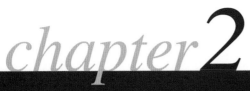

chapter 2

Developing Movement

CHAPTER OBJECTIVES

To identify the basic patterns of child development and adult movement

To understand the key reasons for the loss of movement efficiency

ONTOGENESIS MODEL OF FUNCTION

The development of the human being, otherwise known as 'ontogeny', is based on developing levels of maturation within the nervous, muscle and soft-tissue, and articular systems. This development is based upon programs that are engrained from birth, and advancement to the next level is dependent on the successful completion of each previous stage. The study of ontology is pertinent to the study of movement, as it not only explains what ideal expression and movement should look like, but also helps explain why certain posture and adaptive strategies are adopted by clients and patients with movement disorders.

A child first learns to move through feel: it is a complete proprioceptive experience driven by engrained motor programs, reflexive patterns, and a desire to accomplish a specific goal, i.e. feeding themselves, locomotion, pain avoidance, etc. The patterns the child adopts are typical of each stage and represent a necessary progression to the next major developmental milestone. While many physical and occupational therapy approaches have been adapted based on child development patterns, their use was mostly limited to the children and adult neurological patient population. However, in the early 1900s, Mabel Elsworth Todd utilized several developmental positions such as rolling and crawling to help clients improve balance and regain function in the dancers and athletes she worked with. This training would become instrumental in the development of the field of movement referred to as 'ideokinesis'. Moshe Feldenkrais was known to utilize rolling patterns in his awareness through movement techniques. More recently, Vaclav Vojta, a Czech pediatric neurologist, began utilizing developmental patterns and noted that specific stimulation of key points in children with cerebral palsy elicited characteristic and repeatable responses. He also noted similar responses in the adult population, which could be used to change long-standing movement dysfunction and would eventually become the basis of his Reflex Locomotion Technique.

Pavel Kolar, a student of the Vojta method, developed a system of exercises (Dynamic Neuromuscular Stabilization) based on these developmental positions, to establish normal stabilization and movement patterns in the adult orthopedic population. He utilized each of the child developmental milestones to develop a series of corresponding corrective and advanced exercise patterns designed to restore these primitive patterns in the client with stabilization and movement system dysfunctions.

Listed in the table below are several of the child developmental milestones, which are based on Vojta's Reflex Locomotion and Kolar's Approach to Dynamic Neuromuscular Stabilization. The corresponding corrective exercises that will be utilized in the corrective exercise section are presented and associated with each stage, along with the reasons for their inclusion. Many of these exercise recommendations are modified and adapted from Kolar's Approach to Dynamic Neuromuscular Stabilization, which formed the basis for many of the corrective techniques and strategies in this book.

Time	Developmental Milestone	Corresponding Corrective Exercise Patterns
6 weeks	Child lifts head, supports on forearms and belly	First level of prone thoracic extensions Function: to develop optimal respiration and function of the neck stabilizers, including the deep neck flexors, and the scapular stabilizers, including the serratus anterior
3½ months	Supine with triple flexion of legs (hips, knees, ankles) and co-activation of breathing and abdominal support (IAP)	Breathing and core activation, with legs elevated in triple flexion Function: to develop optimal position of the spine, thorax, and pelvis, as well as develop the optimal stabilization and respiratory strategies of the diaphragm and muscles of the thoracopelvic canister
	Prone – double limb support	Second and third levels of prone thoracic extension Function: to further develop stabilization role of deep neck flexors, scapular stabilizers, and spine extensors
4½ months	Upper extremity differentiation and can reach midline Stabilization in the sagittal plane	Wall plank with arm lift off Quadruped with trunk rotation or reach Function: to progress into unilateral upper extremity support, with neck and thoracopelvic stabilization
6 months	Abdominal chains are formed to allow side lying and turning	Side lying isometric patterns Function: to develop scapular and glenohumeral stabilizers and coordinate unilateral stabilization between trunk and upper and lower extremities
	Supine support on thoracolumbar junction by coordinated activity of diaphragm, psoas, deep anterior and posterior abdominal walls	Modified dead bug Function: to develop optimal stabilization of the thoracolumbar junction

7–8 months	Oblique sit to upright sitting positions Tripod position (support on legs and one arm) Quadruped position and creeping (pulling from arms)	Advanced side lying patterns and oblique sit with reach Quadruped progressions Function: to further develop trunk stability with coordination of limb differentiation
6–9 months	Crawling (contralateral differentiation between arms and legs) Standing up and side-walking with arm support	Advanced quadruped progressions Crab walk and band progressions Function: to develop hip stabilization and verticalization progressions
10 months	Squatting	Squatting progressions Function: to develop trunk stabilization in upright posture with coordination of hip mobility
10–12 months	Independent stance and progression of the gait pattern	Fundamental movement patterns Function: to coordinate respiratory and stabilization activities into fundamental movement patterns
3 years	Single leg stance	Single leg patterns Function: to progress fundamental patterns into sport- or work-specific activities

While these developmental patterns are rarely thought of as part of conventional training, several of them can be seen in many of the common patterns that are part of functional stabilization routines.

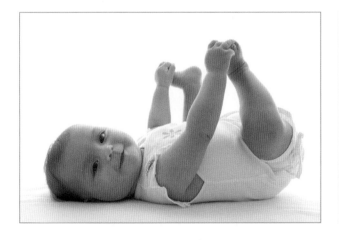
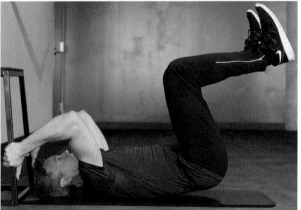

While lying supine, the child often grabs their feet and lifts themselves to stabilize at the thoracolumbar junction (image above left). This strategy helps the child develop the deep stabilization system and alignment of the trunk, spine, and pelvis that will be required to get themselves into an optimal upright posture. This position is trained in the pelvic abdominal lift and this alignment must be maintained during functional movement patterns (image above right).

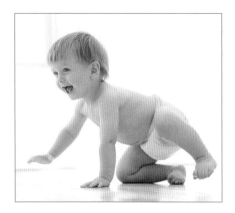 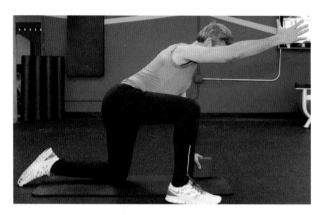

As the child progresses to crawling, they stabilize on contralateral limbs while moving their trunk around the stabilized limbs. The kneeling reach with contralateral stabilization mirrors this pattern as the client stabilizes on contralateral limbs and reaches with the free arm and leg.

The triple support position, referred to as the 'holy triple' (Kolar 2009), is a progression to the upright posture in addition to providing stability for the support limb and mobility for the moving limb. The child's left leg (image below left) is in a centrated position as they reach with their left arm. This position helps the child gain the centrated hip position and trunk stability necessary to achieve the upright posture. The 3-point rotation re-creates many of the same forces through the three points of support: ipsilateral hip and shoulder and contralateral hip.

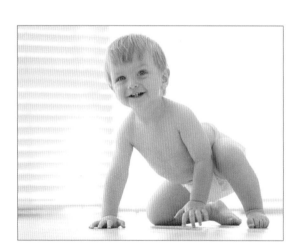 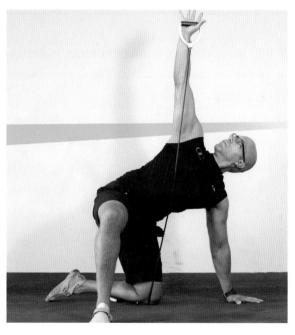

These developmental milestones set the stage for the development of the fundamental movement patterns that are characteristic in the adult population. Correction of movement dysfunction often makes it necessary to revisit some of these more primitive, engrained patterns in the corrective exercise approach. These influences will be seen in many of the patterns leading up to the development of optimal fundamental movement patterns that are presented in later chapters.

FUNDAMENTAL MOVEMENT PATTERNS

The end goal of any corrective exercise, rehabilitative strategy, or conditioning program is to improve performance in the fundamental movement patterns and reduce the likelihood of injury. When working with the general population, the end goal is to improve the efficiency of work, sport, and activities of daily living. Athletes may share these same goals but are generally looking for improved efficiency in motion to enhance their game while minimizing their risk of injury. Regardless of the end goal, improving a patient or client's function in these fundamental patterns is essential because all movement is a combination of five primary patterns.

In the infant, the fundamental movement patterns, sometimes referred to as 'primitive movement patterns', are supine support, rolling, pushing up, quadruped, and crawling. These patterns will eventually develop into the five adult fundamental movement patterns that include gait, level changes, pulling, pushing, and rotation. These patterns will be discussed below.

GAIT: WALKING TO RUNNING

The basic function of our neuromusculoskeletal system is to provide us with the ability to travel from one place to another. Remember, our goals for thousands of years were to survive, find food and shelter, procreate, and avoid being eaten. We were often moving from one area of land to another at varying rates of speed. Our neuromusculoskeletal system is highly efficient and adaptable to enable us to transport ourselves in a walking manner or to move at a more rapid pace such as running or sprinting. To cross over larger areas or uneven terrain, or to increase our foot placement, we can utilize varying positions of running, skipping, hopping, leaping, bounding and jumping.

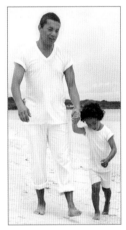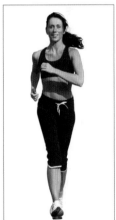

LEVEL CHANGES: SQUATTING, LUNGING, AND CLIMBING

The upright posture of the human body allows us to maintain a center of gravity by distributing our weight across the spine and skeleton. This posture is incredibly efficient and allows us to effectively load our muscles to perform a myriad of motions. From this position we are able to perform squatting, which enables us to lower our center of mass and to lift objects from the ground. The lunging pattern allows us to asymmetrically load our lower extremities to increase our reach, lower our torso towards the ground or maneuver around objects. Using our upper extremities to pull and the lower extremities to push we can move our body up a tree or the side of a mountain, or climb a staircase.

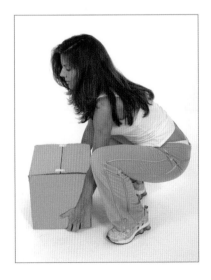

PULLING / PUSHING

By manipulating the extremities, a myriad of tasks can be performed such as lifting and carrying in addition to innumerous fine motor tasks. While muscles on their own can only perform pulling motions, by utilizing the skeleton as a lever system, they are capable of performing pushing motions. Pulling motions allow us to bring objects into our body for greater ease in lifting and carrying. Pushing motions allow us to move objects away from our body, either by lifting them onto another surface or by accelerating them, as seen in throwing. Our body commonly works in a cross pattern where one extremity is pulling while the opposite one is pushing, as seen in walking, running or throwing an object. The contralateral forces act to cancel each other, thus allowing us to maintain our center of gravity.

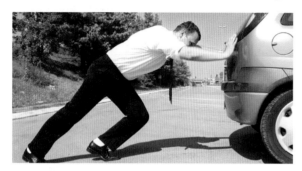 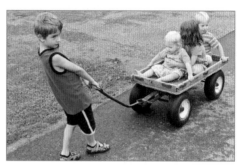

ROTATION

The fifth and final basic movement pattern is perhaps the most inclusive of all movement, as all movement is rotation. As sports conditioning specialist Ben Shear says, "The body does not know sports, it only knows rotation." This movement pattern includes changing of direction, which is performed through rotation and twisting, and also allows motion of the body perpendicular to the force of gravity or against horizontal forces. Through the summation of forces that are generated by the varying regions of the core musculature, the body is able to accelerate and decelerate itself or an object, as seen in throwing or swinging a club. Additionally, rotation allows the body to move and perform a limitless number of complex movements by simple adjustments in the limbs or trunk.

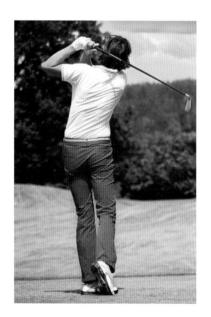

It is important to keep these basic movement patterns in mind when designing general training and rehabilitation programs. It should become obvious after studying the five basic movement patterns that the body is meant to move by combining movement in all three planes of motion, across all the joints of the kinetic chain, at varying levels of speed and with the right amount of control. However, all movements can be broken down into individual components or 'chunks.' For example, even a complex move such as swinging a golf club is a combination of several movement patterns. During the address, there is a change in the center of gravity as the hips are flexed. During the backswing, there is a change in direction of the trunk and pelvis, and a combination of pulling and pushing of the extremities as these regions are loaded. During the swing phase, there is an unloading of the forces as the trunk and pelvis rotate and the club is now pushed through by motion of the trunk and the extremities.

It should also become apparent when looking at the five basic movement patterns that the body never works in isolation. It functions in an integrated manner by selecting various movement patterns, rather than preferentially choosing isolated regions or muscle groups. The body does not like to work in isolation and will attempt to distribute force across as many joints as possible to reduce stress to any one region. This will be the basis of integrative movement training: involve as many muscle groups and joints as possible and teach the body to integrate the movements precisely the way they were designed. This does not suggest that isolated rehabilitation, corrective exercise, or training is unnecessary, rather that once the isolated dysfunction is discovered and improved, it must be reintegrated into the fundamental movement patterns. A final point when taking this view of movement is that, as trainers and health care practitioners, there must be a global view of the entire kinetic chain when attempting to enhance performance or improve causes of dysfunction. Dysfunction anywhere along the kinetic chain can impact distal structures and therefore have significant effects on the overall functioning of the neuromusculoskeletal system.

THE SELF-PERPETUATING PATTERN OF MOVEMENT DYSFUNCTION

The self-perpetuating pattern of dysfunction has been proposed as a means of describing the perpetuation of dysfunctional movement patterns (Liebenson 2007, Rattray and Ludwig 2002, Page et al 2010). It graphically depicts how any stressor to the nervous system – including acute and repetitive trauma, emotional stress, up-regulation of the sympathetic nervous system, and pain – can alter movement strategies that essentially create a self-perpetuating cycle of dysfunction. This model also provides a likely explanation of the incidence of reoccurring injuries in those who have suffered previous injuries such as low back pain and ankle sprains.

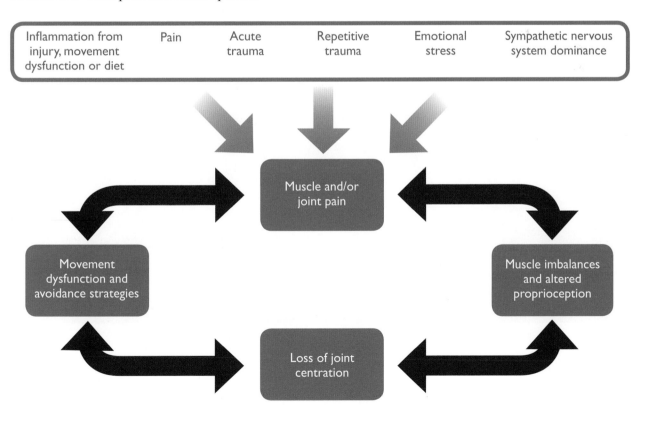

The goal of the corrective strategy is to break this cycle by interrupting some aspect of the dysfunctional cycle. At what point the trainer or therapist enters their particular client's cycle is dependent on several variables, including how long the client has had the dysfunction, the degree of pain the client is in, where the greatest area of dysfunction is, and what the client's 'story' of their dysfunction means to them. In the acute phases of trauma, the primary goal is to control the pain prior to addressing the movement dysfunction. Soft tissue techniques, joint mobilization, ice, anti-inflammatory or analgesics, and rest are the generally accepted methods of treatment during this phase. Specific exercises can often be useful, even in the acute phase; however, the trainer or therapist should ensure that the exercises are specific for the client. With clients experiencing more chronicity with their condition, the trainer or therapist will usually get better results by addressing the greatest source of movement dysfunction, in other words the 'weakest link' in the chain. For clients with chronic pain, it is unlikely that acutely decreasing the painful source will change the client's perception or symptoms, so addressing the biggest 'driver' in the cycle of dysfunction generally fosters greater results. As a general rule, exercise is always indicated during this phase and again must be highly specific to the individual client because they are caught in the chronic cycle of dysfunction and require a corrective strategic solution directed at the cause of their issue.

The stabilization-dissociation model that will be presented later in this section will help shed more light on how these cycles of dysfunction perpetuate movement dysfunction.

Key To Success
Finding the Greatest Driver

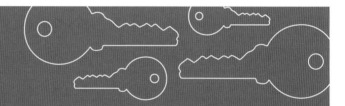

While it is tempting for the clinician to chase the painful area, when dealing with the chronic pain client it is important to look at the area of the greatest dysfunction. Pain of a chronic nature often results from poor stabilization and movement strategies. Therefore, it is helpful to find the greatest 'driver' or region that is driving most of the dysfunction, otherwise referred to as the 'weakest link.' It may be necessary to 'peel back' the proverbial layers of dysfunction, meaning that the region of greatest dysfunction may be merely a compensation of a deeper level of dysfunction. Regardless, attempting to discover the area of greatest dysfunction and 'unpeeling' the layers will serve the clinician well in attempting to improve their client's movement patterns.

KEY: When dealing with the client suffering acute pain, address the pain source and get that under control before dealing with the associated movement dysfunction. In the client with chronic pain, address the region demonstrating the greatest stabilization or movement dysfunction.

JOINT CENTRATION

Developing optimal, efficient movement while placing the least stress on soft tissue and articular structures is reliant on one premise: the achievement of optimal joint centration. Optimal joint centration is the place where there is ideal contact as well as ideal neuromuscular control of the articular surfaces of the kinetic chain. This allows for the maximum length-tension relationships of the functional antagonists of the joint to supply the muscle synergy required to stabilize and bear load across the joint surfaces (Kolar 2009). See Video: Explaining Joint Centration, www.fitnesseducationseminars.com/osar-book

The general principle is that centration is a combination of stabilization and dissociation. The client must be able to stabilize one portion of the articulation as they dissociate the other portion of the articulation. While often used interchangeably, dissociation is much more than simple mobility of a joint. Dissociation is the controlled movement of an articulation. Whereas mobility of a joint is required for effective dissociation, mobility is simply the available range of motion within the joint and does not imply control of this motion. Dissociation includes the neuromotor control of a range of motion while maintaining an optimal axis of control. Therefore, efficient movement requires the coordinated neuromuscular control of both joint stabilization and dissociation. This combined effort is what establishes optimal joint centration and the development of efficient movement patterns.

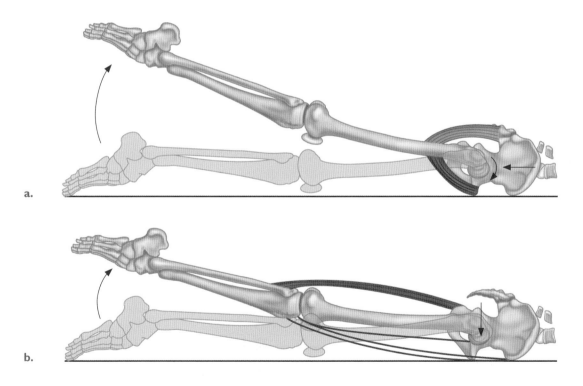

a.

b.

Notice how the muscles closest to the axis of rotation help maintain an optimal axis of rotation (image a) whereas the muscles further from the joint can perform a similar action but are unable to preserve the centrated joint position (image b). In the above example, the gluteus maximus is closer to the axis of rotation and is therefore able to maintain joint centration as it assists hip extension. The hamstrings, inserting further from the axis of rotation, will drive the femoral head forward within the acetabulum when they become the primary hip extensors.

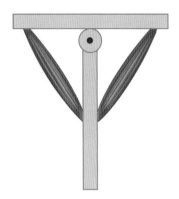 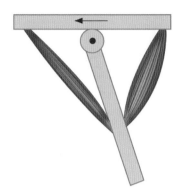

When all the muscle synergists are working optimally, joint centration is maintained (image above left). In the presence of muscle inhibition (thinner muscle), the functional antagonist (thicker muscle) exerts its pull on the joint and centration is lost (image above right).

The hip and shoulder provide great examples of these concepts. For example, the psoas major and gluteus maximus are often labeled as antagonists owing to the fact that the psoas major is a hip flexor and the gluteus maximus is a hip extender. However, the deep medial fibers of both the psoas major and the gluteus maximus help centrate the femoral head in the acetabulum, thereby allowing for an optimal axis of rotation during hip motion (Gibbons 2005). Inhibition of one of the functional antagonists will up-regulate the synergists to help achieve optimum centration. In this example, if the psoas major was to become inhibited by an acute disc irritation for instance, the other hip flexors, including the tensor fasciae latae and rectus femoris, would become the dominant hip flexors. Unfortunately, since they are located further from the axis of hip rotation, they do not provide for optimal joint centration and instead pull the femoral head forward in the acetabulum as the client brings their hip into flexion (Sahrmann 2002, Lee 2008). Similarly, inhibition of the gluteus maximus leads to up-regulation of the hamstrings to support hip extension. Being further from the axis of rotation, the hamstrings drive the femoral head forward in the acetabulum as the client brings their hip into extension.

This is a very common scenario that leads to femoral anterior glide syndrome (Sahrmann 2002) and the loss of optimal hip function and strength.

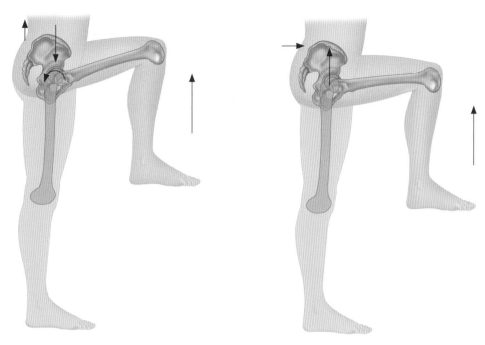

The individual flexes their hip and is able to maintain a centrated joint when there is optimal co-activation of the muscle synergists of the hip complex (left image). When there is muscle dyskinesis, joint centration is lost and activation of the prime movers of the hip drives disruption of the axis of rotation (right image).

A similar scenario exists in the shoulder. The rotator cuff muscles are responsible for maintaining centration of the humerus in the glenoid fossa. The subscapularis is unique in that it helps draw the

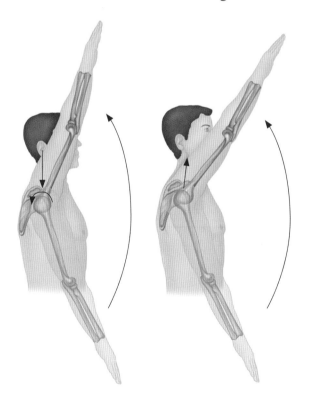

humerus posteriorly in the glenoid fossa. With inhibition of the subscapularis, the other internal rotators of the shoulder, mainly the teres major and latissimus dorsi, are up-regulated to assist control of the glenohumeral joint. Because both muscles lie further from the axis of rotation, they will draw the humerus forward in the glenoid, creating humeral anterior glide syndrome (Sahrmann 2002). The client then uses this strategy in all their functional movement patterns, engraining this pattern with every increasing movement they perform.

The individual raises their arm and is able to maintain a centrated joint when there is optimal co-activation of the muscle synergists of the shoulder complex (left image). When there is muscle dyskinesis, joint centration is lost and activation of the prime movers of the shoulder drives disruption of the axis of rotation (right image).

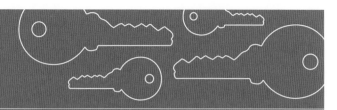

Key To Success

Joint Centration

Joint centration is achieved by the combined neuromotor tasks of stabilization and dissociation. While no single muscle is any more important to function than any other, each muscle does have its own unique action that it is best suited for and if inhibited, it alters the ideal centration and therefore overall movement efficiency of the joint and ultimately the entire kinetic chain. The deeper local muscles likely play a bigger role in the fine, minute control of joint positions during movement and will often require preferential attention when attempting to restore optimal movement patterns.

KEY: One of the keys to improving function is to ensure activation of all joint synergists, and develop ideal stabilization strategies and dissociation patterns to enhance the client's ability to achieve optimal joint centration.

GLOBAL RESPONSES OF INSTABILITY
THAT LEAD TO LOSS OF JOINT CENTRATION

Following an injury, it is common for a client to experience loss of joint centration in the affected region. The nervous system reacts by up-regulating functional synergists in an attempt to protect and stabilize the joint. This up-regulation can also occur when there is a general loss of visual or vestibular input, or an overall general proprioceptive dysfunction following an injury.

'Gripping' patterns can result as the body up-regulates functional synergists to aid support or stabilization in the case of local or global instability. This is often the cause of chronic postural habits and movement patterns, as well as explaining why 'balance-specific' exercises (balance boards, wobble devices, etc.) can actually perpetuate bad habits rather than help clients and patients with poor balance. While this phenomenon can be seen anywhere in the body, there are several compensatory strategies that are common among clients with poor trunk and/or lower extremity stabilization.

- **Shoulder gripping:** The latissimus dorsi, teres major, pectoralis minor, and rhomboids will often show signs of overactivity in an attempt to stabilize the trunk. This pattern will lead to downward rotation of the scapula and contribute to trunk rigidity. These clients will generally demonstrate poor trunk rotation and arm swing during gait, as well as limitations in overhead arm motion.

- **Trunk gripping:** Overactivation of the erector spinae, generally at the level of the thoracolumbar junction, results in thoracolumbar extension. The external abdominal obliques are generally the more common overactive muscles of the abdominal wall and create a posterior tilt of the pelvis and/or trunk flexion and narrowing of the sternal angle of the rib cage. Overactivation of the internal abdominal obliques will lead to a widening and flaring of the rib cage. Generally overactivity of either the abdominal wall or the erector spinae results in a reflexive co-activation of the opposing muscle group, leading to rigidity of the trunk and spine.

- **Hip gripping:** Hip gripping, also referred to as 'butt gripping' (Lee 2008), will result in an anterior femoral head position and general overcompression of the femoroacetabular joint. It may also result in posterior rotation of the ilium on the femur during single leg stance. This is a common substitution strategy especially when individuals lose stability in single leg stance.

- **Toe gripping:** There are essentially two toe-gripping strategies that clients will utilize: toe clawing and toe curling. Toe clawing, more commonly referred to as 'hammer toes', is extension of the proximal metatarsophalangeal joint and flexion of the proximal interphalangeal joint. Toe curling is flexion of both the metatarsophalangeal and interphalangeal joints. This overactivity of the toe flexors results in a decrease in ankle dorsiflexion and leads to compensations through the mid-foot, knee, and/or trunk especially during single leg stance and in situations where balance is compromised.

These substitution patterns are common throughout functional activities and, as mentioned, often occur secondary to injuries that inhibit or functionally compromise a muscle's ability to perform its function. Because the client's will is often greater than their ability to stabilize (due to the instinctive survival mode present in all living beings), as well as the nervous system's compensatory adeptness, the resultant activities require the nervous system to adopt alternative muscle strategies to perform the task at hand. This is a major contributor to movement dysfunction and the reason that it is so easy for clients and patients to perpetuate their habitual patterns. Several of the more common inhibited muscles are listed in the table below, along with their synergistic muscle substitutions and the postural or movement dysfunction that often results in response to this strategy.

Region	Inhibited Muscle	Common Muscle Substitution	Resultant Postural and/or Movement Dysfunction
Shoulder	subscapularis	teres major, latissimus dorsi	anterior humeral head position poor glenohumeral dissociation
	supraspinatus	deltoids	superior humeral head position
	serratus anterior, upper trapezius, lower trapezius	rhomboids, levator scapula, pectoralis minor	downward rotation of scapula lateral flexion of neck towards the side of inhibition
Hip	psoas major and minor	In the hip: rectus femoris, tensor fasciae latae In the trunk and spine: erector spinae, oblique abdominals	In the hip: anterior femoral head position In the trunk and spine: global rigidity of trunk and spine and hyperextension of the thoracolumbar junction
	gluteus maximus	hamstrings, piriformis, lumbar erector spinae	anterior femoral head position, lumbar hyperlordosis (if erector spinae dominant) or posterior pelvic rotation (if hamstrings are dominant)
	gluteus medius and minimus	tensor fasciae latae, rectus femoris, quadratus lumborum	pelvic unleveling (higher on side of positive Trendelenburg's) spinal curvature (compensated Trendelenburg's)
Respiration and trunk stabilization	diaphragm	scalenes, sternocleido-mastoid, pectoralis minor	accelerated respiratory rates, apical breathing patterns, hypertrophy of accessory muscles of respiration, rigidity of neck, trunk, and spine, forward head and neck
	transversus abdominis	oblique abdominals, erector spinae	global rigidity of trunk and spine
	pelvic floor	piriformis, obturator externus, quadratus femoris	'butt gripping,' poor femoroacetabular dissociation

THE STABILIZATION-DISSOCIATION MODEL OF FUNCTION

To perform coordinated, efficient motion, the kinetic chain consists of alternating articular regions requiring stabilization and dissociation. Gray Cook initially proposed the stability-mobility model to describe the function of the various links within the kinetic chain. Adapting his model, it can be determined that stabilization is required at the foot, knee, lumbopelvic complex, scapulothoracic, and cervical spine, while dissociation is required at the ankle, hip, thoracic spine, glenohumeral, and suboccipital regions. This model does not mean to suggest motion is not required in regions of the foot, knee, or scapula, for example, but rather serves as a guideline as to the general function of each segment of the kinetic chain.

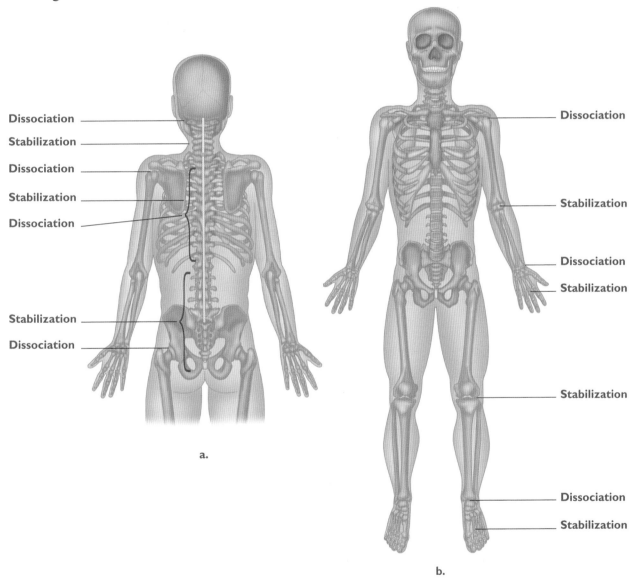

The stabilization-dissociation model of function (a. posterior view, b. anterior view).

Key To Success
Note on the Stabilization-Dissociation Model

While certain regions of the kinetic chain may be better designed for stabilization and others are better designed for dissociation, it is important to note that all regions must at certain times be stable and during others, be able to dissociate. For example, the lumbo-pelvic region must generally be stable when loaded. However, the few degrees of motion that each segment contributes, is important to overall motion of the spine during the gait cycle for example. Similarly, while the knee is designated as a region of stabilization, there must be an ability to dissociate the tibia and femur to provide optimal loading and unloading during the gait cycle.

KEY: All regions of the kinetic chain require a level of stabilization to efficiently load the joints and the ability to dissociate to functionally 'unlock' the joints to allow motion. Both these functions must be respected and respectively conditioned into each region of the kinetic chain.

Dysfunction occurs when there are alterations in these relationships where the joints requiring stabilization become hypermobile and conversely the joint that should be mobile becomes hypomobile. Several common dysfunctional movement patterns that follow the stabilization-dissociation model are described in the following table.

Loss of Dissociation	Common Compensatory Patterns
Ankle	Increased knee abduction (valgus) and/or increased foot pronation
Hip	Posterior rotation of the pelvis and lumbar spine flexion and/or intra-pelvic rotation (loss of sacroiliac integrity)
Thoracic	Posterior rotation of the pelvis and lumbar spine flexion and/or scapulothoracic instability Increased cervicothoracic motion
Glenohumeral	Scapulothoracic instability and/or cervical spine instability

Generally the areas that become hypermobile secondary to poor local stabilization and poor distal dissociation – mainly the knees, lumbopelvic region, and scapulothoracic regions – are the regions where most clients complain of pain first and are the reasons they seek out the services of a trainer or therapist (they will generally pay a visit to their orthopedic surgeon when these areas become intolerable). While hypermobility of the knee and lumbar spine often leads to premature degeneration of these areas, degenerative issues also tend to arise at the overly compressed joints, i.e. at the hips, although it generally takes a longer time for direct manifestation of these dysfunctions. This is generally why the medical and orthopedic world tends to blame 'heredity' for joint degeneration and osteoarthritis for these conditions, rarely attributing them to dysfunctions in patients' movement strategy.

These alterations in joint function will also change muscular control of the region. For example, loss of scapulothoracic stability secondary to thoracic rigidity results in tightness of the rotator cuff as it reflexively up-regulates to help improve stabilization. This results in diminished glenohumeral dissociation, causing glenohumeral motion to drive scapulothoracic motion, perpetuating the scapular dyskinesis. Additionally, as the scapulothoracic articulation becomes more mobile, the neck becomes stiffer as the muscles of the cervical spine also up-regulate in an attempt to stabilize and anchor the scapula. This increases compressive forces through the neck, irritating the peripheral nerves of the cervical spine, leading to muscle inhibition and further perpetuation of the movement dysfunction.

A similar pattern can be seen in the lower extremities. With loss of hip dissociation secondary to a poor hip stabilization pattern such as 'butt gripping' or restrictions in the posterior capsule, the clients will move by means of the lumbopelvic region, either posteriorly rotating the pelvis or flexing the lumbar spine, or a combination of both. This drives hypermobility of the lumbar spine and reflexive tightness of the hip external rotators and/or hamstrings, effectively perpetuating the cycle.

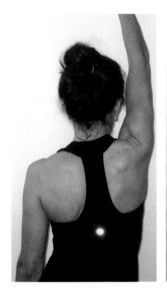 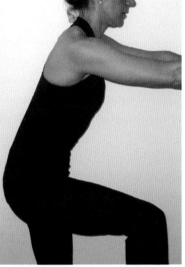

Poor patterns of dissociation: The client does not achieve optimal dissociation of their glenohumeral joint, which causes them to overly abduct and elevate the scapulothoracic articulation (image to left). They do not achieve optimal dissociation of the hip, resulting in posterior rotation of the pelvis and lumbar flexion (image to right).

The key to halting these perpetuating cycles of dysfunction is to identify and correct the key drivers and institute corrective patterns to engrain new movement patterning into the nervous system. While some trainers or therapists may argue the point whether the hypomobility preceded the hypermobility or vice versa, it is often as senseless a discussion as the great chicken or egg debate. The goal of the corrective strategy will be to mobilize the hypomobile regions, stabilize the hypermobile regions, and institute a corrective exercise strategy that respects the relationship between the regions. A general rule of thumb will be to stabilize the proximal structures – the spine in the examples above – and then teach optimal dissociation through the extremities, i.e. the hip and shoulders. This will be the basic premise of the corrective exercise strategy that is presented in the later sections of the book.

The goal of the corrective strategies is to improve joint centration by improving the function of the muscle synergists around the particular dysfunctional joint(s) and then teach the client how to dissociate the appropriate regions of the kinetic chain. They are then provided with a strategy for incorporating the new joint position and control back into the fundamental movement patterns. This approach often requires the use of specific muscle activation strategies to improve the role of the inhibited functional muscle antagonists and will be the discussion of a later section of the book.

PREDICTORS OF INJURY

While it is impossible to predict with a one hundred percent accuracy, there are three factors that have demonstrated clinical consistency in establishing the cause, as well as predicting the potential for injuries: asymmetries in range of motion, previous injury, and aberrant motor control.

Asymmetries in hip range of motion have been found in clients with low back pain (Van Dillen et al 2008). Not only was there a greater loss of total hip rotation in those clients with low back pain, but there was also a greater asymmetry in range of motion between the left and right sides. Similarly, Ellison, Rose, and Sahramnn discovered a predominant loss of internal hip rotation when comparing healthy subjects to patients with low back pain (1990). Loss of internal hip rotation is a common anecdotal clinical finding in clients with low back pain and similarly the loss of internal shoulder rotation accompanies neck and upper back pain. Assessing asymmetries in motion will be a basis for several of the range of motion tests that will be performed in the assessment function.

Previous injury has been suggested as a predictor of injury, although, in a literature review of predictive factors for lateral ankle sprains, Beynnon et al (2002) found no consistent factors on which to base future ankle injury predictions. However, mechanical instability (joint effusion, ligamentous or joint capsule laxity, and impaired arthrokinematics) and functional instability (altered proprioception, muscular activation patterns, and impaired postural control) have been discovered following joint injury and have been suggested to play a role in recurrent injuries (Hertel 2002). Experimental joint effusion (injection of saline solution into a joint) has been shown to create inhibition of the local stabilizers (vastus medialis) of the knee (Hopkins et al 2002). Individuals experiencing low back pain and unilateral sciatica-type symptoms have demonstrated atrophy in multifidus and psoas major (Dangaria et al 1998). Kamaz et al (2007) demonstrated atrophic changes in the psoas major, quadratus lumborum, and multifidus in patients with chronic low back pain, with similar findings discovered by Barker, Shamley and Jackson (2004). Poor performance in balance tests has also been shown to be a reliable predictor of ankle injuries (McGuine et al 2000). While the research may not convincingly indicate a relationship, there is enough empirical as well as anecdotal clinical evidence to suggest that previous injuries and resultant muscle atrophy can be predictors of future injuries when combined with the results of a functional assessment.

Additionally, dysfunctions in motor control and altered muscle activation strategies have been consistently demonstrated in clients with low back pain versus those without pain (Richardson et al 2004). Increased activation of the global muscles rather than the local muscles of the trunk has been demonstrated in athletes with chronic groin pain (Cowan et al 2004), and in patients with pelvic girdle pain there is increased pre-activation of the biceps femoris and adductor longus over the transversus abdominis (Hungerford et al 2003). Deficits in neuromuscular control of the trunk have been shown to be a predictor of knee injury in athletes (Zazulak et al). In a study of 303 college athletes, timing delays in trunk muscles were demonstrated to be a risk factor for developing low back pain. With athletes who reported a previous episode of back pain, there was a greater than twofold increase in the risk for developing future back pain (Cholewicki et al 2005). Thus, identifying movement dysfunction and improving motor control must be components of the corrective exercise strategy when attempting to improve dysfunctional movement patterns.

CONCLUSION

Identifying the components of human movement helps the trainer or therapist understand some of the nuances of movement as well as the causes for movement inefficiencies. Understanding and appreciating the developmental and advancing roles of the neuromusculofascial system enables the practitioner to better design and implement corrective and progressive exercise patterns that are specific to the fundamental needs of the patient or client. The next sections will take a closer look at the shoulder and hip complexes to facilitate better understanding of the intricacies of these regions, as well as improve comprehension of the ideal kinematics a client will require to achieve improved function, decreased likelihood of injury, and enhanced performance.

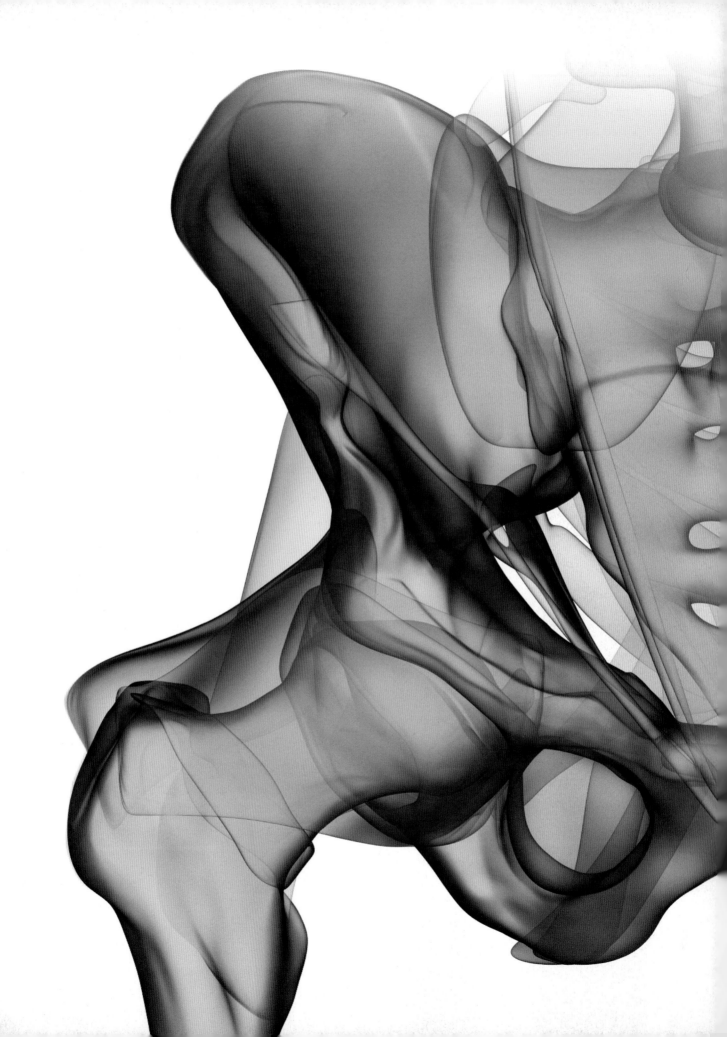

part II

Identifying and Assessing the Hip and Shoulder Complexes

chapter 3

The Shoulder Complex

CHAPTER OBJECTIVES
To identify and understand the functional components of the shoulder complex

To identify the key regions of dysfunction within the shoulder complex

To understand the ideal mechanics of the shoulder complex

The shoulder is a complex system of joints working together to allow for a large range of mobility of the upper extremity. The shoulder complex functions to support the upper extremity to allow for the specific placement of the hand in the actions of pulling, pushing, lifting, and throwing.

STRUCTURE OF THE SHOULDER COMPLEX

The shoulder complex is formed by four joint articulations: glenohumeral (GH), scapulothoracic (ST), acromioclavicular (AC), and sternoclavicular (SC). The collective action of these four joints make the shoulder complex the most mobile joint complex in the body. However, this mobility comes at a price: stability. To understand exactly how stability is created, a basic knowledge of shoulder kinematics and functional anatomy is necessary.

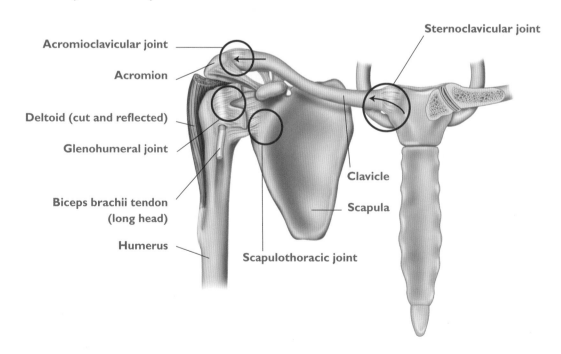

THE GLENOHUMERAL JOINT

The glenohumeral (GH) joint (see below, right arm, lateral view) is an enarthrodial (ball-and-socket) joint formed by the humeral head and the glenoid fossa of the scapula. Although it has traditionally been classified as a ball-and-socket joint, the GH joint can be more correctly thought of as a golf ball on a tee. As mentioned, this arrangement allows for a tremendous amount of motion but it comes at the cost of stability. Therefore, the GH joint relies on the passive support that is provided by the glenoid labrum, joint capsule, and numerous ligaments surrounding the joint, as well as that supplied by the rotator cuff muscles, which add additional dynamic support. Each of these components will be looked at in greater detail below.

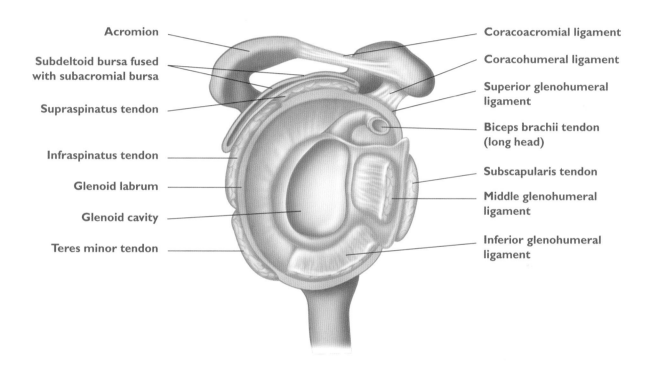

Acromion

Subdeltoid bursa fused with subacromial bursa

Supraspinatus tendon

Infraspinatus tendon

Glenoid labrum

Glenoid cavity

Teres minor tendon

Coracoacromial ligament

Coracohumeral ligament

Superior glenohumeral ligament

Biceps brachii tendon (long head)

Subscapularis tendon

Middle glenohumeral ligament

Inferior glenohumeral ligament

THE LABRUM AND JOINT CAPSULE

The labrum is a fibrocartilagenous lip surrounding the glenoid fossa, creating a greater depth to the fossa, which thereby deepens the contact area for the head of the humerus. Approximately twice the size of the humeral head, the joint capsule is a fibrous structure that surrounds the head of the humerus and glenoid fossa. The joint capsule blends with the three glenohumeral ligaments – the superior glenohumeral ligament, the middle glenohumeral ligament, and the inferior glenohumeral ligament – which add stability and strength.

MUSCLES OF THE ROTATOR CUFF

The muscles of the rotator cuff and long head of the biceps blend intimately with the joint capsule, adding a dynamic component to this structure. The rotator cuff consists of four muscles: supraspinatus, infraspinatus, teres minor, and subscapularis. While each serves a specific function at the GH joint, collectively the rotator cuff muscles, along with the long head of the biceps brachii, depress and stabilize the humeral head in the glenoid fossa. The specific function of the rotator cuff muscles will be discussed below.

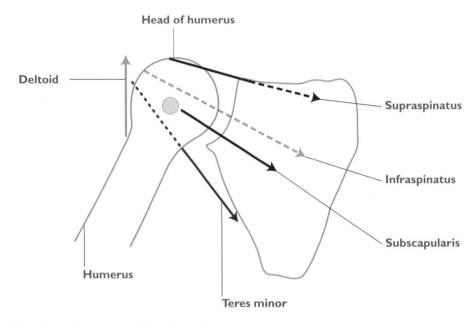

Directions of rotator cuff muscle actions.

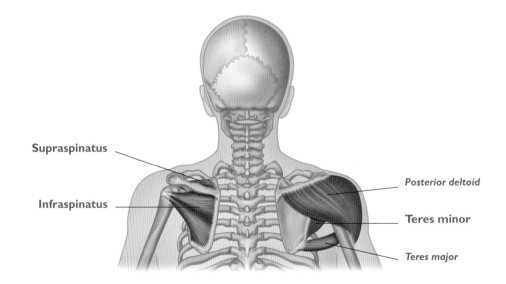

The rotator cuff muscles. Subscapularis is located on the anterior surface of the scapula, between the scapula and the ribs, and attaches to the humerus.

The supraspinatus attaches superiorly from the supraspinatus fossa to the greater tubercle of the humerus. While the action of initiating humeral abduction is generally assigned to the supraspinatus, it is actually the humeral head moving inferiorly on the concave surface of the glenoid fossa that in turn causes abduction. This movement serves to counteract the superiorly directed pull on the humerus created by the deltoid muscle. Weakness or inhibition of the supraspinatus causes a superior humeral glide and a jamming of the supraspinatus tendon and subacromial bursa underneath the coracoacromial roof as the humerus is pulled superiorly by the upwardly directed force of the deltoid.

The infraspinatus attaches from the posterior surface of the scapula to just below the supraspinatus tendon on the greater tubercle. The teres minor attaches from the lateral border of the scapula to the greater tubercle just below the infraspinatus. Collectively, the infraspinatus and teres minor externally rotate the humerus as the humerus nears 60 degrees to 90 degrees of abduction. This acts to rotate the greater tuberosity posteriorly and creates space for the supraspinatus tendon and subacromial bursa. Additionally, the infraspinatus and teres minor aid in humeral head depression during arm elevation thus helping to counteract the superior pull of the deltoid. Weakness in these muscles maintains the greater tubercle in an internally rotated position and may create an *impingement syndrome*, involving the supraspinatus tendon, subacromial bursa, and long head of the biceps coming into contact with the coracoacromial roof. This also occurs if the client begins with an internally rotated humeral position rather than a neutral humeral position. Individuals with this pattern will typically experience pain in the range of 60 degrees to 120 degrees of abduction since this is where there is minimal space between the coracoacromial roof and the greater tubercle. The movement is usually pain free above 120 degrees since the humerus will begin to inferiorly translate at this time. This is known as the *painful arc*.

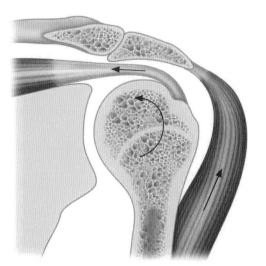 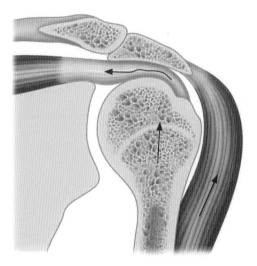

Supraspinatus impingement: with optimal co-activation between the deltoid and rotator cuff muscles, there is optimal joint centration of the glenohumeral joint (image above left). Without an optimal downward pull from the rotator cuff muscles, the humeral head is driven up into the acromion process by contraction of the deltoids and impinges against the supraspinatus tendon (image above right).

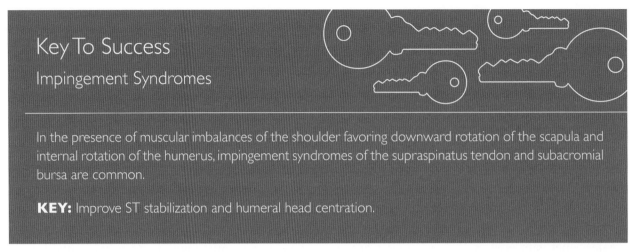

Key To Success

Impingement Syndromes

In the presence of muscular imbalances of the shoulder favoring downward rotation of the scapula and internal rotation of the humerus, impingement syndromes of the supraspinatus tendon and subacromial bursa are common.

KEY: Improve ST stabilization and humeral head centration.

The subscapularis, the often forgotten member of the rotator cuff, attaches from the anterior surface of the scapula to the lesser tubercle of the humerus. It functions to internally rotate, depress, and adduct the humeral head in the glenoid fossa. It has two separate distinct divisions with dual innervations that have differing functions based upon the actions of the upper extremity (Decker et al 2003). It is an important muscle since it is the only rotator cuff muscle to posteriorly pull the humeral head in the glenoid fossa, offsetting the anterior-directed pull of the posterior deltoid, teres minor, and infraspinatus. It acts as a synergist to the other rotator cuff muscles in centration of the humeral head in the glenoid fossa. Weakness or inhibition of the subscapularis leads to anterior humeral glide syndrome as the larger internal rotators, mainly the latissimus dorsi and teres major, dominate and drive the humerus forward in the glenoid fossa. Therefore, weakness or inhibition in the subscapularis can contribute to impingement syndrome and bicipital tenosynovitis of the shoulder.

Key To Success
Anterior Humeral Glide Syndrome

In the presence of scapular dyskinesis and resultant rotator cuff compensation, the humerus can lose its optimum axis of rotation. This often leads to the humeral head gliding forward rather than remaining centrated in the glenoid fossa during pushing and pulling movements. This is the most common cause of bicipital tenosynovitis.

KEY: Improve ST stabilization and centration of the humeral head.

While technically not considered part of the rotator cuff, the biceps brachii deserves special mention due to its attachment through the joint capsule. The long head of the biceps attaches from the superior lip of the glenoid labrum on the supraglenoid tubercle, passes through the joint capsule, inferiorly through the bicipital (intertubercular) groove to insert into the radial tuberosity. In addition to its actions on the elbow, the biceps functions as an anterior stabilizer of the humerus. The bicipital tendon sits along the bicipital groove of the humerus and allows the humerus to glide along it as it moves. Altered position of the shoulder, especially anterior tilting of the scapula or internal rotation of the humerus, creates altered movements of the intertubercular groove around the biceps tendon. Chronic irritation of the biceps tendon as it slides across rather than in the bicipital groove may lead to inflammation of the synovial sheath of the biceps tendon, referred to as 'bicipital tenosynovitis'.

THE SCAPULOTHORACIC JOINT

The scapulothoracic (ST) joint is formed by the pseudo-articulation of the scapula on the thorax. While the ST joint is not a true joint – it lacks ligamentous support, a joint capsule, a synovial membrane, and synovial fluid – its relationship to the integrity of the shoulder complex cannot be disputed. The ST joint functions to place the humerus in space and to position it in optimal alignments that improve the functional support of the GH joint. The anterior surface of the scapula is concave and ideally sits flush on the convex nature of the thorax. Therefore, any postural changes that affect the thorax affect this relationship and compromise the stability of the ST joint.

Neutral position of the scapula is located between the second and seventh thoracic vertebral levels and approximately one to three inches from the midline of the spine (Sahrmann 2002). The scapula sits approximately 30 degrees off the coronal axis, with the glenoid fossa facing anteriorly. This is referred to as the *scapular plane* and motion in this plane is often referred to as *scaption*. Scaption is believed to be a safer way of lifting the arm overhead as it creates less twisting of the joint capsule and impingement of the rotator cuff muscles. It is important to note that the *scapular plane* will change as the functional position of the shoulder changes. Since it lacks both the form closure of a more stable joint, such as the hip joint, and the ligamentous integrity of most joint articulations, the scapula relies heavily on the position of the thorax and scapula stabilizers to maintain its integrity. Understanding normal ST motion will aid in the identification of the functional role of the scapular stabilizers.

SCAPULOTHORACIC MOTION

There are ten cardinal movements available at the ST joint: adduction, abduction, depression, elevation, downward rotation, upward rotation, internal rotation, external rotation, anterior tilting, and posterior tilting. Protraction and retraction have been included in the table opposite and are terms that refer to the collective movement of the shoulder complex.

Terms	Definition
Adduction	Refers to the scapulae approximating each other or moving closer towards the midline of the body. The adductors of the scapula include the middle trapezius and rhomboids.
Abduction	Refers to the scapulae moving away from each other or away from the midline of the body. The abductors of the scapula are the pectoralis minor and serratus anterior
Retraction	Movement of the entire shoulder complex along the transverse plane of motion in a posterior direction. The retractors of the shoulder include the rhomboids, middle, upper and lower trapezius, and the latissimus dorsi.
Protraction	Movement of the entire shoulder complex along the transverse plane of motion in an anterior direction. The protractors of the shoulder include serratus anterior, pectoralis major and minor.
Depression	Lowering of the scapula in an inferior direction along the rib cage. The scapular depressors include the lower trapezius, latissimus dorsi, pectoralis minor, lower fibers of the pectoralis major and lower fibers of the serratus anterior.
Elevation	Raising of the scapula in a superior direction along the rib cage. The elevators of the scapula include the upper trapezius, levator scapula and rhomboids.
Downward rotation	Rotation of the scapula in a downward direction along the frontal plane of motion so that the glenoid fossa points towards the floor. The downward rotators of the scapula include the pectoralis minor, rhomboids and levator scapula.
Upward rotation	Rotation in an upward direction along the rib cage so that the glenoid fossa points towards the ceiling. The upward rotators of the scapula include the upper and lower trapezius and the serratus anterior.
Internal rotation	Internal scapular rotation occurs when the scapula tilts anteriorly along a vertical axis. This motion is primarily a function of the pectoralis complex.
External rotation	External scapular rotation occurs when the anteromedial aspect of the scapula approximates the thoracic cage along a vertical axis. All three divisions of the trapezius and the serratus anterior are primarily responsible for this motion.
Anterior tilting	Anterior tilting is movement along a coronal plane axis where the superior angle approximates and the inferior angle comes away from the thorax. Pectoralis minor and the short head of the biceps brachii are most responsible for anterior tilting of the scapula.
Posterior tilting	Posterior tilting is movement along a coronal plane axis where the superior angle moves away and the inferior angle of the scapula approximates the thorax. The lower trapezius and lower fibers of the serratus anterior are most responsible for posterior tilting of the scapula.

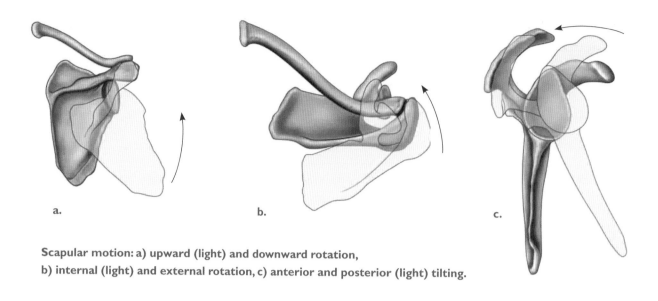

Scapular motion: a) upward (light) and downward rotation,
b) internal (light) and external rotation, c) anterior and posterior (light) tilting.

Scapular force couples: the serratus anterior and the upper and lower trapezius work together to produce upward rotation and control downward rotation.

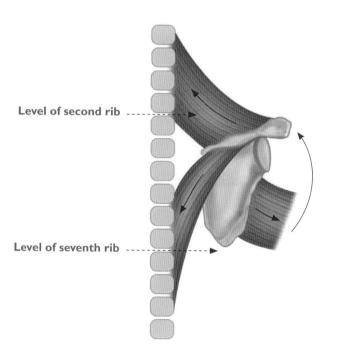

Level of second rib

Level of seventh rib

ACCESSORY MOVEMENTS

It is the lack of optimal posterior tilting that creates the all-too-familiar winged scapula posture. *Winging* of the scapula typically refers to an excessive anterior tilting of the scapula, where the inferior angle is pulled away from the thorax while the superior aspect of the scapula remains in relative contact with the thorax. *Flaring* of the scapula refers to the entire medial border of the scapula being lifted away from the thorax while the lateral aspect of the scapula remains in relative contact with the thorax. Both of these positions result from poor ST joint stabilization, and strategies to improve the integrity of the ST joint will be discussed later in this book.

COUPLED MOTIONS OF THE SHOULDER

To move the GH joint through its cardinal planes of motion, there must be respective movements of the ST joint. These coupled movements are listed below.

- **Sagittal plane motion:** Flexion of the arm requires upward rotation and posterior tilting at the ST joint, while extension of the arm requires downward rotation and anterior tilting of the ST joint.

- **Frontal plane motion:** Abduction of the arm requires upward rotation of the ST joint, while adduction of the arm requires downward rotation of the ST joint.

- **Transverse plane motion:** Internal rotation of the arm requires ST joint protraction, while external rotation requires ST joint retraction.

The lack of optimal ST motion will subsequently affect all motions of the upper extremity.

THE THORAX

While not technically part of the shoulder complex, it would be negligent to avoid discussing the thorax and its role in ST integrity. The thorax is made of twelve thoracic vertebrae and twelve pairs of articulating ribs. The thorax forms a mobile yet stable base for the scapula to rest upon. The thoracic spine (T spine) should have a gentle posterior curvature (kyphosis), where the apex is approximately around vertebral level of T4–T6. Recall the importance of this convex posture as a base for the concave anterior surface of the scapula. Proper biomechanics requires the upper T spine to extend as the shoulder goes into flexion, flex as it goes into extension, and laterally flex away from the direction of motion as it goes into abduction. Altered alignment, joint fixation, and/or changes in thoracic motion will result in compensatory motions of the shoulder complex.

THE ACROMIOCLAVICULAR JOINT

The acromioclavicular (AC) joint aids in the optimal positioning of the scapula for overhead motion, although its contribution is often overlooked. It is classified as an arthrodial (gliding) joint and is formed by the distal end of the clavicle and the medial aspect of the acromion process of the scapula. Although significantly less stable than the SC joint, the AC joint is passively stabilized by the acromioclavicular and coracoclavicular ligaments and actively stabilized by the anterior deltoid, upper trapezius, and subclavius muscles. These muscles will be discussed in further detail below.

MUSCLES OF THE ACROMIOCLAVICULAR JOINT

ANTERIOR DELTOID

The anterior deltoid attaches from the medial aspect of the acromion process of the scapula and distal end of the clavicle to the deltoid tuberosity of the humerus. The anterior deltoid aids anterior stabilization of the AC joint and aids in overhead motion of the humerus.

UPPER TRAPEZIUS

Attaching from the posterior aspect of the skull, the upper seven cervical vertebrae, and ligamentum nuchae to the distal aspect of the clavicle and acromion process, the upper trapezius functions to pull up on the AC joint to assist in upward rotation of the scapula. Therefore, inhibition of the upper trapezius significantly affects the ability to raise and stabilize the arm overhead.

SUBCLAVIUS

An often forgotten muscle of the shoulder complex, the subclavius attaches from the inferior aspect of the first rib and acromion process to the middle one-third of the clavicle. Its stated action of clavicular depression and first rib elevation minimizes its role in overhead motion. As the subclavius contracts, it draws the clavicle inferiorly and anteriorly. This motion on the 'S'-shaped clavicle creates an upward rotation of the clavicle and subsequently the scapula through the ligamentous attachments at the AC joint. Inhibition of the subclavius significantly diminishes the range and stability of overhead motion.

Activation strategies for improving function of these important muscles will be demonstrated in a later section.

THE STERNOCLAVICULAR JOINT

The sternoclavicular (SC) joint is the only bony attachment of the appendicular skeleton to the axial skeleton. It is a saddle joint consisting of the proximal end of the clavicle and the manubrium of the sternum. Of the four joints in the shoulder complex, the SC joint is the most stable, yet its' contribution is essential for optimal overhead motion. The SC joint is passively stabilized by sternoclavicular, interclavicular, and costoclavicular ligaments and dynamically stabilized by the sternocleidomastoid and pectoralis major.

MUSCLES OF THE STERNOCLAVICULAR JOINT

STERNOCLEIDOMASTOID

The sternocleidomastoid (SCM) attaches from the mastoid process of the skull to the manubrium of the sternum and proximal end of the clavicle. In addition to its action on the head and neck, the SCM stabilizes the SC joint and elevates the clavicle and sternum. In the presence of altered respiratory mechanics, the SCM becomes a dominant respiratory muscle, increasing the compressive loads on the neck and potentially altering the axis of rotation at the SC joint.

PECTORALIS MAJOR

The sternal portion of the pectoralis major (PMj) attaches from the anterior surface of the proximal half of the clavicle and half of the anterior surface of the manubrium of the sternum to the outer lip of the bicipital groove of the humerus. The sternal fibers of the PMj function to adduct the clavicle and thereby stabilize the SC joint as the upper trapezius, subclavius, and clavicular fibers of the pectoralis major elevate the clavicle.

THE CERVICAL SPINE

In relation to shoulder mechanics, the cervical spine deserves special mention. Several key scapular stabilizers – including the upper trapezius, rhomboid minor, and levator scapula – have attachments on the cervical spine. Instability of the scapula often causes increased activation of the levator scapula and rhomboids in an attempt to improve stability. The increased activity in these muscles disrupts optimal centration of the ST joint and increases compressive loads on the cervical spine. Because the brachial plexus, derived from cervical nerve root levels of C5–T1, innervates many of the muscles of the upper extremity, motor function can often be compromised. The chronic irritation on the cervical spine is often the leading cause of muscle inhibition of several of the key scapular stabilizers, including the serratus anterior, which is innervated by the long thoracic nerve. Most disc herniations in the neck occur at the C5–C6 disc level, and the long thoracic nerve is derived from cervical nerve roots C5–C7, thereby affecting motor function of the serratus anterior. Because of the loss of scapular stability, resulting in downward rotation, inhibition of the serratus anterior creates increased stress on the cervical spine, perpetuating the pattern of shoulder-neck dysfunction.

MUSCLES OF THE CERVICAL SPINE

While neck stabilization is intimately tied to scapular stabilization, there are several key muscles that are responsible for direct postural control of the cervical spine. These are the longus colli, longus capitis, and multifidi.

LONGUS CAPITIS AND LONGUS COLLI

The longus capitis attaches from the anterior aspects of the transverse processes of C3–C6 to the inferior, anterior portion of the occiput. The longus colli attaches from the anterior aspects of the transverse processes, vertebral bodies of levels C3–T3 to insert onto the similar regions of the vertebrae several levels above. Collectively, these muscles will flex the head on the neck and the neck on the trunk, as well as assist rotation of the head and neck. However, their true function is stabilization and via their deep, intersegmental attachments, they assist elongation of the cervical spine to counteract the compressive pull of muscles such as the cervical erector spinae, levator scapula, and sternocleidomastoid.

MULTIFIDI

The cervical multifidi attach from the articular processes of levels C4–C7 to the spinous processes 1–4 levels above. While its assigned function is extension and rotation, similar to its counterparts in the thoracic and lumbar regions of the spine, the cervical multifidi resist forward translation of one vertebra on another, which aids stability of the cervical spine during head and neck extension as well as movement of the shoulder complex.

In addition to the suboccipitals and other deep intersegmental muscles, these three muscles have the important role of providing proprioceptive sense of the cervical spine and head. Similar to deep stabilizers in the rest of the body, they also have a feed-forward role to help stabilize the head and neck prior to motion of the arm. Injury often results in inhibition of these key stabilizers, necessitating the increased activation of the superficial cervical erector spinae, levator scapulae, scalenes, and sternocleidomastoid to aid in the stability of the head and neck. The goal of corrective exercise is to improve the activation of the deep stabilizers while diminishing the overactivity of the superficial musculature.

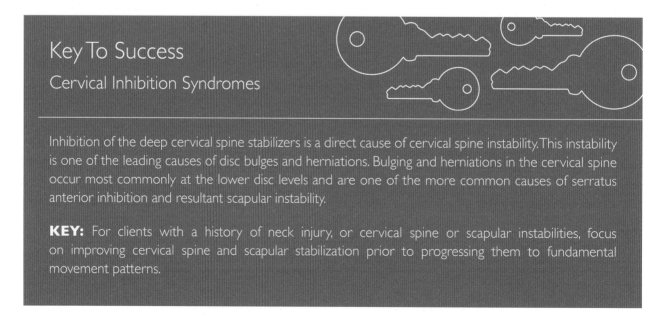

Key To Success
Cervical Inhibition Syndromes

Inhibition of the deep cervical spine stabilizers is a direct cause of cervical spine instability. This instability is one of the leading causes of disc bulges and herniations. Bulging and herniations in the cervical spine occur most commonly at the lower disc levels and are one of the more common causes of serratus anterior inhibition and resultant scapular instability.

KEY: For clients with a history of neck injury, or cervical spine or scapular instabilities, focus on improving cervical spine and scapular stabilization prior to progressing them to fundamental movement patterns.

MUSCLES OF THE SHOULDER COMPLEX

Given the range of motion and subsequent stability requirements of the shoulder complex, many muscles are responsible for maintaining this precision control. While several of the muscles controlling the shoulder complex have been previously discussed, muscles of the shoulder complex can essentially be categorized as spinoscapular, thoracoscapular, spinohumeral, thoracohumeral, and scapulohumeral, depending upon their specific attachments.

SPINOSCAPULAR

The spinoscapular group of muscles originates from the spine to attach to the scapula. These include the levator scapula, upper trapezius, rhomboids minor and major, middle trapezius, and lower trapezius. The upper trapezius has been discussed earlier. The levator scapula attaches from the posterior aspects of the transverse processes of C1–C4 to the superior angle of the scapula. As well as elevating the shoulder complex, the levator scapula functions to ipsilaterally flex and rotate the neck. It is a synergist to the upper trapezius in shoulder elevation (shrugging) and lateral flexion; however, it is an antagonist not only as it downwardly rotates the scapula while the upper trapezius upwardly rotates the scapula, but also as it ipsilaterally rotates the neck as the upper trapezius contralaterally rotates the neck. These last two functions enable smooth and coordinated actions during motion of the head, neck, and shoulder.

The rhomboids – major and minor – attach from the nuchal ligament, supraspinous ligaments, and spinous processes of C7–T5. The rhomboid functions to adduct and downwardly rotate the scapula, thereby acting as a synergist to the levator scapula and an antagonist to the upper and lower trapezius. It is an important medial stabilizer of the ST articulation.

The middle trapezius attaches from C7–T3 to the acromion and the posterior border of the spine of the scapula. It functions to adduct and stabilize the medial border of the scapula and thereby acts as a synergist to the rhomboids.

The lower trapezius attaches from spinous processes and supraspinous ligaments of T4–T12 as well as the thoracolumbar fascia, to the smooth triangular surface on the medial end of the spine of the scapula. This muscle is an important depressor of the scapula, thereby opposing the upper fibers of the trapezius, levator scapula, and rhomboids. In the role of upwardly rotating the scapula, it acts as a functional agonist to the upper trapezius and serratus anterior, thereby opposing the levator scapula, rhomboids, and pectoralis minor.

Collectively, the spinoscapular muscles will contralaterally rotate the spine towards the fixed arm which is one strategy for improving dysfunctional spinal curvatures.

THORACOSCAPULAR

The serratus anterior and pectoralis minor are the only muscles attaching directly from the scapula to the thorax and each deserves special mention. While no muscle works in isolation, the serratus anterior may be the muscle most responsible for scapular stabilization, whereas the pectoralis minor may be the muscle most responsible for the anteriorly tilted scapulae and resultant forward shoulder posture.

Attaching from the first nine ribs to the anteromedial border of the scapula, the serratus anterior is most responsible for stabilizing the scapulae on the thorax. Additionally, it assists overhead motion by upwardly rotating and abducting the scapulae. The lower fibers have the important function of anchoring the lower aspect to the thorax as the scapula upwardly rotates. Weakness in these fibers results in scapular elevation as the arm goes overhead and scapular winging as the arm returns from an overhead position. With the upper limb fixed, the serratus anterior can also assist trunk motion.

The pectoralis minor attaches from the coracoid process to ribs 3–5. It is responsible for stabilizing the scapula; however, when overactive and unchecked by the lower trapezius and serratus anterior, it anteriorly tilts the scapulae, contributing to the forward shoulder position. Additionally, the pectoralis minor is an accessory muscle of respiration. In the presence of poor diaphragmatic breathing the pectoralis minor becomes overactive as it attempts to elevate the rib cage. This contributes to the elevated thorax position and wide sternal angle that is prevalent with dysfunctional breathing. Given the approximately 22,000 breaths taken daily, dysfunctional breathing has been clinically found to be the most common cause of hypertonicity of the pectoralis minor as well as the scalenes and sternocleidomastoids. With the upper arm fixed as in crawling, the pectoralis minor can assist the parascapular muscles in pulling the scapula over the fixed humeral head.

SPINOHUMERAL

The latissimus dorsi is a unique muscle as it is the only one directly attaching the spine to the humerus, making it analogous to the psoas major of the hip. It takes its origin from the pelvis, thoracolumbar fascia, and lumbar and thoracic vertebrae to attach on the humerus. While its actions include extension, adduction and internal humeral rotation, its role is much more expansive. The oblique fibers of the latissimus dorsi run nearly parallel to the lower fibers of the lower trapezius, and even has a fascial connection to the inferior aspect of the scapula. These oblique fibers contribute to bringing the scapula down and around the thorax – similar to the combined action of the serratus anterior and lower trapezius.

As part of the posterior oblique chain, the latissimus dorsi is a primary stabilizer of the sacroiliac joint, lumbar spine, and thorax in addition to its role in accelerating and decelerating rotational motions of the trunk and spine. When stiff and/or short, it can contribute to anterior rotation of the pelvis and hyperextension of the thoracolumbar junction. Additionally, because of its unique attachment to the medial side of the intertubercular groove, in the presence of poor scapular stability, the latissimus dorsi will pull the scapula into further anterior tilt and depression, often necessitating its release prior to instituting corrective exercise. During closed-chain activities or those in which one arm is fixed, the latissimus dorsi can pull the trunk towards the hands and contralaterally rotate the spine.

THORACOHUMERAL

The pectoralis major, the only muscular connection from the anterior thorax directly to the humerus, attaches from the clavicle, sternum, and ribs to the lateral lip of the intertubercular groove of the humerus. While not directly attaching to the scapula, it affects the ST articulation through its action on the humerus. The clavicular fibers will adduct and flex, while the sternal fibers are most responsible for bringing the arm across the body (horizontal adduction). The sternal fibers assist GH extension and adduction. Collectively these muscles will internally rotate the humerus and contribute to stabilization of the SC joint and costochondral articulations (the area where the rib articulates with the cartilage). During closed-chain activities or those in which one arm is fixed, the pectoralis major and minor function to pull the trunk towards the fixed humerus. When overactive, the pectoralis major will contribute to anterior humeral glide syndrome and forward shoulder position by pulling the humerus forward as it internally rotates. However, the pectoralis major is often inhibited and subsequently over-lengthened in many clients with shoulder dysfunction. When the pectoralis major is inhibited, the pectoralis minor becomes shorter and stiffer and the latissimus dorsi and teres major become the primary internal rotators and contribute to pull the shoulder complex inferiorly and anteriorly.

SCAPULOHUMERAL

The scapulohumeral muscles originate from the scapula and attach to the humerus. These include the anterior, middle, and posterior fibers of the deltoid, the rotator cuff muscles (including the supraspinatus, infraspinatus, teres minor, and subscapularis), the teres major and the coracobrachialis.

The posterior fibers of the deltoid assist GH external rotation and extension. When the posterior fibers become the prime movers of external rotation, they contribute to the anterior humeral glide syndrome by pulling the humerus forward in the socket and limiting posterior glide. The middle deltoid assists abduction and, in the presence of supraspinatus inhibition, creates a superior glide of the humerus in the glenoid fossa, which is a contributing factor to impingement syndromes. The anterior deltoid is responsible for flexion, adduction, and internal rotation of the GH joint and contributes to the forward internal rotation shoulder position when there is an imbalance with the external rotator cuff muscles.

The rotator cuff muscles are most responsible for precise stabilization and maintenance of the GH axis of rotation and were discussed in an earlier section.

Teres major has similar functions as the latissimus dorsi, assisting GH extension, adduction, and internal rotation. When the scapula anteriorly tilts by the pull from the latissimus dorsi and pectoralis minor, the teres major contributes to the anterior humeral glide syndrome by pulling the humerus forward in the socket and limiting posterior glide of the humerus. The coracobrachialis attaches from the coracoid process of the scapula to the middle of the humerus. It assists the anterior deltoid in flexion and adduction of the humerus. Shortness in the coracobrachialis contributes to the anteriorly tilted scapula by pulling the scapula towards the humerus.

ADDITIONAL MUSCLES

While often thought of as elbow muscles, the biceps brachii and triceps brachii have a much greater functional role than merely flexing and extending the elbow. Along with the ipsilateral latissimus dorsi and teres major, the triceps brachii is part of the posterior chain that is responsible for pulling the trunk over the stationary arm in the developing child. In addition to extension of the shoulder and elbow, the triceps brachii attaches to the posterior capsule and functions as a GH stabilizer.

Similarly, the biceps brachii is much more than a flexor and supinator of the elbow. Biceps curls, while great for developing the flexion function of the elbow, are totally opposite of its actual functional role. In the developing child, the biceps brachii functions to pull the scapula over the stationary humeral head. Like the triceps brachii, the biceps brachii functions primarily as a GH stabilizer, helping to prevent anterior gliding of the humeral head.

So how are these developmental patterns trained in the adult population? While crawling would be effective, progressive patterns – such as reclined pull-ups, traditional pull-ups, cable push and pull patterns, and plank patterns – can help restore primitive function of these muscles as part of the muscle chains system. These will be discussed further in the corrective exercise and training sections.

SCAPULOHUMERAL RHYTHM AND OVERHEAD MECHANICS

Overhead mechanics, both flexion and abduction, require precise interaction of each articulation of the shoulder complex. The following mechanics relate to overhead mechanics and, while there will be relatively varying amounts of motion given each client's physical attributes and history, the ideal mechanics will be relatively similar.

Movement between the GH and ST joints is often referred to as the *scapulohumeral rhythm*. A range of 180 degrees of shoulder motion is considered normal for both flexion and abduction. Of this motion, 120 degrees is at the GH joint, while the SC, AC, and ST joints collectively contribute the remaining 60 degrees. The ratio of GH–ST motion is often referenced as a ratio of 2:1, where there are 2 degrees of GH motion to every 1 degree of ST motion. These numbers are not always agreed upon by all experts in the field and may be purely theoretical as loading the arm often alters this ratio, as do individual differences. Motion at the respective joints is described below.

During the initial 90 degrees of shoulder elevation, the arm abducts 60 degrees at the GH joint and the scapula upwardly rotates 30 degrees, where 25 degrees of this scapular motion is at the SC joint and the AC joint contributes the remaining 5 degrees.

During the final 90 degrees of shoulder elevation, the GH joint abducts an additional 60 degrees and the scapula upwardly rotates an additional 30 degrees. These final 30 degrees of scapular motion are a combination of 5 degrees of SC elevation and 25 degrees at the ST joint.

What becomes most evident when looking at the preceding mechanics is that analysis of overhead motion requires much more than just looking at GH motion. Movements at the SC, AC, and ST joints are integral components to both the actual movement as well as the stability of the upper arm during overhead movement. Therefore, muscles controlling these joint motions must be considered in both the rehabilitation and corrective exercise strategy and the conditioning of the upper extremity.

DYSFUNCTIONS IN UPPER EXTREMITY PATTERNS

The lack of optimal scapular stabilization leads to compensatory patterns during overhead motion. There are several common movement dysfunctions that can be noted as clients raise their arms overhead: these dysfunctions are depicted in the image (right):

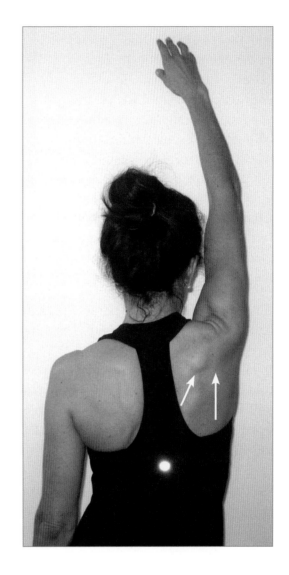

- **Non-optimal scapulothoracic stabilization:** The scapula is moving up over the thorax rather than around it (vertical arrow).

- **Excessive elevation and scapula activity:** At the superior angle insertion of the levator scapula there is increased tone (arrow) and the neck is pulled into right rotation by the levator scapula.

- **Non-optimal cervical and thoracic spine stabilization:** The cervical spine moves into excessive right lateral flexion and the trunk moves into left lateral flexion due to poor stabilization at the left cervical and right thoracolumbar regions respectively.

This lack of optimal stabilization is often the cause of pain at the compensatory joint segments. The loss of optimal stabilization creates hypermobile segments that tend to be where the client will experience pain. The nervous system responds by compensating with areas of hypertonic muscles that are the corresponding locations of myofascial trigger points. This example also illustrates why myofascial approaches that focus on trigger point release often fail to produce long-term results because the primary problem is a stabilization issue and the trigger points are the compensatory issue.

Many clients with scapular instability or dyskinesis are able to move their scapulae into upward rotation; however, they have a poor ability to control this motion as they bring their arms back down to their sides. The scapula can be seen to be moving into anterior tilt and downward rotation, producing the winged scapula look. The problem is twofold: the scapula moves excessively into downward rotation and/or it moves faster than the humerus. Both situations drive accessory muscle stabilization and are common causes of the downward rotation syndrome.

Notice how this client's right scapula is fairly well controlled in the overhead motion (image left). Then note the scapular winging and downward rotation (arrow) as the client eccentrically lowers his arm (image right). In clients with scapular control issues, this winging generally occurs around 45 degrees of shoulder elevation, where the scapular stabilizers are at their most disadvantaged point (longest length-tension).

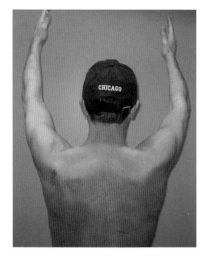
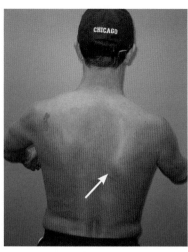

Consider the consequences on this client's neck and subacromial structures if he was to then perform front dumbbell raises or upright rows. Winging is often common in clients with up-regulation of the glenohumeral muscles (deltoids and rotator cuff) and poor dissociation between the humeral head and the glenoid fossa.

The downward rotation syndrome and anterior humeral glide syndrome are two additional dysfunctional patterns of the upper extremity. These two dysfunctional movement patterns will be discussed below.

In clients with a downward rotation syndrome, the levator scapula and rhomboids assume the primary role of scapular stabilization. During many common exercises – such as cable rows, lat pull-downs, pull-ups, biceps curls, and triceps cable push-downs – the levator scapula will become prominent because there is inadequate inferior stabilization of the scapula by the serratus anterior and lower trapezius. The 'levator scapula sign' (arrow) will be present as the client loads their shoulder.

Notice the increased levator scapula activation as the client performs shoulder extension against a relatively light theraband (see right).

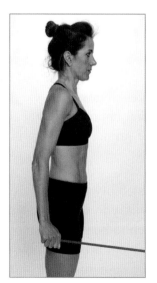
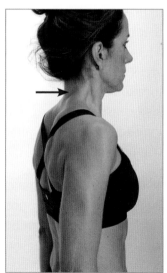

The levator scapula sign is common in many patterns where there is poor scapular stabilization. The therapist or trainer can palpate increased hypertonicity in the lateral aspect of the neck during many common exercises, indicating overactivity of the levator scapula. The levator scapulae should be relatively quiet and there should not be palpable overactivity during functional movement patterns. This client will often complain of neck tightness and/or headaches following resistive training because they are using their neck as the anchor for the shoulder complex rather than anchoring at the thorax.

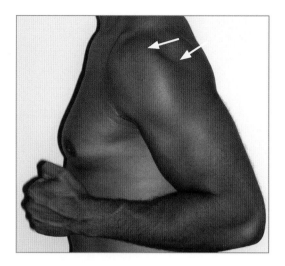

The anterior humeral glide syndrome (Sahrmann 2002) is a common result of muscle imbalances of the glenohumeral joint and is commonly observed as the shoulder moves into extension. A divot will be noted at the posterior aspect of the joint due to the loss of joint centration (right arrow), and the head of the humerus can be observed (left arrow) or palpated as it translates forward, moving on the fossa. This occurs most often as the arm moves into extension during patterns such as the concentric phase of pulling patterns (e.g. cable rows and pull-downs) and the eccentric phase of pushing patterns (e.g. horizontal cable chest presses).

In the anterior humeral glide syndrome, more than one-third of the humeral head can be palpated in front of the acromion process, and the posterior aspect of the humeral head will be palpated forward of the posterior aspect of the acromion process.

There are four main causes of anterior humeral glide syndrome:

1. **Short posterior joint capsule:** To remain centrated in the glenoid fossa, there must be proper extensibility of the joint capsule. Shortness in the posterior joint capsule does not allow the humerus to move posteriorly in the glenoid fossa, causing an anterior shift in the humeral resting position.

2. **Short posterior rotators:** As mentioned above, the humeral head must remain centrated in the glenoid fossa. Shortness and/or stiffness of the posterior rotators, infraspinatus, teres minor, and/or posterior deltoid causes a shift in the axis similar to the short posterior joint capsule.

3. **Muscle imbalances:** Recall, the function of the subscapularis and pectoralis major is to draw the humeral head back in the socket. Weakness or inhibition of the subscapularis and/or dominance of the latissimus dorsi and teres major as internal rotators will drive the head of the humerus forward.

4. **Dysfunction in the stabilization-dissociation relationship:** Verbal cuing that favors instructions such as 'pull your shoulder blades down and back' or 'squeeze your shoulder blades together' during pulling patterns functionally 'lock' the scapula, which results in compensatory increases in glenohumeral motion. In an attempt to move the resistance, the only available motion for the shoulder is by anteriorly gliding the humerus in the glenoid cavity.

During ideal patterning, the humeral head remains centrated in the glenoid fossa. There should be no anterior migration of the humeral head and no gapping or divots observed in the posterior aspect of the shoulder. Poor patterning is common with biceps curls in the presence of poor ST and/or GH stabilization, and the humeral head is consequently driven forward during the eccentric phase of the exercise.

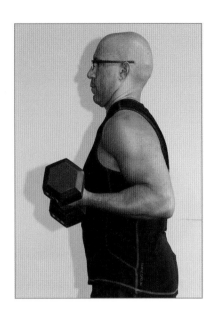

Note the anterior shoulder position (right image) during the eccentric phase of the biceps curl, due to the loss of both GH and ST stability. These clients will often complain of pain over the anterior aspect of the humeral head secondary to irritation of the bicipital tendon.

It is important to observe and correct this position during functional movement patterns because every repetition that the individual is allowed to perform incorrectly brings them one step further in establishing a permanent movement dysfunction. While the short posterior joint capsule is usually a soft-tissue restriction secondary to repetitive injury, the short posterior rotators are usually a result of poor motor patterning or up-regulation secondary to poor motor control of the GH joint by the scapulohumeral muscles. Mobilization of the posterior capsule, release of the posterior rotators, and activation of the subscapularis, in addition to movement retraining, will help reverse this problem. It is helpful to palpate the head of the humerus as well as the scapula during corrective exercise and functional patterns, to help monitor and cue proper humeral head and scapular positioning.

COMMON INJURIES OF THE UPPER KINETIC CHAIN

SHOULDER INSTABILITY SYNDROME

Anterior instability syndrome includes many of the common conditions that affect shoulder stability. These include multi-directional instabilities (instability in more than one direction) and subluxation/dislocation of the shoulder. The most common direction of instability is anteriorly, which correlates to the higher percentage of anterior shoulder dislocations than posteriorly. While common in traumatic injuries such as a fall on an outstretched arm or a motor vehicle accident, a frequent cause of instability is an altered motor control that results in anterior displacement of the humeral head in the glenoid fossa. Although capsular laxity and impaired proprioception have been suggested as causes, altered patterns of muscle activation have also been shown to create anterior instability (Myers et al 2004). The pectoralis major, short head of biceps brachii, coracobrachialis, anterior deltoid, and the subscapularis provide anterior support to the shoulder joint and have been shown to be inhibited in individuals with anterior instability. This instability may be a predisposing cause of impingement syndromes as well as tears of the supraspinatus tendon and glenoid labrum.

SHOULDER IMPINGEMENT SYNDROME

Impingement syndromes of the shoulder generally involve the supraspinatus tendon as it crosses under the acromion to attach onto the greater tubercle; the subacromial bursa beneath the anterior portion of the acromion process and coracoacromial ligament; and the long head of the biceps brachii as it passes underneath the anterior aspect of the acromion process to insert into the superior lip of the glenoid fossa. Impingement syndromes are generally related to scapular dyskinesis and the lack of scapular stabilization, upward rotation, and posterior tilting. While impingements can occur during many shoulder motions, abduction and flexion around 60 degrees to 120 degrees (the point where there is the least amount of subacromial space and the lever arm is the longest) is generally the range where clients will experience the most amount of symptoms. Inhibition of the rotator cuff diminishing the ability to depress the head of the humerus during overhead motion will additionally contribute to impingement syndromes of the shoulder.

Decreases in posterior tilt and increases in internal rotation of the scapula during humeral elevation have been demonstrated in subjects with shoulder impingement as compared to those without shoulder impingement (Lukasiewicz et al 1999). Tears of the rotator cuff tendons have been proposed as both a result and a cause of impingement syndromes. Interestingly, in a study of 96 asymptomatic individuals by Sher et al (1995), 34% of individuals with no report of shoulder pain had MRI findings that were diagnostic for a tear of the rotator cuff.

LABRAL TEARS

Labral tears of the glenoid labrum are common with traumas such as a fall on an outstretched arm. They are also common with repetitive injuries of the shoulder often related to poor scapular stabilization as well as poor humeral head centration of the upper arm. Anterior humeral head migration is a common movement pattern found anecdotally in clients with labral tears. Tightness of the posterior joint capsule, myofascial contractures of the posterior rotator cuff, and inhibition of the subscapularis (in posterior humeral head glide) are also contributing factors to labral tears of the glenohumeral joint.

BICIPITAL TENDONOSIS

Bicipital tendonosis is a degenerative change of the biceps tendon. It is often confused with tendonitis, which is an inflammatory condition affecting a tendon. With tendonosis there is degeneration and thinning of the collagen fibers of the tendon (Khan and Cook 2010) and it generally occurs secondary to overuse. Bicipital tendonosis typically occurs with poor scapulohumeral mechanics and the anterior humeral head position. The biceps tendon sits in the bicipital groove and functions as an anterior stabilizer of the humerus within the glenoid fossa. Postural alterations – such as an anterior tilt of the scapula, forward position of the humeral head in the glenoid fossa secondary to a tight posterior capsule, and muscle inhibition favoring the muscles that pull the humeral head forward in the glenoid fossa – contribute to increased friction between the anterior aspect of the humerus and the bicipital tendon.

Excessive use of exercises such as bicep curls, bench presses, and dips, as well as any upper extremity exercise performed with non-optimal glenohumeral positioning, can lead to overloading of the bicipital tendon. Micro-fraying of the biceps tendon can lead to pain and decreased strength in its stabilization role of the humeral head.

THORACIC OUTLET SYNDROME

Thoracic outlet syndrome is caused by entrapment of the brachial plexus as it exits the neck in between the anterior and middle scalenes, under the clavicle or underneath the pectoralis minor, and makes its way down the arm. This condition is characterized by radicular symptoms (numbness and tingling) in the arm and/or digits number four and five of the hand.

Thoracic outlet syndrome has multiple causes including:

- altered respiratory patterns favoring the accessory muscles of respiration, especially the scalenes, sternocleidomastoid, and pectoralis minor;

- postural alterations including Janda's Upper Crossed Syndrome and the scapular downward rotation syndrome;

- sleeping postures where the arm is abducted and placed under the head;

- repetitive stress injuries such as working on a computer;

- exercises that stress a chronic forward position of the trunk and shoulders such as bench presses, dips, and bike riding.

MEDIAL AND LATERAL EPICONDYLITIS

Medial and lateral epicondylitis, more commonly referred to as 'golfer's elbow' or 'throwing elbow' and 'tennis elbow' respectively, are overuse injuries from a variety of causes including golf, tennis, and throwing. They are also common cumulative impact injuries in individuals who work at a computer, on a phone device, or in activities such as knitting. An underlying cause of lateral epicondylitis is a cervical radiculopathy from the C7 nerve root. The C7 nerve innervates the muscles of the triceps and extensor muscles of the arm and irritation of this nerve from a space-occupying lesion in the neck (disc bulge or osteophyte) can mimic lateral epicondylitis.

CONCLUSION

While each of these conditions discussed above are separate entities with multiple and varying etiologies, there is one common thread among them. Each generally stems from variations of the following issues:

• poor centration of the glenohumeral joint;

• poor motor control of the shoulder complex, especially the scapulothoracic articulation;

• poor eccentric control of the upper extremity.

While this may seem like an oversimplification of the upper extremity injury process, it identifies the key factors in the development of most movement dysfunctions of the upper extremity. These factors will form the basis of the corrective exercise approach that will be presented in the next section of the book.

Given the aforementioned dysfunction, improving function of the shoulder complex lies in retraining the motor system in three key areas. These include:

1. improving stabilization of the cervical spine and thorax;

2. improving stabilization and upward rotation of the scapula;

3. improving eccentric control as the arm is lowered.

DEVELOPING A WINNING STRATEGY

Several key concepts regarding shoulder function and dysfunction were revealed during the Scapular Summit (Kibler et al 2009) and, in combination with the information presented throughout this section, contribute to the corrective exercise strategy that will be presented in later chapters. These concepts are summarized below.

1. There must be upward rotation and posterior tilting of the scapula, together with posterior rotation of the clavicle and acromioclavicular joints, for a client to produce normal overhead motion. Improving these functions is the goal of several of the early corrective exercise strategies that will follow.

2. Scapular kinematics is affected by fatigue of the shoulder muscles and may persist even after the task. Improving tolerance of the scapular stabilizers is a primary strategy early in the corrective exercise strategy.

3. Dyskinesis (alterations in overall scapular movement patterns) and dysrhythmia (altered motion during movement such as poor eccentric control and 'stuttering' during lowering of the arm or poor coordination between the humerus and scapula) of the scapula can be picked up during observation of overhead motion. This is a key component in the assessment process and can pick up movement and stabilization dysfunction, even before the client perceives or reports a problem.

4. The trainer or therapist can place the scapula in the correct position and/or aid upward rotation and posterior tilting of the scapula, and determine if this improves the client's ease of motion and/or diminishes their pain. This test was first proposed by Sahrmann (2002) and has shown clinical reliability in determining scapular relationships to shoulder dysfunction. Since most dysfunctional shoulders have a scapular component, improving scapular mechanics will be an important first-step process of the corrective exercise strategy.

5. Manual muscle tests are a valuable part of the assessment process and will be briefly introduced in the assessment section.

6. Tightness in the posterior shoulder region is related to scapular dyskinesis, impingement syndromes, and labral tears so a strategy to improve glenohumeral range of motion and posterior glide of the humeral head is provided in the corrective exercise section.

7. Improving muscle activation timing, joint position, and co-activation of shoulder muscles is important when providing corrective exercises. These components are included in the corrective exercise strategy to improve joint centration, muscle co-activation, and timing of the optimal shoulder mechanics.

8. Side lying positions tend to favor activation of the lower scapular stabilizers over the elevators and this concept is included in the early corrective exercise strategies.

9. Following injury or surgery, activity of the scapular elevators is increased. This has been anecdotally to be the case both post-surgically and in those clients with chronic shoulder dysfunction. The primary goal of the corrective strategy is to improve the scapular stabilizers that both depress and posteriorly rotate the scapula (serratus anterior and lower trapezius) while limiting the activity of the scapular elevators (levator scapula and rhomboids).

10. An integrated approach involving an accurate assessment, interventions including improving soft tissue extensibility, muscle activation patterns, and corrective exercise patterns is useful in correcting scapular dyskinesis and restoring optimal shoulder mechanics.

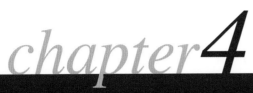

chapter 4

The Hip Complex

CHAPTER OBJECTIVES

To identify and understand the functional components of the hip complex

To identify the key regions of dysfunction within the hip complex

To understand the ideal mechanics of the hip complex

While structurally one of the simplest joints in the human body, functionally the hip complex is anything but simple. Ironically, the magnitude and complexity of the hip joint and its relation to low back and knee dysfunction often go unnoticed in rehabilitation and training environments. Likewise, the significance of achieving ideal hip mechanics in generating power for athletic performance is commonly neglected in lieu of force production, often to the detriment of the athlete needing to both generate and decelerate maximum force. This section will introduce basic anatomy, biomechanics, and kinematics of the hip, while introducing its relation to the pelvis and lower extremity.

STRUCTURE OF THE LUMBOPELVIC-HIP COMPLEX

Just as a discussion of the shoulder is not complete without inclusion of the thoracic spine, a discussion of the hip is not complete without the inclusion of the lumbar spine and pelvis. Analogous to the shoulder complex, the lumbopelvic-hip (LPH) complex consists of several joint complexes that contribute to both the stability and mobility of the lower extremity. These include the lumbosacral (LS), sacroiliac (SIJ), and femoroacetabular (FA) regions.

THE LUMBOSACRAL AND SACROILIAC JOINTS

The pelvis, comprising two innominates joining with the sacrum, forms a stable foundation for the trunk as well as a relay station between the upper and lower extremities. Each innominate is formed by the union of three bones: the pubis, ilium, and ischium. Each of the three bones contributes to the formation of the acetabular fossa and they are joined posteriorly with the sacrum and anteriorly at the pubic symphysis. The wedge-shaped sacrum is formed by the union of the five or six fused segments and articulates with each ilium to form a solid joint articulation. While stable enough to withstand three to ten times body weight that occurs during the single leg stance in running, its few degrees of rotation are critical to the function of both the spine and lower extremity. While many have argued as to whether or not there is motion at the SIJ, the presence of articular cartilage on both the articular surfaces of the sacrum and ilium, synovial fluid, and a joint capsule demonstrates that motion is both present and, more importantly, needed for proper biomechanics to occur, effectively putting this argument to rest. Anyone experiencing a lack of SIJ motion secondary to articular fixation (subluxation), joint arthrosis, and/or capsular restriction can attest to the biomechanical ramifications they will note in their lumbosacral region, hips and/or knees.

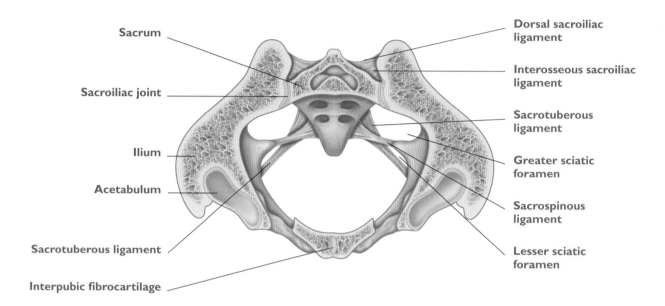

Sacrum

Sacroiliac joint

Ilium

Acetabulum

Sacrotuberous ligament

Interpubic fibrocartilage

Dorsal sacroiliac ligament

Interosseous sacroiliac ligament

Sacrotuberous ligament

Greater sciatic foramen

Sacrospinous ligament

Lesser sciatic foramen

a.

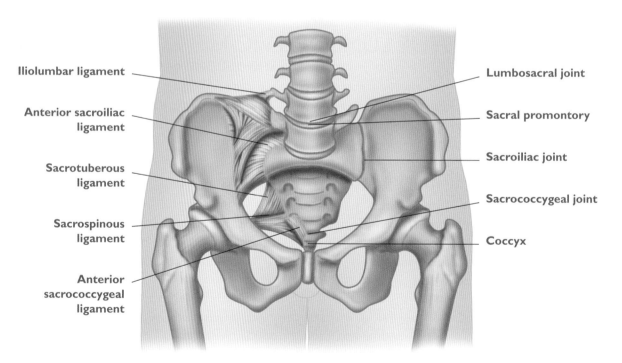

Iliolumbar ligament

Anterior sacroiliac ligament

Sacrotuberous ligament

Sacrospinous ligament

Anterior sacrococcygeal ligament

Lumbosacral joint

Sacral promontory

Sacroiliac joint

Sacrococcygeal joint

Coccyx

b.

The lumbopelvic-hip complex; a) transverse view, b) anterior view.

The L5 vertebrae articulating with the sacrum forms the lumbosacral articulation. Due to its intimate relationship, movement of the lumbar spine causes movement of the sacrum, and likewise movement of the sacrum causes obligatory movement of the lumbar spine and is referred to as the 'lumbopelvic rhythm'. The angle formed between these structures is known as the 'sacral base angle' and determines the degree of lumbar lordosis that is present. While 30 degrees is considered to be a normal sacral base angle, motor control of this articulation is a much greater issue and will be discussed further in the muscle section below. A decreased angle, occurring during prolonged sitting, is often a leading contributor to destabilization of the lumbar spine that then reciprocally contributes to compensatory femoroacetabular motion.

SACRAL NUTATION AND COUNTERNUTATION

Nutation is the anterior inferior motion of the sacral base, while counternutation is the posterior superior motion of the sacral base. Nutation is necessary for the locking of the SIJ during unilateral stance. The inability to nutate the sacrum is a leading cause of unilateral stance instability and one cause of the classic Trendelenburg's gait. Counternutation, on the other hand, is required to unlock the SIJ to allow anterior rotation of the innominate and extension of the hip. Inability to unlock or counternutate the sacrum leads to compensatory increases in lumbopelvic flexion, which leads to and perpetuates lumbar instability.

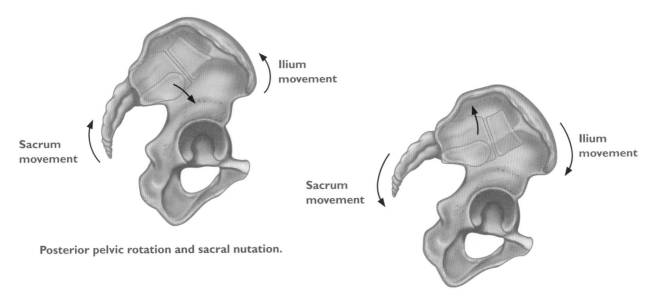

Posterior pelvic rotation and sacral nutation.

Anterior pelvic rotation and sacral counternutation.

LIGAMENTS OF THE SACROILIAC AND LUMBOSACRAL JOINTS

A complex network of ligaments is required to stabilize the sacroiliac and lumbosacral joints. Most notably these are the anterior and posterior longitudinal, anterior and posterior sacroiliac, interosseous, supraspinous, sacrospinous, sacrotuberous, and iliolumbar ligaments. Of particular interest, each of these ligaments has special fascial attachments to the muscle chains to improve stabilization of the pelvis, spine, and SIJ in addition to the upper and lower extremities. These functional attachments will be discussed further overleaf.

THE FEMOROACETABULAR JOINT

The femoroacetabular (FA) joint, more commonly referred to as the 'hip joint', is a classic example of a ball-and-socket articulation. It is made up of the head of the femur and the acetabulum of the pelvis. Similar to the glenohumeral articulation of the shoulder, the FA joint is multiaxial, referring to its multiplanar motion. These movements include flexion and extension in the sagittal plane, abduction and adduction in the frontal plane, and internal and external rotation in the transverse plane. Additionally, it has oblique motion that is a combination of two or three of the above planes. While structurally similar to the shoulder joint, it sacrifices mobility for the benefit of stability. Stability of the hip is derived from several sources, most notably the depth of the acetabulum and the presence of the lunate-shaped *acetabular labrum*, a fibrocartilagenous structure that surrounds and deepens the fossa. Because the labrum is not a complete ring, the transverse acetabular ligament supports the inferior surface of the acetabulum. In addition to its role in deepening the acetabular fossa, the labrum is important in shock absorption, joint lubrication, and force distribution, resisting both vertical and lateral motion of the femoral head in the acetabulum (Groh and Herrera 2009).

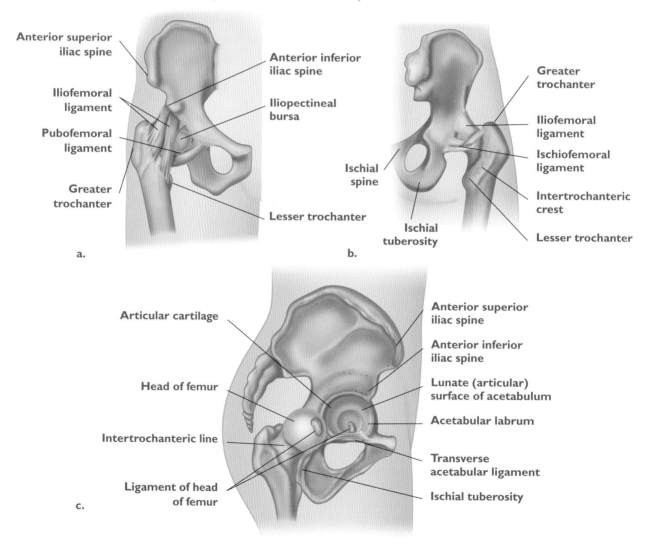

The hip joint; a) right leg, anterior view, b) right leg, posterior view, c) right leg, lateral view.

THE JOINT CAPSULE AND LIGAMENTS OF THE FEMOROACETABULAR JOINT

The hip joint capsule surrounds the articular surfaces and spans from the surrounding regions of the acetabular fossa to the neck of the femur, passively stabilizing the hip joint. The joint capsule blends with several strong ligaments that aid hip support. These include the iliofemoral, pubofemoral, and ischiofemoral ligaments and the ligamentum teres, which are described below.

- **Iliofemoral ligament:** The iliofemoral ligament, also known as the *Y ligament*, lies in an inverted Y-position, attaching from the anterior inferior iliac spine and then dividing to attach distally to the superior and inferior aspects of the intertrochanteric line (in between the greater and lesser trochanters of the femur). It is the anterosuperior thickening of the joint capsule and is one of the strongest ligaments in the body. It limits hip extension and posterior rotation of the ilium on the femur (posterior tilt).

- **Pubofemoral ligament:** The pubofemoral ligament extends from the superior pubic ramus of the pubic bone to attach laterally on the anterior aspect of the intertrochanteric line. It is an anteroinferior thickening of the hip capsule and limits hip abduction and lateral tilting of the pelvis on the femur.

- **Ischiofemoral ligament:** The ischiofemoral ligament originates from the ischium just posterior to the acetabulum then wraps over the femoral neck to attach to the trochanteric fossa. This ligament assists in controlling internal rotation and extension of the hip as well as ipsilateral ilium rotation on the femur.

- **Ligamentum teres:** The ligamentum teres is located within the joint and runs from the internal surface of the acetabulum to attach to the fovea capitis of the femoral head. While it may assist stability of the femoral head within the acetabulum, it functions to transmit blood and nerve supply to the head of the femur.

FEMORAL ANGLE OF INCLINATION AND TORSION ANGLE

The proximal aspect of the femur comprises the shaft, the head, and the neck. Two distinct angles are formed between the femoral neck and the shaft. The first, known as the 'femoral neck angle', represents the angle between the neck and shaft in the frontal plane. The normal femoral angle is approximately 125 degrees; an increase in the angulation is referred to as 'coxa valga', while a decrease is referred to as 'coxa vara'. While coxa valga and vara can be acquired, they are more commonly congenital variants in the femoral angle and can alter the stability and limit the mobility of the FA articulation. Coxa valga can result in an increase in the Q-angle (quadriceps angle). This angle is formed by a bisected line drawn from the anterior superior iliac spine, through the mid-patella, and from the mid-patella through the tibial tubercle. An increase in the Q-angle is often related to patellar tracking issues and increased medial knee instability. Females generally have a larger Q-angle due to a relatively wider pelvis and increased femoral angle, which is thought to be one cause of the increased incidence of anterior cruciate ligament tears in this population.

The 'femoral torsion angle' is the angle of the femoral neck relative to the shaft of the femur in the transverse plane. The generally accepted ideal position is 15 degrees of anteversion, or when the angle is relatively anterior or forward of the frontal plane. An increase in anteversion results in a toe-in posture, commonly referred to as 'pigeon-toed'. Retroversion is when the angle is less than 15 degrees and generally results in a toed-out posture, resulting in a duck-type or waddle gait.

FEMOROPELVIC RHYTHM

The femoropelvic rhythm is the coordinated movement between both femurs and the pelvis to move through greater ranges of motion without overstressing any one joint. As the femur flexes, as in the swing phase of gait, the ipsilateral ilium goes through posterior rotation. The contralateral femur is extending and the ilium goes through anterior rotation. For example, prior to the toe-off phase, as the femur is extending, the ipsilateral ilium is anteriorly rotating. The contralateral femur and ilium are going through similar, albeit opposite, motions during the similar phases of the gait cycle. During external hip rotation, the ipsilateral ilium will move externally in the transverse plane; during internal hip rotation, it will move internally. During hip abduction, the superior aspect of the ipsilateral ilium will tilt medially in the frontal plane; during hip adduction, it will tilt laterally. The lack of proper femoropelvic dissociation and/or canister stabilization alters this normal rhythm, leading to compensatory changes.

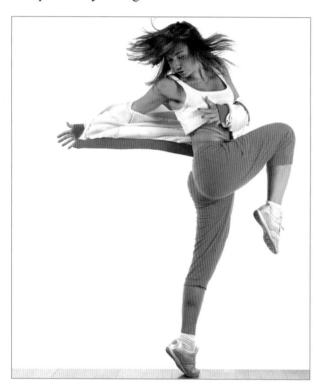 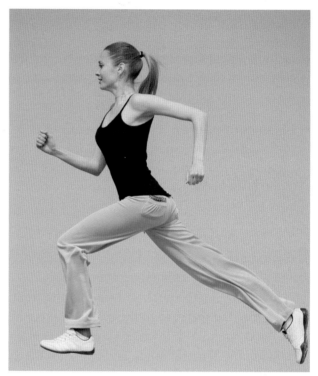

Notice that as the dancer moves into right hip flexion there is associated posterior rotation of the ipsilateral ilium and relative extension at the contralateral hip (left image). During the toe-off phase of the running gait, the runner's left hip is moving into flexion as the ilium rotates posteriorly (right image). Her right hip is extended and there is anterior rotation of the innominate.

FUNCTIONAL CONTROL OF THE PELVIS

Pelvic alignment directly affects the hips by altering the position of the femoral head within the acetabular fossa. Anterior rotation of the pelvis results in relative flexion of the hip, while posterior rotation of the pelvis results in relative extension. Attaining and stabilizing the pelvis in a neutral position is key to maintaining a centrated FA joint.

It is optimal length-tension relationships of the LPH complex force couples that create a neutral pelvic alignment. The pelvis is in neutral alignment when the anterior superior iliac spine (ASIS) and pubic symphysis (PS) are in the same vertical plane (dotted line).

The pelvis is in an anterior tilt (rotation) when the ASIS is anterior to the PS. The pelvis is in a posterior tilt (rotation) when the ASIS falls posterior to the PS. Neutral positioning of the pelvis is important in maintaining centration of the hip joint.

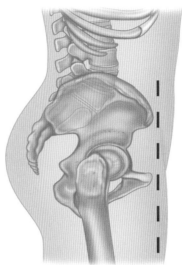

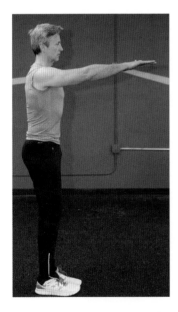
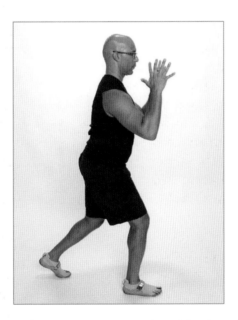

The individual in the left image demonstrates neutral positioning of the pelvis, while the individual in the right image demonstrates a slight anterior tilt of the pelvis. The slight anterior tilt is often a very safe posture to perform exercise, as the flexed hip position preloads the hip extensors and is the athletic stance that can be utilized for many sport-specific drills. Additionally, many experts recommend a slight anterior pelvic tilt when attempting to maximize running speed and agility. The key, however, lies in maintaining a neutral spine position over the pelvis so the motion is at the femoropelvic joints and not at the thoracolumbar or lumbosacral junctions.

Several force couples are responsible for maintaining proper positioning of the pelvis. Shown below is a schematic representing the force couples responsible for controlling the sagittal plane position of the pelvis.

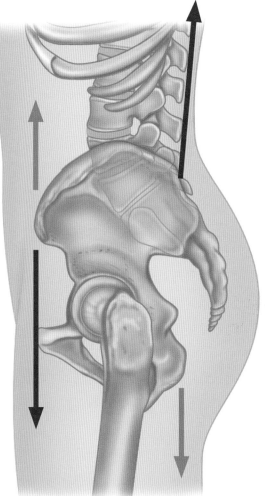

Rectus abdominis
External abdominal obliques
Internal abdominal obliques
Psoas minor

Lumbar erector spinae
Multifidus
Latissimus dorsi

Rectus femoris
Tensor fasciae latae
Sartorius
Iliacus
Psoas major

Gluteus maximus
Hamstrings
Muscles of the pelvic floor

Force Couples	Actions
Abdominals, gluteus maximus, hamstrings, and pelvic floor muscles	Posterior rotation of the pelvis
Lumbar extensors and hip flexors	Anterior rotation of the pelvis

MUSCLES OF THE HIP AND PELVIS

Various muscle and fascial attachments work to provide both the static and dynamic stability required to not only stabilize but also move the hip and pelvis. The forces placed upon the hip and pelvis during many routine activities can be quite formidable, even during seemingly mundane activities such as walking. For example, standing on one leg, such as during the stance phase of gait, increases the weight on the hip by two and a half times the body weight, while walking up stairs increases it by a factor of three. Forces during running may result in four and a half times one's body weight, necessitating a complex interplay of the muscles that directly cross and those that support the trunk and lower extremities.

Muscles of the hip and pelvis rarely act alone, functioning more as muscular chains rather than isolated muscle units. Among others, Vleeming and Meyers have both described the fascial interconnections between the muscles of the thorax, pelvis, and extremities. Generally speaking, these chains run in an alternating muscle-fascia connection that then correspondingly attach to the surrounding ligament/ joint capsule structures of the adjoining joints. This relationship turns the (often thought of as passive) ligaments and joint capsules into active stabilizers of their adjoining joints while enabling the central nervous system instantaneous feedback regarding joint position. These chains provide the stability and mobility required by the hip and pelvis and will be described below.

THE ANTERIOR AND POSTERIOR OBLIQUE CHAINS

As their name suggests, the anterior and posterior obliques run obliquely across the thorax and pelvis, connecting the contralateral extremities in the process. The anterior oblique chain consists of the rhomboids, serratus anterior, external obliques, abdominal fascia, contralateral internal obliques, and adductor fascia. This chain stabilizes the pubic symphysis and controls rotation of the thorax and pelvis. Similarly, the posterior oblique chain runs obliquely over the posterior aspect of the thorax and pelvis, stabilizing the LS junction and SIJs in addition to controlling rotation of the trunk, pelvis, hips, and entire lower extremity. The posterior oblique chain consists of the latissimus dorsi, thoracolumbar fascia, contralateral gluteus maximus, iliotibial band (ITB), and peroneus longus to insert into the fascial sling at the base of the first metatarsal. This chain additionally helps to stabilize the medial arch of the foot and knee, making this a rigid lever necessary to support the body weight in single leg stance (see overleaf).

THE POSTERIOR LONGITUDINAL CHAIN

The posterior longitudinal chain connects the peroneus longus at the base of the first metatarsal to the lateral aspect of the fibular head, to the long head of the biceps femoris, to the ischial tuberosity, to the sacrotuberous ligament, to the fascia and ligaments of the SIJ, and crossing the pelvis to an attachment on the contralateral erector spinae of the lumbar spine. This chain helps to stabilize the ipsilateral lower extremity during heel strike by pulling the fibula inferiorly, which effectively locks the lateral aspect of the ankle and foot complex. Additionally, the tension created through the sacrotuberous ligament locks the SIJ, which is necessary as the weight is progressed over the foot during single leg stance (see overleaf).

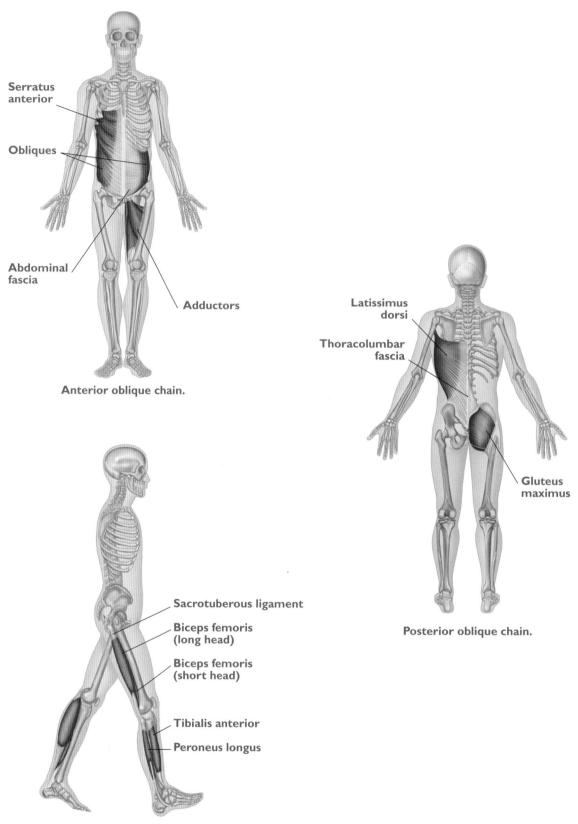

Serratus anterior

Obliques

Abdominal fascia

Adductors

Anterior oblique chain.

Latissimus dorsi

Thoracolumbar fascia

Gluteus maximus

Posterior oblique chain.

Sacrotuberous ligament

Biceps femoris (long head)

Biceps femoris (short head)

Tibialis anterior

Peroneus longus

Deep longitudinal chain.

THE LATERAL STABILITY MECHANISM OF THE HIP AND PELVIS

Because so many individuals demonstrate instability in single leg stance, lateral or frontal plane stability of the hip and pelvis is an important consideration in rehabilitation and conditioning of the LPH complex. Allison Grimaldi (2009) describes the lateral stability mechanism in three layers: the superficial layer comprising the upper fibers of the gluteus maximus and tensor fasciae latae; the intermediate layer comprising the three divisions of the gluteus medius and piriformis; and the deep layer comprising the gluteus minimus. Her research demonstrated that during imposed bed rest there was atrophy of the deep stabilizers of both the hip and the knee; however, no changes were found in the superficial fibers of either the gluteus maximus or the tensor fasciae latae. These findings were similar for clients with degenerative joint disease of the hip (Grimaldi 2009). This suggests that similar to the core, atrophy of the deep stabilizers leads to alterations in the ability to centrate the hip and pelvis. The muscles of the lateral stability mechanism will be further discussed below.

MUSCLES OF THE LATERAL STABILITY MECHANISM

GLUTEUS MAXIMUS

The gluteus maximus (GMx) is the largest muscle in the body, suggesting it plays an important functional role in movement. It is the only muscle that contains fibers that are perpendicular to the SIJ, suggesting its role in SIJ compression. Taking its origin off several bony attachments – including the ilium, sacrum, and coccyx – the GMx attaches fascially to the thoracolumbar fascia, sacroiliac ligaments, and gluteal tuberosity.

Its attachment to the posterior aspect of the ITB makes the GMx the key muscle in the stabilization and control of lower extremity pronation. Through its attachment to the contralateral latissimus dorsi via the thoracolumbar fascia, it functions as part of the posterior oblique chain, serving to compress the SIJ and transfer rotational loads between the spine and the upper and lower extremities. Gibbon's (2005) research suggests that the deeper coccygeal fibers are pivotal in pulling the femur posteriorly in the acetabulum, aiding centration and functional control of the hip joint.

GLUTEUS MEDIUS

The gluteus medius attaches from the anterior two-thirds of the outer surface of the ilium to the greater trochanter of the femur. Its three divisions blend with the gluteal fascia and it functions similarly to the middle deltoid of the shoulder. It is the primary hip abductor and one of the primary frontal plane stabilizers in single leg stance. The anterior fibers assist internal rotation and flexion, while the posterior fibers assist external rotation and extension. Inhibition of the gluteus medius leads to overactivation of the tensor fasciae latae in frontal plane stabilization of the pelvis.

GLUTEUS MINIMUS

The gluteus minimus lies beneath the gluteus medius on the outer surface of the ilium and attaches to the greater trochanter and joint capsule of the hip. While it assists both abduction and internal rotation of the hip, the gluteus minimus resists both the superior and anterior pull of the femoral head and pulls the joint capsule superiorly to avoid impingement during hip abduction.

TENSOR FASCIAE LATAE

The tensor fasciae latae (TFL) is important during functional movements such as squats and lunges and especially during unilateral stance. It attaches at the anterolateral aspect of the ilium to the anterior aspect of the ITB. It functions as part of the lateral stability mechanism along with the ipsilateral gluteus medius and gluteus minimus and the contralateral quadratus lumborum to provide frontal plane stabilization of the LPH complex. During the heel contact phase of the gait cycle, the TFL serves to counteract the posterior pull of the gluteus maximus, which has vast attachments along the posterior aspect of the ITB. It additionally assists the iliacus during the swing phase in flexing the hip. The TFL will often become a dominant hip flexor when there is weakness of either the iliacus or the psoas. It will additionally become overactive as a frontal plane stabilizer when there is weakness or inhibition of the gluteus medius. Since it is also an internal rotator of the hip, if either one of the aforementioned functions becomes dominant, it can produce increased internal rotation of the hip during single leg stance, compensatorily driving increased pronation of the lower extremity. As the hip internally rotates, there tends to be an increased lateral pull on the patella and fascia of the lateral thigh, often leading to patellar tracking dysfunctions and iliotibial band syndromes. In certain cases of extreme external rotation of the hip, the TFL can become an extensor of the knee, as the ITB migrates anteriorly over the lateral femoral condyle.

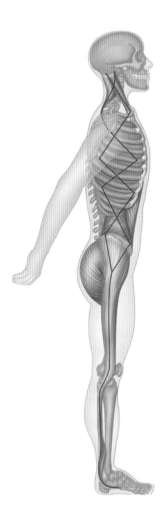

The myofascial lateral lines (Myers).

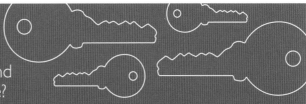

Key To Success

Gluteus Medius-Adductor Imbalances and the Valgus Knee – Is It Really That Simple?

Increased valgus knee position is a common postural and movement fault. Tight adductors and weakness in the gluteus medius is suggested as the primary muscle imbalance causing the valgus knee position. However, is it really as simple as a tight muscle and a weak functional antagonist? And if so, then why does stretching the hip adductors and strengthening the hip abductors only work on some of the clients with this postural-movement fault? Looking a little deeper at the mechanics required for normal gait may provide some light on this debate.

During the loading phase of gait, the metatarsals spread, thereby stretching the interossei muscles of the foot and thus creating a reflexive activation of the extensor chain of the lower extremity (Michaud 1997). The goal during the loading of the foot is to spread the metatarsals in order to create a reflexive response and optimally load the first ray of the foot (first phalanx, first metatarsal, and medial cuneiform). If this motion is blocked by a varus or rigid arch foot, an orthotic insert, or a shoe with relatively stiff instep (to prevent excessive pronation), the nervous system will recognize this and make compensations to help improve the medial loading and metatarsal spreading of the foot. One common way is to drive the knee through the frontal plane into a more valgus position to help load the medial aspect of the foot.

Additionally, studies have demonstrated decreased gluteus medius activation in the presence of ankle instability (Beckman & Buchanan 1995). This will increase the tonus of the adductor complex, as these muscles substitute to provide frontal plane stability during single leg stance.

KEY: Assess the client with the valgus knee movement fault in bare feet to determine how well they load the foot and ankle complex. If they have difficulty maintaining the medial component of the foot tripod through single leg stance and as they perform a series of functional assessments (squat, lunge, or gait), suspect the dysfunction may be coming from the foot and ankle complex and address those imbalances before resorting to stretching the adductors and strengthening the abductors.

THE PIRIFORMIS AND THE DEEP ROTATORS OF THE HIP

The piriformis is important in deceleration of internal rotation of the hip during the loading phase of gait (pronation). Through its attachment on the anterior surface of the sacrum to the greater trochanter, it functions as an important stabilizer of the sacroiliac joint. Stiffness of the piriformis is often a cause of sacroiliac joint dysfunction in individuals who are utilizing a deep rotator stabilization strategy, regarded as 'butt gripping' by Lee (2008).

The deep hip rotators (DHR) include the piriformis, gemellus superior/inferior, obturator internus/externus, and quadratus femoris. Although external rotation of the hip is performed primarily by the piriformis and gluteus maximus, there is a contribution by the DHR. There is little research to date on the 'true' function of the DHR; however, their size and location suggests that they have a significant role as supporters of the pelvic floor and as local stabilizers of the sacroiliac and hip joints. The literature confirms the obturator internus functions as part of the pelvic floor, supporting the pelvic organs and providing stabilization of the LPH complex. Overactivation of the deep rotators is common secondary to poor control of the LPH by the local stabilization system that often results during pregnancy, trauma, surgery and/or pelvic pain syndromes. This over compression leads to alterations in hip centration that may be direct contributors to the nearly 250,000 complete hip joint replacements that occur each year in the United States.

ADDITIONAL MUSCLES OF THE LUMBOPELVIC-HIP COMPLEX

While the muscular chains were discussed above, there are many additional muscles lending support to the LPH complex. Several of these muscles will be discussed below.

HAMSTRINGS

Four muscles make up the hamstring complex: the two divisions of the biceps femoris, the semitendinosus, and the semimembranosus. The biceps femoris (BF), originating from the superomedial aspect of the ischial tuberosity, shares an adjacent common origin with the semitendinosus. This arrangement increases the stabilization of the sacroiliac joint, likely acting as a 'check rein' and creating greater control over distal motion at the knee. Fascial attachments connect the BF to the sacrotuberous ligament, which together with the contralateral erector spinae and deep lamina of the thoracolumbar fascia constitute the deep longitudinal chain. The deep longitudinal chain functions to increase the stabilization of the sacroiliac joint by tensing the thoracolumbar fascia. The BF, through its attachment to the sacrotuberous ligament, decelerates and if short and tight, it limits the degree of sacral nutation.

The semitendinosus (ST) attaches from the ischial tuberosity and shares a common tendinosus attachment with the sartorius and gracilis on the anteromedial aspect of the tibia. These are the only muscles that directly cross the medial aspect of the knee joint and therefore likely contribute to medial stability to the knee.

The semimembranosus (SM) has several fascial slips that run posteriorly and support the posterior aspect the capsule of the knee (oblique popliteal ligament), laterally to cover the popliteus muscle (popliteal fascia), and anteromedially to blend with the medial aspect of the joint capsule. Michaud (1997) reports that the SM additionally has fascial attachments to the posterior horn of the medial meniscus and prevents impingement by pulling it posteriorly during knee flexion.

The hamstrings have been classically described as knee flexors; however, their functional role is much more significant during gait. During the gait cycle, the hamstrings are instrumental in decelerating hip flexion and knee extension during the end of the swing phase. They will additionally assist the propulsive phase of gait by accelerating extension of the hip and assisting extension of the knee. Although prone and seated leg curls have been the traditional exercises of choice for strengthening the hamstrings, their significant functional role make these exercises limiting and potentially counterproductive. See the exercise section for more on this subject.

RECTUS FEMORIS

The rectus femoris originates from two tendons – the straight head from the anterior inferior iliac spine and the reflected head from just above the brim of the acetabulum – to insert on the common patellar tendon. The rectus femoris is a two-joint muscle that functions both as a flexor and internal rotator of the hip, and additionally extends the knee and anteriorly rotates the pelvis. Eccentrically, it decelerates extension of the hip, flexion of the knee, and posterior tilting of the pelvis. It often becomes a dominant hip flexor and pelvic stabilizer when there is inhibition of the psoas major and is the muscle that is commonly responsible for hip flexor 'tightness.'

VASTI

The muscles of the vasti group – lateralis (VL), medialis (VM), and intermedius (VI) – are known for their role as knee extensors while eccentrically controlling knee flexion. However, functionally these muscles play more significant roles in lower extremity mechanics.

- **Vastus lateralis:** The VL arises from an aponeurosis attachment on the intertrochanteric line, gluteal tuberosity, and upper lateral aspect of the linea aspera to insert into the lateral aspect of the patella and lateral patellar retinaculum. It lies underneath the ITB and contraction of the VL pushes out into the ITB, helping to stabilize the lateral knee and lower extremity during single leg stance (hydraulic amplifier or fascial gain effect). While not directly crossing the hip, through its fascial connection to the pelvis, and its distal attachment on the knee, contraction of the VL contributes to internal rotation of the hip.

- **Vastus medialis:** The VM arises from an aponeurosis attachment on the medial aspect of the linea aspera and intermuscular septum to attach to the medial aspect of the patella and patellar retinaculum. The VM fascially blends with the adductor complex to aid medial stabilization of the knee. Studies have demonstrated that the VM is most active during the last 10 degrees, which led to the development of rehabilitation strategies that stress terminal knee extension (TKE) as a means of improving medial patellar tracking. While the VM seems to be important in controlling the medial tracking of the patella, TKEs rarely improve VM activity, necessitating a more functional approach to improving lateral patellar tracking issues. This topic will be expanded upon in the exercise section. Similar to the VL, the VM does not cross the hip joint; however, through fascial connections and its distal function on the knee, activation of the VM contributes to external rotation of the hip.

- **Vastus intermedius:** The VI arises from the anterolateral surface of the upper two-thirds of the femur to insert into the patellar tendon. The VI assists the other knee extensors in knee extension and decelerating knee flexion.

ADDUCTORS

The function of the adductor complex – including the pectineus, gracilis, and adductor brevis (ABr), longus (ALg) and magnus (AMg) – has been classically defined in anatomy texts as adductors of the hip joint. There seems to be little agreement between the texts as to whether these muscles additionally assist internal or external rotation of the hip. However, a closer look at the size and complexity of this muscle complex suggests it has a much greater functional role than has been previously assigned.

Giving credence to this point are the vast attachment regions of several of the adductor muscles. For example, the proximal portion of the AMg serves as the origin of the vastus medialis, and the ALg has attachments via its aponeurosis to the AMg and ABr posteriorly and the VM anteriorly, suggesting its role in stabilization of the medial knee. The adductors also have a significant role in functional activities such as gait. The adductor complex, along with the gluteus medius/minimus and the contralateral quadratus lumborum, makes up the lateral chain. The lateral chain is responsible for frontal plane stabilization of the LPH complex during unilateral stance, such as during the gait cycle, in addition to squatting and lunging movements. The adductor complex additionally serves as part of the anterior oblique chain (ipsilateral internal oblique and adductor complex with the contralateral external oblique and hip external rotators), providing transverse plane stabilization during rotational movement patterns such as seen during the gait cycle and in throwing. During gait, the adductors show increased activity during the swing phase of gait, indicating that they may assist flexion and both external and internal rotation of the hip. The adductor magnus seems to have constant activation throughout the gait cycle – the anterior fibers assist in hip flexion, the oblique fibers assist in hip adduction (stance phase), and the posterior fibers aid in deceleration of hip extension during the terminal phase of gait.

PSOAS MAJOR, PSOAS MINOR, AND ILIACUS

Perhaps no muscles are more misunderstood and have more dysfunction attributed to them than the psoas muscles. Similar to the gluteus maximus, the psoas major (PMj) has vast attachments and functions on the spine, pelvis, and hip, lending credence to its important functional role. The PMj arises from fascial attachments on the diaphragm, anterior aspects of the transverse processes, vertebral bodies, and intervertebral discs of levels L1–L5, to attach to the lesser trochanter of the femur as well as blend fascially with the pelvic floor. It has several important functional roles, including but not limited to:

- flexion, abduction, and external rotation of the hip;

- eccentric control of extension, adduction, and internal rotation of the hip;

- maintenance of hip centration and an optimal axis of rotation (key role);

- as part of the deep muscle system of the TPC, it aids compression and stabilization of the lumbar spine (key role).

Since the muscle is located very close to the axis of rotation, it contributes only minimally to spinal motion (Bogduk 2005). However, it produces a significant compressive force upon the spine, especially during a sit-up-type maneuver. A benefit of the spinal compression produced by the contraction of the psoas is the creation of spinal stiffness, which counteracts the anterior pelvic rotation that is created by contraction of the iliacus (McGill 2004). Additionally, the PMj provides spinal stability, which is necessary to provide a counterforce during lower extremity motion. McGill also suggests that the psoas and iliacus are separate muscles with separate tendons and nerve innervations. Research by Dangaria and Naesh (1998) has demonstrated that there tends to be unilateral atrophy of the psoas in the region of disc herniations, most likely occurring secondary to inhibition by pain. Barker, Shamley and Jackson (2000) noted similar unilateral atrophy in both the multifidus and psoas on the side of low back pain.

The psoas minor arises from the anterior surface of the T12 and L1 vertebral bodies to attach on the front of the innominate at the innominate line and iliopectineal eminence. While it is said to be absent in nearly 40% of the population, the psoas minor may appear as fascial slips from the psoas major (Gibbons 2005). It functions to posteriorly rotate the pelvis, resisting the anterior pull of the other hip flexors, which act to anteriorly rotate the pelvis.

The iliacus lies inside the iliac fossa and attaches via its own tendon to the lesser trochanter of the femur. It is the only true hip flexor and will also externally rotate and abduct the hip. With the foot fixed on the ground it becomes a powerful anterior rotator of the pelvis. It decelerates extension, adduction, and internal rotation of the hip as well as posterior rotation of the pelvis.

DYSFUNCTIONS IN LOWER EXTREMITY PATTERNS

There are several common movement dysfunctions that can be noted in common lower extremity patterns. These include loss of neutral spinal stabilization and ability to anteriorly rotate the pelvis during forward bending, loss of hip stability in frontal plane patterns, loss of the squared pelvis, and general loss of stability during unilateral or single leg stance.

LOSS OF NEUTRAL SPINAL STABILIZATION

During forward bending it is common for clients to be unable to maintain a neutral lumbopelvic alignment. They will often flex through the most mobile area of the spine as they reach forward in the lunge position. This will also tend to be the area where they already have or will develop pain. Notice the thoracic spine flexion in the client to the left because he does not attain enough anterior pelvic rotation. Also notice the cervicothoracic hyperextension because he is cued to keep looking up as he reaches forward.

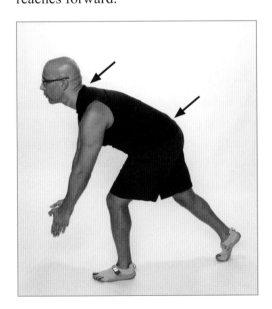

Correction: Cue the client to maintain a neutral spine position as they reach forward, especially if they are lifting a significant load and/or are experiencing back or spinal pain. This may limit their overall range of motion: it will however spare their spine from flexion-related forces.

LOSS OF HIP STABILITY

While it is common in most unilateral patterns, loss of hip stability can be seen most easily in the frontal plane pattern. The function of the lateral stabilization chain is to maintain stability in the frontal plane. In this plane, the hip must remain inside the loaded leg. Instability can be noted when the body weight shifts too far laterally outside the stance leg. Note in the image below, the individual's body weight shifts outside their base of support.

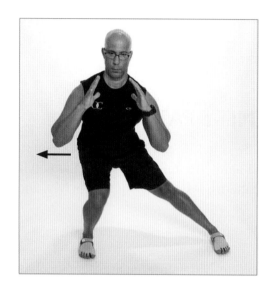

Correction: Limit the individual's range of motion so that their body weight remains within their base of support. They should feel the weight on the inside rather than the outside of the foot that they are loading, and the ipsilateral knee must remain in line of the foot and hip.

LOSS OF THE SQUARED PELVIS

In the squared pelvis, control of the pelvis is maintained by the medial stabilization chain, and the iliac crests remains level while alignment is maintained in the hip, knee, and ankle/foot complex (left image). When medial control is lost, the pelvis laterally shifts on the support side and there is subsequent internal rotation and adduction of the lower extremity (left image below).

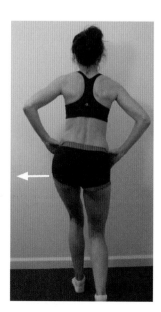 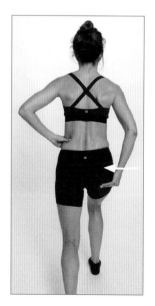

The squared pelvis must be maintained during functional patterning. The client places their hands on the pelvis to help monitor this position as they lower themselves in the split squat position (right image). When they lose control, their pelvis tilts and shifts towards the forward leg (left image).

Correction: The client should be cued to activate the deep gluteus maximus and deep hip rotators to pull their pelvis back into position. If they cannot be cued out of this position, the lower fibers of gluteus maximus and the deep external rotators may need to be activated.

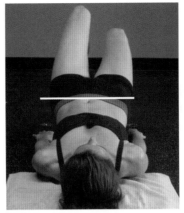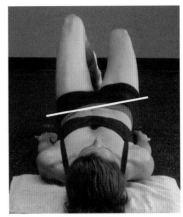

The squared pelvis must also be maintained during single leg patterns such as single leg and marching bridges. Notice how the client maintains a level pelvis as the leg is lifted to perform a single leg bridge (left image). As they fatigue, they lose control, allowing the pelvis to tilt towards the raised leg (right image). The client should be cued to maintain optimal hip positioning by placing their hands on their pelvis and focusing on core activation. The trainer or therapist should also have the client connect their medial stabilization chain – the medial column of the foot, vastus medialis, adductor complex, and deep medial gluteus maximus – to help them maintain ideal hip alignment. If these cues do not make a significant difference, the trainer or therapist can try an activation strategy, and if this fails to help, then the pattern must be regressed until the client is able to sufficiently stabilize the pattern.

LOSS OF STABILITY IN SINGLE LEG STANCE

Many clients in the gym setting are instructed to perform unilateral lower extremity patterns – everything from performing upper body exercises to single leg activities performed on labile equipment. Unfortunately, most of these individuals are not cued properly and do not have adequate stability to support themselves in this position. The premise that is held in the fitness and rehabilitative industries alike is that if life and sports occur mostly on one leg, clients must perform lower extremity patterns on one leg. Again, rarely are the clients and patients cued or evaluated for their ability to be on one leg other than by the fact that they are able to do it. There are four main indicators that demonstrate instability during single leg loading:

1. **Non-compensated Trendelenburg:** A positive Trendelenburg's sign is where the pelvis drops on the unsupported side or the side of hip flexion (image below left). This is generally accompanied by hip abduction and internal rotation and results in the classic model gait. It is also the gait pattern that feeds into injuries of the meniscus, medial collateral, and anterior cruciate ligaments of the knee.

2. **Compensated Trendelenburg:** A compensated Trendelenburg's gait occurs when the client has compensated for the lack of stability by shifting their trunk over the stance hip (image to right). This individual usually demonstrates a waddling-type gait as their trunk shifts excessively in the frontal plane.

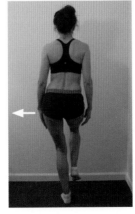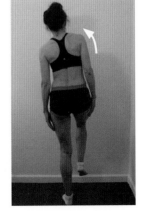

Non-compensated (left), compensated (right).

3. **Butt gripping and anterior hip shear:** This occurs when the client attempts to stabilize themselves in a single leg stance by over-gripping their deep hip rotators, which posteriorly rotates the ilium and drives the hip anteriorly in the socket. This client will present with a huge divot in the lateral aspect of the pelvis in a standing posture, which will increase as they shift their weight onto the stance leg. Generally, this client will hold their center of gravity behind their support leg and also have concurrent abdominal gripping.

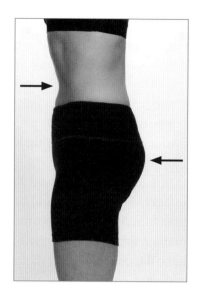

Correction: The client should be cued to relax their hips while performing activities of daily living and to spread through their ischial tuberosities or sink the hip back in the socket as they perform squatting and lunging patterns.

4. **Foot gripping:** Excessive toe gripping occurs when the client attempts to stabilize themselves by overutilizing the long toe flexors and muscles of the posterior compartment rather than by the foot intrinsics (images below). When lying in a relaxed position, they will generally demonstrate flexion of the interphalangeal joints, clawing, or hammering of the toes because of the chronic overutilization of this strategy.

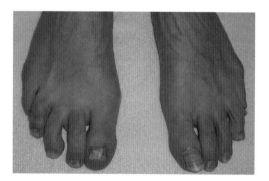 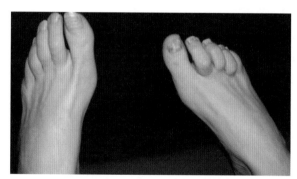

Correction: The client must be regressed to a pattern where they can be successful and demonstrate good stability until they show improved stability. Proper cuing should also be utilized but if a client is demonstrating one of the above patterns, it is likely they are showing signs of instability that they cannot be cued out of. Improve their areas of functional deficit and their stability in split and supported positions prior to moving them to single leg patterns.

THE OVERACTIVE POSTERIOR HIP COMPLEX

Overactivation of the deep hip rotators, otherwise referred to as 'butt gripping' by Diane Lee and Linda-Joy Lee, is a common cause of hip dysfunction. As the name suggests, this pattern is caused by a contraction of the deep hip rotators and superficial gluteus maximus and looks as if the individual is standing or walking in a perpetual contraction. In actuality, they are. This stabilization pattern is a result of several causes, including trying to make the rear end look smaller (generally females are guilty of this); weakness in the pelvic floor, causing reflexive overactivation of the deep hip rotators and adductors; instability anywhere in the lower extremity, causing overactivation of the posterior hip musculature; and learned cuing techniques from trainers and therapists who stress to 'squeeze the glutes as hard as possible.'

Palpation over the lateral hip region just behind the greater trochanter will reveal an indentation or hollowing, created by overactivation of the deep external rotators of the hip (see image below). In supine position, the head of the femur can be palpated by placing the hands just medial to the anterior superior iliac spine (ASIS) and pushing lightly posteriorly. It is common to palpate increased tone or 'fullness' in the tensor fasciae latae (just lateral to the ASIS). With this 'gripping' pattern, the head of the femur will generally be pushed forward and superior in the acetabulum. Not so ironically, the superoanterior aspect of the femoral head is the most common region of cartilaginous degenerative changes of the hip.

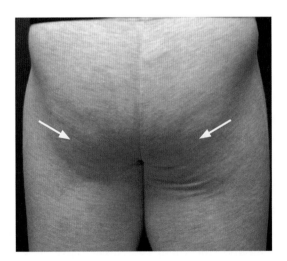 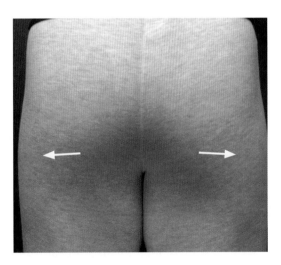

Butt gripping (left); the client is cued to relax through the hips (right).

By cuing the individual to relax the hips and spread the sit bones (arrows), there is a change in the tone in the posterior hip region (image to the right). Palpation over the anterior hip region will reveal the head of the femur has been centered in the socket secondary to the relaxation of the posterior hip muscles.

While the previous technique is extremely effective for releasing butt-gripping patterns, some individuals require more specific techniques for decreasing activation of the deep hip rotators and/or the posterior hip capsule. The next section demonstrates a release technique effective for releasing the posterior hip capsule as well as reducing myofascial restrictions.

COMMON CONDITIONS OF THE LOWER EXTREMITY

In a 2002 study of approximately 2,000 individuals who reported injuries as a result of running, patellofemoral pain syndrome was the most common overuse injury, followed by iliotibial band friction syndrome, plantar fasciitis, meniscus injuries, and patellar tendinopathies (Taunton et al 2002). These injuries are also common in many cardiovascular-type exercises that require repetitive motion, including cycling, walking on the treadmill or outdoors, and using an elliptical-type training machine. There are several common overuse injuries affecting the lower kinetic chain and various causes for these conditions, although many of them tend to have overlapping etiologies. These conditions include iliotibial band syndrome, patellofemoral pain syndrome, labral tear, hamstring strains, hip impingement and groin pain, and anterior cruciate ligament tears, which will be discussed below.

ILIOTIBIAL BAND SYNDROME

Iliotibial band syndrome is common in athletes such as runners who perform repetitive activities that involve load bearing through the lower extremity. It is characterized by pain at the distal aspect of the iliotibial band as it crosses the lateral condyle of the femur to insert into both the lateral patellar retinaculum and Gerdy's tubercle of the tibia. It is commonly referred to as a friction syndrome, as repetitive contractions of the tensor fasciae latae, in addition to movement of the hip and knee, cause the band to rub across the lateral condyle. There are two primary contributing factors for this condition.

1. Both the gluteus maximus and the tensor fasciae latae insert into the iliotibial band and are responsible for stabilization of the lower extremity during the support phase of the gait cycle or when squatting, lunging, climbing stairs, etc. In the presence of gluteus maximus inhibition, the tensor fasciae latae is unchecked, creating a more anterior pull of the iliotibial band over the lateral condyle. The tensor fasciae latae can also be up-regulated as a frontal plane stabilizer with inhibition of the gluteus medius, or as a hip flexor with psoas major inhibition. Because of synergist dominance, the tensor fasciae latae will become more adept at stabilizing the lower extremity; however, it will also drive more internal of the lower extremity and therefore cause friction of the iliotibial band.

2. The hip abductors must support approximately two and a half times the body weight in single leg stance (Fagerson 1998) and significantly more when running. Inhibition of the hip abductors, which has been related to ankle instability (Beckman and Buchanan 1995), can cause a synergist dominance of the tensor fasciae latae in frontal plane stabilization of the lower leg. This leads to similar biomechanical changes as noted above, leading to iliotibial band friction syndromes.

PATELLOFEMORAL PAIN SYNDROME

Patellofemoral pain syndrome (PFPS) is a painful condition that results from cartilaginous changes of the articular surfaces between the patella and the femoral condyle. The client generally experiences the most pain when walking down stairs or performing deep squats. While there are many etiologies, excessive forward shear of the knee or internal rotation of the knee that creates lateral tracking of the patella are two common causes. These patterns are generally set up by poor ankle dorsiflexion and/or hip flexion during squatting, lunging, or walking down stairs, as well as uncontrolled internal rotation.

Increased valgosity and internal knee rotation is also related to increases in the quadriceps angle or Q-angle (angle formed by an intersecting line drawn from the anterior superior iliac spine through the mid-patella and one drawn from the mid-patella through the center of the tibial tubercle) and has been suggested as a contributing cause of lateral tracking of the patella and increased degenerative changes of the knee. Because of a relatively greater Q-angle and deficits in eccentric control of the lower extremity, patellofemoral pain syndrome tends to be more common in females.

Females with PFPS have demonstrated poor eccentric control and increased adduction positions as compared to control participants (Baldon et al 2009). It is believed that poor eccentric control of the hip by the hip abductors leads to this increase in frontal plane mechanics. Training of eccentric control of hip abduction is therefore recommended as a preventative for repetitive functional activities (Baldon et al).

LABRAL TEARS

Tearing of the acetabular labrum was first diagnosed in 1957 (Groh and Herrera 2009). Due to advances in MRI technology and clinical awareness, there has been a recent increase in the diagnosis and treatment of acetabular labral tears in recent years. A tear of the acetabular labrum is generally a result of repetitive trauma; however, a sudden acute trauma such as a fall with legs split can also result in labral injuries. These tears are generally more common in the athletic population, especially those who are performing high level activities such as running, activities requiring significant internal hip rotation such as tennis, golf, and baseball, and sports requiring sharp cutting motions such as martial arts, soccer, and basketball. General clinical signs include stiffness of the hip joint, especially in internal rotation and abduction, clicking or catching in the joint, and pain at the end ranges of motion. Poor centration of the femoroacetabular joint and lack of optimal muscle activation synergies around both the hip and the lumbopelvic-hip junction are common predisposing factors in clients experiencing labral tears relating to repetitive traumas. Most labral tears in the United States tend to be anterior, suggesting that forward displacement of the femoral head within the acetabulum secondary to a 'butt-gripping' strategy is likely a common etiology (Groh and Herrera 2009).

HAMSTRING STRAINS

Hamstring strains are a common injury affecting athletes involved in running, sprinting, and jumping. The 'pulled' or, more accurately, strained hamstring muscle is a common ailment found in almost any sport or activity that requires explosive speed, rapid deceleration, or jumping. Various studies demonstrate that the biceps femoris seems to be the most commonly injured of the hamstring muscles and that the injury itself tends to occur during the eccentric terminal swing phase of gait, while others suggest injuries to the semitendinosus and semimembranosus. Pre-activation of the biceps femoris and adductor longus rather than the transversus abdominis and multifidus was found in individuals with sacroiliac joint pain, as compared to those with no pain during the single leg stance test (Hungerford et al 2003). This suggests that control of the lumbopelvic-hip complex is critical in both the etiology as well as the rehabilitation and prevention of hamstring injuries.

HIP IMPINGEMENT, GROIN PAIN, AND SNAPPING HIP SYNDROME

Hip impingement is characterized by pain in the inner groin and/or hip region during internal rotation and adduction of the hip. It has been discussed as a precursor to labral tears, groin pulls, and 'snapping' hip syndrome. Hip impingement, and the resultant maladies of labral tears, groin pulls and snapping hip syndrome, were found to be related to the lack of optimal joint centration and the resultant forward migration of the femoral head within the acetabulum (Sahrmann 2002). In fact, labral tears have been found in more than 90% of patients presenting with groin pain (Groh and Herrera 2009). Posterior capsular restrictions of the hip and myofascial contractures of the posterior hip muscles, otherwise referred to as 'butt gripping' (Lee 2008), have also been suggested as causative factors of the loss of joint centration and resultant forward femoroacetabular positioning that predisposes an individual to impingement and groin pain.

Another common complaint involving the hip is the 'snapping,' 'clicking,' or 'popping' hip syndrome. It is characterized by an audible or palpable click as the individual attempts to extend the leg from a bent hip position. This can occur in either standing or supine positions and is most commonly experienced near or at the end range of eccentric hip extension. There have been several proposed theories as to the origin of this clicking, including the tendon of the psoas flipping over the lesser trochanter or hip bursa, crepitus from an unstable lumbar vertebrae or sacroiliac joint, or instability at the pubic symphysis. This clicking has anecdotally been found to be related to poor hip centration and inhibition of the local system of the lumbopelvic-hip complex. Specifically, the deep fibers of the psoas major and gluteus maximus are necessary for proper centration of the femoroacetabular joint (Gibbons 2005). It has also been clinically noted that the audible sound may be related to an instability at one of the vertebral attachments of the psoas. Clinically, stabilizing the thoracolumbar junction (attachment of the psoas major) tends to decrease or eliminate the 'click'. This suggests that snapping hip syndrome is related in part to poor TPC stabilization as well as poor centration and lack of optimal muscle synergies around the femoroacetabular joint.

ANTERIOR CRUCIATE LIGAMENT INJURIES

Injuries involving the anterior cruciate ligament (ACL) in addition to the medial collateral ligament (MCL) and medial meniscus (MM) are rampant in both the athletic and non-athletic population. Women seem to be at a greater risk as evidenced by the higher incidence of these types of injuries that occur in this population, regardless of sport or occupation. As with many musculoskeletal conditions, there are a number of perpetuating myths surrounding the origins of these injuries as well. To simplify the discussion, injuries to the ACL, MCL and MM will be grouped together since they often have a similar mechanism and are frequently injured in unison.

The ACL consists of two bands that run from the posterior aspect of the femoral condyle to attach to the medial tibial eminence. It functions as the primary restraint to anterior shear of the tibia and secondary to internal rotation and valgus forces on the knee (Moeller and Lamb 1997). It acts with the posterior cruciate ligament (PCL) as axes of rotation for knee movement (Moeller and Lamb 1997).

Females experience a 3.6 times greater ACL injury rate, as compared to their male counterparts (Myer et al 2008). Females participating in soccer, volleyball, and basketball tend to have a higher incidence of ACL injuries, as compared to other sports. Interestingly, most injuries involving the ACL are non-contact injuries, meaning that there is no direct trauma that results in the injury. The mechanism of injury to the ACL tends to be flexion, adduction, and internal rotation of the knee and can often occur as the individual attempts to decelerate her momentum and/or quickly change direction. If that is the case, then what are the underlying causative factors behind these injuries? There are several purported theories behind the increased incidence of injuries in females and several are discussed below.

1. Women have a greater Q-angle: The most common reason given as to why women have an increased incidence of knee injuries is that they have a greater Q-angle (or quadriceps angle) than men. Recall, the Q-angle is the angle that is formed between a straight line drawn from the ASIS to the mid-patella and from the mid-patella to the tibial tubercle. The angle in women averages around 18 degrees, whereas in men it tends to average around 13 degrees. An increase in the Q-angle typically tends to occur with an increase in genu valgum (knock-knee), potentially leading to several conditions involving the knee. These include alterations in the positioning of the patella (usually superior and lateral), leading to patellar tracking problems and chondromalacia patellae, and external rotation of the tibia, which increases the torsion on the ACL, MCL, and MM. The reasons for the increased angle in women include:

- a wider pelvis, which positions the ASIS more laterally;

- a decrease in the angle of the femoral neck;

- a slightly greater degree of ligament laxity of the MCL and ACL of the knee and spring ligament of the foot.

2. Biomechanical alterations: Factors such as alignment issues of the lower extremity, including hip anteversion, external tibial rotation and forefoot pronation, seem to be related to greater incidences of knee injuries in females.

3. Hormonal factors: Increase in hormones, especially around the premenstrual and menstrual phases of the cycle, tend to increase susceptibly of female soccer players to injuries (Biondino 1999). However, taking oral contraceptives seemed to decrease the incidence of injuries in female soccer players.

So what does the literature have to contribute to the cause and prevention of ACL injuries? Research has demonstrated deficits in feed-forward (anticipatory) motor control in individuals experiencing low back pain, leading to altered stabilization patterns of the lumbopelvic-hip region (Richardson, et al. 2004) which thereby alters lower extremity stabilization. Another study looked at changes in ground reaction forces during jump landing in individuals who demonstrated ankle instability. Interestingly, multi-directional instabilities were detected in individuals who experienced previous ankle injuries, which lead the authors to conclude these individuals were experiencing deficits in motor control. This information is incredibly valuable to the rehabilitation and conditioning specialist, as it points to the importance of evaluating previous lower extremity injuries and their potential contribution to alterations in neuromotor control and resultant compensations in an individual's movement patterns.

Additional studies have demonstrated that females tend to exhibit greater internal rotation forces and higher knee stiffness values than males during single leg landing (from single leg jumping). Females possessing higher levels of joint laxity in the knee tend to demonstrate increased activation of the gastrocnemius and biceps femoris in response to lower extremity perturbations, which may contribute to higher stiffness values that were noted earlier. Much of the literature suggests variations between male and female biomechanics in landing from jumping. While some researchers have demonstrated that female athletes landed with accelerated and greater degrees of knee flexion, others have demonstrated that female athletes exhibit significantly lower knee and hip flexion angles and higher ground reaction forces, as compared to male athletes. Similar studies have shown differences in muscle activation patterns, including decreased gluteal activity and increased quadriceps activity in female collegiate athletes, as compared to their male counterparts. The quadriceps act as an antagonist to the ACL, creating an anterior shear force on the tibia and when over-activated, can increase stress on the ACL. The hamstrings and soleus in contrast act as agonists to the ACL by providing posterior checks to anterior movement of the tibia and when inhibited, allow increased anterior shear of the tibia under the femur.

Poor eccentric control of frontal plane mechanics has also been cited as a major contributive factor (de Marche Baldon et al 2009). Increased abduction of the knee, secondary to poor functional control from the gluteus maximus and medius, increases stress across the ACL as well as the MCL.

While each of these conditions discussed above are separate entities with multiple and varying etiologies, there is one common thread among them. Each generally stems from variations of the following issues:

- poor centration of the femoroacetabular, knee, and ankle-foot complex;
- poor motor control of the lumbopelvic-hip complex;
- poor eccentric control of the lower extremity.

While this may seem like an oversimplification of the lower extremity injury process, it identifies the key factors in the development of most movement dysfunctions of the lower extremity. Addressing these factors, improving centration of the hip and ankle-foot complexes, and improving motor control of the lower extremity will form the basis of the corrective exercise approach that will be presented in the corrective exercise section of this book.

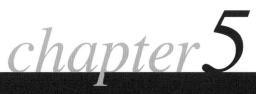
chapter 5

Assessment

CHAPTER OBJECTIVES

To identify and understand the functional components of the shoulder and hip assessment

To identify the key regions of dysfunction within the shoulder and hip complexes

To identify the key drivers of shoulder and hip dysfunction

"People only see what they are prepared to see." (Ralph Waldo Emerson)

Proper assessment is important prior to working with a client, regardless of their prior training or current functional goals. The assessment will drive the corrective exercise strategy the trainer or therapist will use and allow them to determine when the individual can be appropriately progressed. Additionally, the assessment will dictate the client's home exercise, and proper education in the assessment process will help the trainer or therapist educate the client in self-awareness and feedback. In other words, if the client will not be back to therapy or training for a while because of financial, geographical, insurance, or other reasons, the self-assessment aspect can help the individual monitor their own progress, independent of the therapist or trainer.

THE FUNCTIONAL ASSESSMENT

While there are any number of valid assessments that can be used, the ones given below have been chosen because of the type of information they provide. More specifically, they have been selected to look at a few of the biggest causes of shoulder and hip dysfunction, including loss of optimal breathing and trunk stabilization, inability to maintain joint centration with subsequent loss of internal rotation in both the shoulders and hips, and poor loading strategies through the shoulder complex, trunk, and hip complex. These tests have been chosen based upon their ability to accurately evaluate for these dysfunctions. A description of each test will be provided, along with the common signs of inefficient stabilization and movement patterns.

The purpose of the assessment is not to test the individual for an entire hour, running them through a battery of tests to discover every single movement fault. The goal of the assessment is to help the trainer or therapist determine the biggest driver of the client's dysfunction. In other words, what is the greatest movement or stabilization dysfunction that is causing this individual's dysfunction. While there can be several causes, one is likely to be the primary, while the others are likely to be secondary compensatory problems.

After performing a thorough assessment, what if the therapist or trainer chooses the wrong primary driver and chooses a corrective exercise approach based on this faulty premise? The worst case scenario is that the client does not improve, while the best case scenario is that the client improves a little, which for some clients will be all they need to resume their activities or accomplish their functional goals. Unfortunately, this strategy will not help many chronic pain sufferers or elite athletes, the two groups of individuals at the extreme ends of the functional continuum. These individuals will need a specific approach to improving their performance, which is why the tests and evaluations must be precisely administered and their results efficaciously interpreted to determine the priority of the intervention.

At times, despite the trainer's or therapist's best intentions, an incorrect corrective approach may be administered. While corrective strategies can take weeks, months, or even years depending upon the severity, complexity, or intensity of the presenting issues, if the chosen approach is not demonstrating any functional progress within two weeks, it is likely not the correct approach or perhaps not the appropriate time for that part of the intervention, provided the trainer or therapist is confident that the client is doing their part in the process by performing their homework. Therefore, a new approach should be instituted and reassessed for its efficacy within the next two weeks following the introduction of the new strategy.

It is common to have clients present with several layers of dysfunction or multiple compensation strategies. It is often necessary to 'peel back' the proverbial layers by addressing the major complaint first, even though this may not be the primary driver of the dysfunction. For example, a client presents with acute exacerbation of low back pain after playing tennis. Upon evaluation, the trainer or therapist discovers a lack of internal rotation of their left hip (their lead leg if they are a right-handed tennis player), poor respiratory patterns, stiffness in their thorax, and decreased ankle dorsiflexion and determines a lumbar flexion lesion to be the source of the client's back pain. While the poor hip rotation or loss of ankle range of motion following a fracture of the ankle several years ago may be the root of the problem, the more immediate issue is the acute low back pain and instability. It may be necessary to stabilize the low back and improve the respiratory patterns prior to addressing the ankle and hip issues to provide the client more immediate relief. If the same client is presenting with identical symptoms and results during their functional assessment, although their pain is chronic, now the approach may switch to improving the greatest driver of the dysfunction whether the trainer or therapist feels it is the ankle, the hip, or respiratory issues. The direction the trainer or therapist takes is dependent upon the client's presenting issues and goals, the results of their functional assessment, and the trainer's or therapist's intuition.

How can the corrective exercise approach be based on intuition? Unfortunately, when dealing with the human body, not everything can be based upon empirical evidence. Both the information the assessment provides and the corrective strategy utilized are based upon multiple factors, only one of which is empirical evidence. As Collins discusses in his provocative novel *How The Mighty Fall*, the lack of evidence to support something does not invalidate its occurrence. He uses the example of cancer and how the lack of evidence of cancer in the body does not mean the patient does not have cancer, only that the methods used to test for cancer did not show any signs of it. Similarly, in his book *The Black Swan*, Taleb discusses how the lack of evidence of a black swan, otherwise supported by the common thought process of 'I have never seen nor has anyone I know ever seen a black swan' mean that there is no such thing as a black swan (Taleb 2007). In his groundbreaking work on the adaptive unconscious and through a process termed 'thin slicing,' Gladwell (2005) describes how an expert's unconscious mind can make reasonably accurate assessments, even when given very little time or information about a particular topic, and at times when too much information is presented, the decision-making process can be overloaded, a term described as 'analysis paralysis.' This notion of less is sometimes more is supported by Taleb. Taleb describes how an increase in information does not necessarily lead to an increase in correct predictions, just an increase in the confidence that the individual feels about those predictions.

"… in another telling experiment, the psychologist Paul Slovic asked bookmakers to select from eighty-eight variables in past horse races those that they found useful in computing the odds. These variables included all manner of statistical information about past performances. The bookmakers were given the ten most useful variables, then asked to predict the outcomes of races. Then they were given ten more and asked to predict again. The increase in the information set did not lead to an increase in their accuracy; their confidence in their choices, on the other hand, went up markedly. Information proved to be toxic." (Taleb p. 145)

On the other hand, this is not to say that one test will yield all the information necessary to provide a rationale for a specific corrective strategy. For example, some individuals will choose to look at the overhead squat as the basis of their corrective approach, claiming that hip adduction (knees going into a valgus position) is a sign of tight adductors and weak hip abductors. The arms moving forward signifies poor length of the latissimus dorsi or extensibility of the thoracolumbar fascia. If the heels come off the floor, then a tight Achilles tendon and gastrocnemius is to blame. While each of these are valid assumptions based on the overhead squat assessment, they are just that – assumptions. Without proving the assumption with a more direct follow-up test, for example, a range of motion assessment on the adductors, and a strength test on the hip abductors in the case of valgus knees, the tester is making a faulty premise based upon their own biases.

Therefore the assessment is a combination of objective testing, clinical intuition, and experience while limiting personal biases. While all assessments have a level of bias, the goal of the assessment screen should be to eliminate as many of the personal biases and to have additional tests that either confirm or refute the findings. The other purpose of the selection criteria is to make each test easy to administer while providing relatively consistent evaluation of the results despite the tester. These tests were chosen with that goal in mind, although the functional muscle testing has some challenges with inter-tester reliability if the tester has never performed precision muscle testing before. In these cases, the trainer or therapist can omit the muscle tests and allow the other tests to drive the corrective, rehabilitative, or training strategy that is implemented. Where necessary, the trainer or therapist can perform additional tests to clear up the clinical picture.

Functional Assessment	
Standing	Posture Single leg stance Good morning
Seated	Seated hip flexion Seated shoulder flexion and abduction
Supine	Thorax: position, mobility, and respiration Internal range of motion: shoulders and hips Ankle range of motion Manual muscle tests
Additional test	Push-up: on the floor, against a table, or against a wall

POSTURE

Posture is the positioning of the bones, joints, and soft tissue of the body. Normal resting posture requires little muscular contraction or energy and thus is regarded as physiologically efficient. Proper posture is the synchronization of the contractile and the non-contractile tissues to achieve optimal joint centration over a balanced center of gravity.

Achieving neutral posture is important for maintaining proper length-tension relationships throughout the kinetic chain. This is considered the length at which the muscles can develop maximum tension due to the optimization of cross-bridging of the actin and myosin filaments. If this relationship changes, the nervous system will be required to recruit a different muscle synergy or strategy to create the desired stabilization or movement pattern.

A postural assessment is one component in the analysis of the musculoskeletal system, as it provides an overall presentation of the client's stabilization strategy. Additionally, the postural assessment provides the trainer or therapist a starting point from which to initiate the corrective exercise strategy while providing a tool for monitoring client progress. While the postural assessment is part of a thorough evaluation, it is not intended to replace a functional assessment. The postural assessment shows the examiner the result of the client's particular strategy, whereas the functional assessment begins the process of figuring out why the client has adopted this strategy.

For example, if a client is standing in a posterior pelvic tilt with overactivation of the deep posterior hip and their hip positioned anteriorly within the acetabulum, it is safe to assume that when they load their hip during functional movement patterns such as squatting and lunging, they will use this type of 'gripping' strategy (image to right). This finding should be confirmed by palpating the greater trochanter and acetabulum and monitoring their relationship during the assessment of their single leg stance.

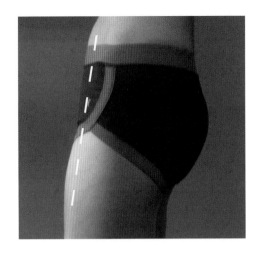

Notice the ASIS is posterior to the pubic symphysis in the image to the right.

The postural assessment begins with observing the client from the front, back, and both sides. The trainer or therapist notes the client's alignment as well as the particular strategy the client is using to hold themselves in that posture. The client's particular commitment to their strategy can be determined by gently trying to move the client from their position. For example, with the client standing, facing away from the therapist, the client can be pushed gently side to side to determine how rigid they are holding their body. In normal relaxed posture, the client should be primarily using an ankle stabilization strategy so there should not be much overall rigidity in their system. If the therapist cannot easily move the client, they are likely utilizing a gripping or bracing strategy. This procedure can be performed in the following regions:

- The tester gently pushes the client's thorax side to side to note how rigid the client is holding their thorax.

- The tester gently tries to bend the client's knees one at a time to determine how rigid the client is holding their lower extremity and how easily they can move the knee through the sagittal plane while dorsiflexing their ankle. The tester can also move the patellae – they should move freely. Lack of mobility of the patellae in quiet standing indicates over-contraction of the quadriceps for stabilization.

- The tester gently attempts to rotate the pelvis around the lower extremity to see how easily the client can dissociate their pelvis from their hips.

Another postural assessment strategy that can be a useful tool for the trainer or therapist is repositioning the client's posture to determine their commitment to that posture and how effectively it changes the other postural issues (Lee 2008). For example, the therapist notes forward head posture, a depressed scapula on the right, lateral flexion through the thorax, a high right pelvis, internal rotation of the right hip, and a flattened longitudinal arch on the right foot. The therapist can help the client achieve a better foot position by re-establishing the foot tripod and seeing what effect that has on the rest of the postural alterations. If this adjustment corrects the majority of the postural faults, this is the likely place to enter the client's system and begin corrective exercise. If this process does not dramatically change or if it worsens the client's posture, the therapist moves to another region of the body and repeats the procedure.

POSTURAL ASSESSMENT

The goal in this section is not to describe all the nuances of ideal posture but rather to point out some of the key alignment landmarks and common postural faults that directly affect the hip and shoulder. This is not to suggest that other areas of the body do not have a direct effect on the hip and shoulder, but rather to point out the relationship between the shoulder, trunk, and hip complexes. See Video: Postural Assessment of the Spine and Pelvis, www.fitnesseducationseminars.com/osar-book

SPINE, THORAX, AND PELVIS

The spine and thorax should stack up vertically over the pelvis with the lower ribs in a relatively caudal position. There should be a gentle kyphotic curve in the thorax and gentle lordotic curves in the cervical and lumbar regions of the spine. The shoulders and pelvis should be level with no excessive unleveling, anterior or posterior rotation, or intra-pelvic rotation. The pubic symphysis should line up vertically with the anterior superior iliac spines. The neck should be long with the eyes level with the horizon (see images below).

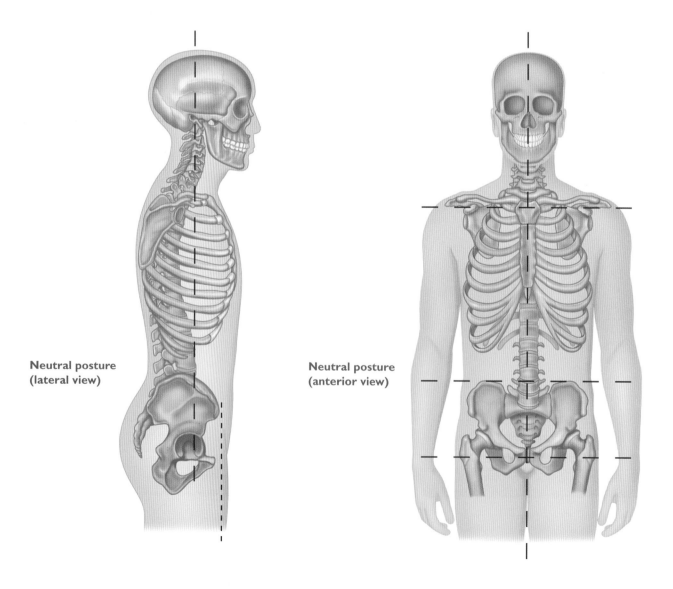

**Neutral posture
(lateral view)**

**Neutral posture
(anterior view)**

SCAPULA AND GLENOHUMERAL JOINT

The scapulae should be positioned approximately between the vertebral levels of T2–T7. The medial border should be relatively parallel to the spine and approximately two to three inches equidistant from it. If the inferior angle of the scapula can be palpated closer to the midline of the spine than the superior angle, the client is said to have downward rotation of the scapula. The scapulae should rest completely flush on the thorax. Flaring of the scapula is when the entire medial border moves away from the thorax, while scapular winging is when just the inferior angle of the scapula comes off the thoracic cage. The humerus should sit in the glenoid fossa, where approximately one-third of the humeral head can be palpated directly under the anterior aspect of the acromion process. If greater than one-third can be palpated, the individual is considered to have an anterior humeral head position. The shoulders should be in neutral alignment with no excessive internal or external rotation. Generally the elbow fossae should face forward and the palms of the hands should face the body in resting posture. The client is in internal rotation when the elbow fossae face towards the body and the palms face posteriorly. One way to assess if the shoulder and elbow alignment originates from poor scapular positioning or overactivity of the forearm pronators is to passively reposition the scapulae into a more ideal position and check the position of the elbow fossae and hands. If scapular repositioning changes the alignment of the shoulder and elbow, it is a scapular stabilization issue and the trainer or therapist can begin working on that. However, if this strategy does not change the position, it is a local problem of glenohumeral and elbow restriction and the client likely needs specific release strategies to the glenohumeral and elbow regions.

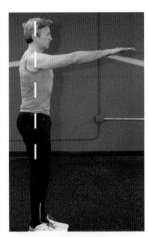

NEUTRAL ALIGNMENT OF THE THORAX AND SPINE

The individual in this alignment presents with neutral spinal curvatures in the thoracic and lumbar regions, even with 90 degrees of shoulder flexion. The head is stacked over the thorax and there is maintenance of the thoracopelvic canister.

JANDA'S UPPER AND LOWER CROSSED SYNDROME

This individual presents with the classic Upper and Lower Crossed Syndromes as described by Janda. There is an increased thoracic curvature (middle arrow) and forward head and shoulder position, as well as an increase in the lumbar lordosis (bottom arrow). Note the superior position of the humeral head (top arrow). This posture is more common in middle-aged individuals, those who have manual labor jobs, and people with over-developed muscles of the superficial stabilization system.

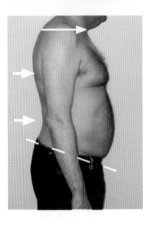

THORACIC LORDOSIS

The individual in the image to the right presents with a lordotic curve from the mid lumbar spine through the upper thoracic spine. This is a common posture in younger individuals and those who exercise regularly. It is common for fitness professionals and therapists to cue this posture into their clients by using verbal instructions such as "lift the chest" or "stand up tall." These individuals will also present with a forward head and shoulder position and often use thoracic extension as a strategy for improving this posture. While this may seem like good alignment, the increase in erector tone can lead to decreases in thoracic mobility and in the ability of these individuals to achieve ideal posterior diaphragm excursion.

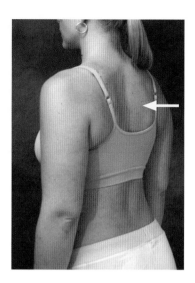

POSTERIOR PELVIC TILT

The individual in the image to the right presents with a posterior tilt of the pelvis and lower lumbar flexion. She is overactivating her abdominal wall, indicated by the sharp indentation at this location (image to right). Palpation over the lateral pelvis indicates a forward femoral head position and a hollowing of the lateral gluteal musculature. This is a common strategy that clients adopt, and one that trainers and therapists cue into their clients. These individuals must be taught to relax both their abdominal wall and 'spread' their hips or they will perpetuate their movement dysfunctions.

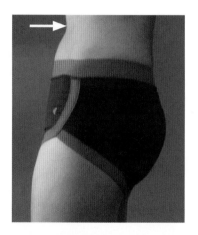

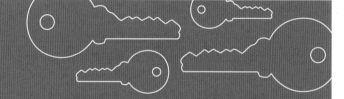

Key To Success
Posture and Avoidance Strategies

Postural alterations can cause decreases in movement efficiency and set up potentially damaging movement patterns. Faulty posture can be a result of muscle imbalances but can also perpetuate muscle imbalances. These imbalances can lead clients to avoid certain movements because of muscle inhibition or pain. These clients commonly do not even realize that they are avoiding a certain movement pattern because this has become their 'normal' strategy. It is not a question of *if* postural alterations can cause faulty biomechanics or tissue damage but rather *when*.

KEY: The goal of corrective exercise is to identify the client's stabilization as well as avoidance strategy, improve the 'weak' link, and re-establish ideal postural, stabilization, and movement patterns.

SINGLE LEG STANCE

PURPOSE: To evaluate the client's ability to balance as well as their stabilization strategy in single leg stance.

CLIENT: Standing with the arms at the sides and the legs together, preferably in bare or stocking feet.

TEST: The client lifts one leg to approximately 90 degrees, holds it for a second and puts it back on the floor, repeating the procedure on the other side. They can perform this several times to allow the tester to get a sense of their transition from leg to leg.

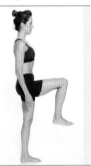

INTERPRETATION: The client should be able to lift their leg with minimal weight shift over the stance leg.

Hips and pelvis: The pelvis should remain level and centrated over the femur. Loss of frontal plane stabilization will result in the classic positive Trendelenburg's test. A client can compensate by laterally flexing their trunk over the stance leg (compensated Trendelenburg's). 'Butt-grippers' will drive the femoral head forward in the acetabulum as they attempt to stabilize their hip, creating a hollowing or divot behind their greater trochanter. The tester can palpate for this by placing their fingers lightly in front and their thumbs lightly behind the client's greater trochanter of the stance leg during the test. In the flexed hip, the tester can also determine the client's ability to dissociate their hip as they bring the hip into a flexed position. Internal rotation of the stance leg is another common sign of poor hip stabilization during the single leg stance.

The client's patella will tend to rotate medially when viewed from the front, and the patella fossa likewise rotates laterally when observed posteriorly. These clients will additionally demonstrate increased activity of the tensor fasciae latae and decreased activity in the posterior fibers of the gluteus medius during palpation of the stance leg. The tester may note hypertrophy of the tensor fasciae latae and atrophy in the gluteus medius upon palpation in the client with chronic knee or hip pain.

Spine: There should be an elongation of the spine and relatively little rotation of it as the hip is flexed. Excessive lumbar spine flexion or thoracolumbar extension in the sagittal plane or transverse plane rotation indicates loss of spinal stability.

Foot: The foot should remain in a relatively stable tripod position on the floor with no excessive toe gripping or excessive ankle wobble. Excessive toe gripping is considered a dysfunctional strategy.

GOOD MORNING

PURPOSE: To evaluate the client's ability to extend their thoracic spine and externally rotate their shoulders.

CLIENT: Standing with the head and spine flat against the wall, shoulders abducted to 90 degrees, and elbows flexed to 90 degrees.

TEST: The client maintains the spine position and externally rotates the shoulders. The tester monitors for the client's ability to maintain a long spine and rotate their shoulders, while noting any asymmetries in range of motion.

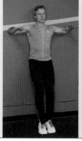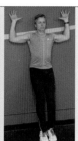

INTERPRETATION: The client should be able to maintain the spine against the wall while rotating the shoulders.

Head and spine: Many clients will be unable to achieve a flat spine against the wall. The goal is not to necessarily maintain the spine in a flat position against the wall, but rather to see where the client is unable to lengthen their spine. They may be in excessive forward head and suboccipital extension, increased thoracic flexion, and/or thoracolumbar hyperextension that prohibits them from achieving this position. The tester should cue them to see how adaptive that position of the spine is – if they can modify the position with cuing, that area is not the key driver. The key regions are those regions that the client is unable to be cued out of.

Shoulder: The goal is to get the scapula to posteriorly tilt and slide around the thorax to enable the client to reach a relatively flat forearm position against the wall. Rarely is a lack of external glenohumeral rotation the reason that a client is unable to achieve this position. Generally it is an inability to achieve enough thoracic extension in addition to their lack of ability to posteriorly tilt, depress, and abduct the scapula.

SEATED HIP FLEXION

PURPOSE: To evaluate the client's ability to flex their hip while stabilizing their spine in single hip support.

CLIENT: Sitting on the edge of the table with the legs hanging off the edge and the arms bent to 90 degrees.

TEST: The client lifts one leg off the table, holds it for a second, and puts it back on the table, repeating the procedure on the other side. They can perform this several times to allow the tester to get a sense of their transition from leg to leg.

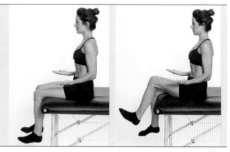

INTERPRETATION: The seated posture limits the lower legs in the evaluation of spinal stability. The client should be able to lift their leg with minimal weight shift over the stationary hip. They will tend to sway and/ or laterally flex their spine in the presence of poor hip flexion dissociation or stability in the stationary lumbopelvic-hip complex.

Spine: There should be an elongation of the spine and relatively little spinal rotation of it as they flex their hip. Excessive spine flexion in the sagittal plane, lateral trunk flexion, or transverse plane rotation indicates loss of spinal stability and/or poor hip dissociation.

SEATED SHOULDER FLEXION AND ABDUCTION

PURPOSE: To evaluate the client's ability to dissociate their glenohumeral joint and stabilize their scapulothoracic joint during flexion and abduction of the shoulder. To evaluate the mobility and stability in the upper thorax while making a bilateral comparison of range of motion.

CLIENT: Sitting on the edge of the table with the legs hanging off the edge and the arms straight.

TEST: The client lifts one arm straight overhead (flexion), holds it for a second, and puts it down, repeating the procedure on the other side. They perform this test both unilaterally and bilaterally. They repeat this test for abduction, performing both unilateral and bilateral versions.

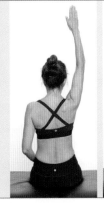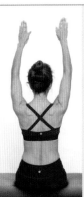

INTERPRETATION: The client should be able to lift their shoulder with minimal change in spinal or head position. Unilaterally, the spine should remain relatively straight during flexion and laterally flex slightly away from the side of the arm being lifted during abduction. The spine should extend slightly in the sagittal plane during both bilateral flexion and abduction. The motion should be fairly symmetrical on both sides. A difference in range of motion of 10 degrees or greater is considered significant.

Eccentric considerations: The client must be able to control their scapula eccentrically as they lower their arm. Therefore, it is particularly important to directly observe the scapula with the shirt off in males and with a sports bra in females. If the tester cannot see the scapulae they must palpate lightly around the medial and lateral borders of the scapula as the client goes through the motion. Lower scapular angle prominence and a rapid, uncoordinated descent of the scapula as the client lowers their arm are common signs of poor scapular control.

THORAX: POSITION, MOBILITY, AND RESPIRATION

PURPOSE: To determine the position and mobility of the client's thorax, in addition to their respiratory patterns. These assessments will help dictate both the client's stabilization and respiratory strategies.

CLIENT: Lying supine on the table with the legs straight and the arms at the sides.

TEST: The tester first observes the position of the thorax and the client's resting respiratory strategy. Then the client is asked to take a maximum inhalation and exhalation, during which the client's strategy is again observed. Finally the tester performs the rib cage mobility test by placing their hands on the client's rib cage and gently rocking it side to side along its length.

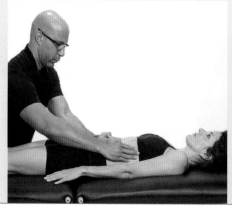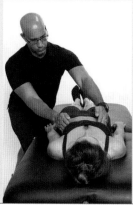

INTERPRETATION: Thorax: The rib cage should lie symmetrically flat on the table, with gentle lordotic curves noted in the cervical and lumbar spines and a gentle kyphosis in the thoracic spine. During the rib cage mobility test, the thorax should be pliable and demonstrate relatively equal mobility side to side. The lack of ease in the mobility test indicates rigidity, either secondary to global stiffness from a 'gripping' strategy or global lack of joint mobility in the thorax. This is common in individuals with chronic back pain, weight lifters, smokers, and those with asthma, allergies, and similar chronic respiratory disorders who develop relatively wide and immobile thoraxes. The client can also be tested for a diastasis recti by having them perform a mini-crunch and either noting midline distension or palpating a gap within the two sides of the rectus abdominis muscles. While common in partum and post-partum women, it is also found in many overweight males due to widening of the lower costosternal angle as well as an overutilization of a poor intra-abdominal stabilization strategy.

Respiration: During respiration, there should be three-dimensional breathing, meaning the ribs should move superior to inferior, laterally, and anterior to posterior. The presence of upper airway and abdominal breathing with the lack of rib cage motion are common signs of respiratory dysfunction. These individuals will also generally demonstrate hypertrophy of the scalenes and sternocleidomastoid as they tend to overuse their accessory muscles of respiration. They will present with forward head posture and suboccipital extension because they are overutilizing the neck muscles both for respiration and for elevation of the thorax. This strategy also leads to the increased rib cage angle and flaring of the lower ribs.

Shoulder: The shoulders will rest off the table due to shortness of the pectoralis minor as a result of its' overuse as an accessory muscle of respiration. Chronic use of this strategy will lead to the pectoralis minor pulling the scapula up and over the thorax and result in scapular winging.

INTERNAL RANGE OF MOTION: SHOULDERS AND HIPS

PURPOSE: To. evaluate the client's ability to dissociate their glenohumeral and femoroacetabular joints and compare side-to-side range of motion.

CLIENT: Lying supine on the table with the arms and legs straight.

TEST: Shoulders: The client abducts the shoulder to 90 degrees and flexes the elbow to 90 degrees position. The client actively rotates the shoulder, repeating the procedure on both sides. The tester can guide the arm lightly to ensure pure axial rotation. The tester then passively rotates the client's shoulder internally, palpating over the anterior and posterior aspects of the humeral head, noting the range of motion and whether or not the client maintains a pure axis of rotation. The client's range of motion and glenohumeral control side to side is then compared. External rotation can be checked as well.

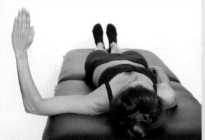 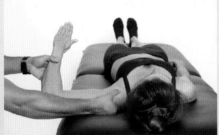

Hips: The client actively internally rotates the hips one at a time and the tester notes the range of motion bilaterally. The tester stands facing the client and grasps the client's ankle just above the malleoli and passively internally rotates the hip (images right). This is repeated on the other side, comparing both the range and relative end-feel of the movement. External rotation can be checked as well.

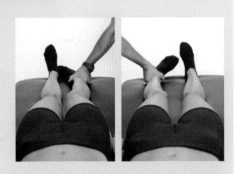

INTERPRETATION: The client should be able to maintain an ideal axis of rotation and demonstrate relatively symmetrical range of motion. A 10 degrees or greater difference in range of motion is considered significant.

Shoulders: It is common to see the humerus glide anteriorly in both the active and passive phases of the exercise in the presence of a stiff posterior joint capsule and/or shortness of the external rotators (teres minor and infraspinatus). In these cases, the tester actively reseats the humeral head in the glenoid fossa and repeats the test. Generally, there is a significant restriction in the available range of motion and the asymmetries become more apparent.

Hips: The client with internal hip restriction may flex the knee and/or rotate the pelvis in the presence of limited hip rotation.

ANKLE RANGE OF MOTION

PURPOSE: To evaluate the client's available range of ankle motion while making a bilateral comparison of their range of motion.

CLIENT: Lying supine on the table with the legs straight.

TEST: The client actively inverts and dorsiflexes one ankle and repeats on the other side (left and centre images). The tester then passively inverts and dorsiflexes the client's ankle to their end range, comparing the range of motion to the individual's active range as well as between left and right ankles (right image).

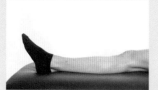 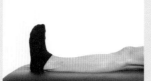 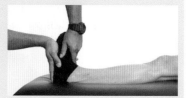

INTERPRETATION: The client should be able to achieve a minimum of 10 degrees of ankle dorsiflexion, which is required for uncompensated gait (Michaud 1997). The tester compares bilateral ranges of motion and notes whether the restricted side has an end-feel that is either stiff and abrupt or elastic. A stiff, abrupt end-feel generally indicates a joint fixation, whereas an elastic end-feel is usually the result of posterior compartment stiffness. The former requires joint mobilization by a chiropractic physician, osteopathic physician or physiotherapist, while the latter will respond to a direct soft-tissue release strategy. Decreased ankle dorsiflexion is a common cause of compensatory motion at the knee and/or foot.

Key To Success
Muscle Testing and the Muscle Chains

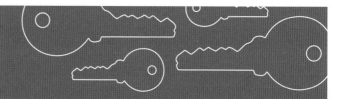

Muscles, fascia, and ligaments are intimately connected, forming chains throughout the human body. Just as a chain is only as strong as its weakest link, these tissue chains are only as strong as their weakest link. The value of muscle testing is that individual 'weak' or inhibited links in the chain can be discovered through specific muscle testing.

KEY: Muscle testing should be included as a valuable component of the assessment process.

PUSH-UP

PURPOSE: To evaluate the client's ability to stabilize their thoracopelvic canister, in addition to loading, centrating, and dissociating the shoulder complex.

CLIENT: Assuming a push-up position on the floor. Can be modified to the side of a table or a wall for clients who do not possess the strength or stability to get down on the floor.

TEST: The client performs a push-up, lowering themselves to the floor and pushing back to the starting position. If one push-up is performed well, the client performs a set of 3–10 repetitions (depending upon their ability) to determine how many can be performed before losing form. Indicate at what number and where the client breaks down.

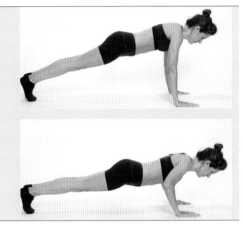

INTERPRETATION: The client should be able to maintain a stable spine and scapulae throughout the pattern.

Head and spine: The client will protract their head and/or go into suboccipital extension during the test, indicating possible loss of deep stabilization by longus capitis and colli.

Trunk and spine: The client can hyperextend through the thoracolumbar junction and flex through the thoracic and/or lumbar regions of the spine indicating that they have lost intrinsic ability to stabilize the thoracopelvic canister.

Scapulae: The scapulae should remain flush with the thorax during the pattern. They should adduct slightly during the eccentric or lowering phase and abduct slightly during the concentric or lifting phase of the test. Excessive scapular adduction during the eccentric phase, or abduction during the concentric phase, accompanied by winging, flaring, or downward rotation during any part of the test is an indication of poor scapular stability.

Hips and legs: Hip flexion and/or knee flexion can indicate tightness in these areas but are also signs of poor thoracopelvic stabilization.

FUNCTIONAL MUSCLE TESTING

"Virtually every condition … involves some form of muscle dysfunction and inhibition. MMT (manual muscle testing), when properly taught and executed, gives practitioners the unique ability to diagnose these problems." (Cuthbert 2009)

Functional muscle testing (FMT) can be utilized as an important evaluation tool in developing a corrective exercise, training, or therapeutic strategy. While it is beyond the scope of this book to discuss all the nuances or the multitude of manual muscle testing (MMT), its use as an evaluation tool is unparalleled. While some question the validity, accuracy, and usefulness of muscle testing, if performed properly, precision MMT can give the tester valuable information about the function of the nervous system and integrity of the clients stabilization system.

Many readers are familiar with traditional MMT, which is taught in medical, chiropractic, and physical therapy schools. Manual muscle testing as part of a functional assessment is demonstrated in the acclaimed book *Muscles: Testing and Function, Fifth Edition* by Kendall, McCreary, Provance, Rodgers, and Romani, 2005. This type of MMT tests the specific strength of a muscle to an applied force.

MMT was later expanded upon by George Goodheart through its use in Applied Kinesiology. Rather than testing the overall strength of a muscle, Dr. Goodheart used what would later be termed 'muscle testing as functional neurology' as an evaluation of how efficiently the nervous system was in controlling the muscle system (Walther 2000). This system of muscle testing did not test for strength or weakness but rather how the muscle reacted to an applied force.

"In most cases, the results of a test do not depend on whether or not the muscle is strong or weak, but how the nervous system controls the muscle." (Walther 2000)

A student of Goodheart, the late Alan Beardall, DC, would expand on the use of MMT and was the first to demonstrate over three hundred muscle tests, one for each specific division of a muscle (Beardall 1982). Believing muscles were the display units of the body (Buhler 2004), Beardall demonstrated that, even in the presence of a strong manual muscle test, a muscle could test weak if each individual muscle division was tested individually. He went on to develop a system of evaluation and correction of this muscle inhibition that eventually formed the basis of Clinical Kinesiology.

Additionally, Beardall pioneered testing each muscle division in its respective shortened position or positions that best approximated the origin and insertion. It was his opinion that the muscle mechanoreceptors were the most sensitive in the lengthened position and the least sensitive in the shortened position (Buhler 2004). He therefore created a series of specific muscle tests to examine each individual muscle division in its respective shortened position. Several of Goodheart's and Beardall's muscle testing concepts can be found in FMT – specifically, the use of the shortened muscle position, the two-second consistent resistance rather than steadily increasing resistance that is applied to the muscle, and the interpretation of a strong, intact muscle versus a weak, inhibited muscle.

PURPOSE OF FMT

FMT evaluates the functional ability of the nervous system to react to an applied force. In other words, it is testing the reaction of the nervous system to an imposed demand. A force is applied to a specific joint position and the response of the nervous system is noted. The principle behind FMT is that if the neuromusculofascial system (NMS) cannot demonstrate adequate stabilization strength in the controlled test positions, it will be forced to utilize substitution and compensatory strategies when asked to perform functional movement patterns. As mentioned, in addition to a thorough history and movement screen, FMT can help formulate a very consistent evaluation of a client's overall nervous system function.

FMT can be performed as part of, as well as before and after, a training or therapy session. Generally speaking, if a client presents to a training or therapy session and passes all three muscle tests (see muscle test section below), they are generally considered to be in a good position to be progressed in that session. However, if the client presents with overall instability or pain in one or more of these tests, further loading with functional exercise is likely to overload their neuromusculofascial system. They will require some type of activation strategy (see later section on activation strategies) before they are progressed to functional exercise. It is important to note that an optimal corrective exercise, training, or therapy session should never cause a previously tested strong muscle to subsequently test weak.

At the end of the session, FMT is performed to ensure that the corrective exercise, training program, or therapy session had its intended response, namely an improvement of function. If the client remains strong, it is likely that they have responded well to the stimuli of that session. However, if the client tests weak after the session, it is possible that either the training or the corrective strategy was incorrect or that the load was too great for the current state of their NMS, causing inhibition. Testing weak after previously testing strong is an indication that the NMS did not accept the intervention in a positive way. In these cases, the trainer of therapist must reassess first the type of intervention that was utilized (were the exercises too intense, did they cause the client to fatigue, were they the right exercises, etc.) and next, the type of strategy the client was using to perform the exercises (were they breathing correctly, were they able to maintain optimal joint centration during the corrective exercises, did they stop the exercises once they were unable to maintain ideal breathing and joint centration, etc.). The previous considerations are very important factors to consider, especially during the rehabilitative and corrective exercise phases of a program, and muscle testing can help formulate the answers to those questions when performed before and after the client performs the exercise.

FUNCTIONAL STRENGTH AND FUNCTIONAL STABILITY

The terms 'weak' and 'strong' are often used to determine the results of a muscle test and are appropriate for traditional MMT. However, FMT does not evaluate muscle strength but rather the ability of the nervous system to hold a determined test position. In other words, FMT tests stability rather than strength. Therefore, a 'strong' test will indicate the nervous system can generate optimal stability, whereas a 'weak' test will indicate muscle inhibition of that particular muscle and/or instability of the stabilizing joint. For example, inhibition of the supraspinatus allows the humeral head to rise superiorly during shoulder abduction, which decreases the ability to generate adequate force, causing a weakness in the shoulder abduction test because the humeral head does not remain centrated in the glenoid fossa.

Similarly, cervical spine instability can create a weak muscle test because the nervous system will be protecting the cervical spine from the force that is being driven into it through the shoulder. One way to differentiate between these two scenarios is to perform a cervical spine distraction technique. This can be any combination of light traction, spinal manipulation, and breathing, and/or having the client visualize lengthening their neck and relaxing the upper shoulder and neck tightness, based upon the therapist's or trainer's scope of practice and knowledge of the technique. The shoulder abduction test is then repeated and if it improves the client's ability to hold the test, it is likely a proximal spinal stabilization issue. If the client is still unable to hold the test position, it is possibly a more localized shoulder problem that requires further testing to determine the dysfunction. This procedure can be utilized in the trunk with the lateral trunk flexion test and in the lower extremity with the hip abduction test. The important thing to note is that muscles can often test weak in the presence of proximal instabilities. In other words, inability to breathe correctly and stabilize the TPC can lead to inhibition of the extremities, which is another reason why FMT can be a valuable part of the assessment process.

SUBSTITUTION PATTERNS
The additional benefit of muscle testing is that it allows the trainer or therapist to detect substitution patterns. It is common to have a client who cannot maintain stability during a particular movement pattern and for whom cuing does not help to correct their position. Take, for example, the client who cannot maintain the squared pelvis position during a split squat pattern. The trainer or therapist attempts to verbally and kinesthetically cue the client, which provides no change to the client's ability to maintain the correct alignment. Testing the muscles that help maintain the squared pelvis, mainly the hip rotators and abductors, can help the trainer or therapist look for the test positions that the client has a hard time getting into and/or maintaining, as these will likely be the regions contributing to the movement dysfunction.

Common substitution patterns include global rigidity and bracing, bending of the neck, overextension or flexion of the spine, and abdominal hollowing.

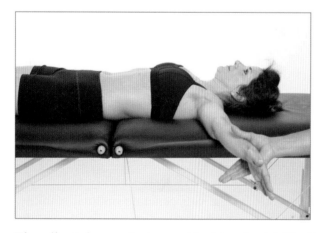 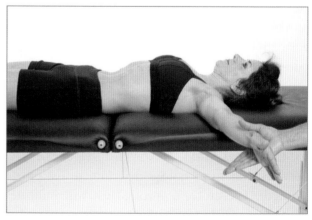

The client demonstrates an ideal trunk stabilization pattern during the upper extremity muscle test; notice how an inferior position of the rib cage is maintained (left image). Note the abdominal hollowing and elevation of the rib cage, indicating poor trunk stabilization pattern, to an applied force (right image).

RESISTANCE

As mentioned above, FMT is testing the reaction of the nervous system, not the overall strength of the muscle. Therefore, the trainer or therapist will apply a direct and steady pressure to the muscles and not attempt to overpower the client. The client applies a perpendicular force to the testing limb or trunk in an even, steady manner. The trainer or therapist applies a force to match the client's resistance for two seconds (counting 'one-one thousand, two-one thousand') and then relaxes their force. The client should be able to maintain the test position against the resistance with no change in position. If they are unable to hold the test position, they can be given up to three attempts. Any further attempts will likely fatigue the client, producing inaccurate results.

GRADING

FMT is graded on a pass/fail scale. It is considered a 'passed' or 'strong' test if the client maintains the test position for two seconds with no alterations in the test position. It is considered a 'failed' or 'inhibited' test if the client cannot achieve or maintain the test position or if there are compensatory movements of the limbs or trunk. Pain during the test is always considered a failed test. If the client fails the test, further testing on that region should be administered to determine the causative factors.

CLIENT POSITION

The client lies supine on the table to help ensure stabilization as well as to diminish the contribution of poor proximal stability to the test. For example, the hip abductors can be tested with the client lying on their side. However, the individual has to hold the weight of their leg against gravity as well as stabilize the lumbar spine and sacroiliac joints. Proximal joint instability in either the lumbar spine or the pelvis can contribute to distal (hip abductor) weakness even in the presence of strong hip abductors. The supine lying position diminishes some of these proximal stability issues so the test more accurately monitors the intended muscles.

THE MUSCLE TESTS

While there are any number of specific muscle tests that can be used, FMT of hip and shoulder abduction as well as lateral trunk flexion will be utilized to provide a general impression of an individual's overall hip and shoulder strength as well as trunk stabilization patterns. Group muscle tests will be carried out in lieu of individual muscle testing as part of the general assessment. While some may question the validity of this approach over isolated muscle tests, Beardall (1982) noted "group muscles represent a consensus of opinion of an area of the body." These tests are therefore used as a representative of an area of the body. If dysfunction is observed, then further attention and assessment is warranted for that area of the body. If it is clear of dysfunction, the trainer or therapist will move on to another region of the body, always rechecking these three regions at the end of any corrective session.

Shoulder abduction is used to test the influence of the neck on the upper limb as well as for looking at the client's trunk and neck stabilization strategy to an imposed resistance on the upper extremity. Hip abduction is used to test the influence of the lumbar spine on the lower extremity as well as trunk stabilization during imposed resistances on the lower extremity. Lateral trunk flexion is used to determine lateral trunk stability and stabilization strategies during direct resistance applied to the trunk. While these three muscle tests have been chosen for their sensitivity (as an expression of a client's general functional stability) and ease of performance, this is not to suggest that other muscle tests cannot be used and produce similar results. It should be noted that these tests are not testing specific muscles but, more accurately, how the nervous system is reacting to the imposed demand.

SHOULDER ABDUCTION

Prime muscles being tested: upper and lower trapezius, serratus anterior, middle deltoid.

Synergists: Subclavius, supraspinatus, clavicular fibers of pectoralis major, cervical and thoracic spine stabilizers.

Procedure: The client lies supine on the table with one arm abducted to 135 degrees and in a neutral position – the palm should be facing away from the head and the elbow remains straight throughout the test. The tester grasps the arm just proximal to the wrist so the tester's forearm is perpendicular

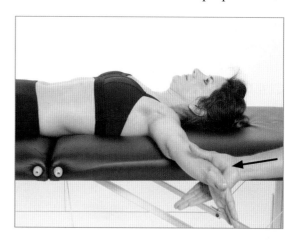

the client's upper arm. The client is instructed both in the direction of the applied force and as to the start of the test. The tester applies a two-second force, attempting to adduct the arm through the frontal plane of the body. The force is steady and not intended to overpower the client.

A passed test is one in which the client resists the force and there is no change in upper extremity or trunk position. It is a failed test if the client cannot maintain the test position of the upper extremity or stabilize the trunk, or if there is pain during the test.

HIP ABDUCTION

Prime muscles being tested: gluteus medius, tensor fasciae latae, upper fibers of gluteus maximus.

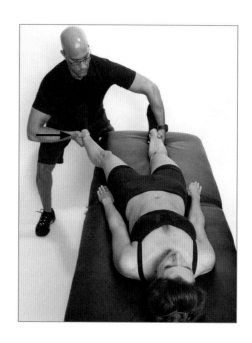

Synergists: gluteus minimus, lumbar and thoracic stabilizers.

Procedure: The client lies supine on the table with one hip abducted to 20 degrees. The hip is neutral, with no rotation, and the knee remains straight throughout the test. The tester contacts the ankle above the lateral malleolus so the tester's forearm is perpendicular to the client's lower leg. The tester's opposite arm braces the client's contralateral leg. The client is instructed both in the direction of applied force and as to the start of the test. The tester applies a two-second force, attempting to adduct the leg through the frontal plane of the body. The force is steady and is not intended to overpower the client.

A passed test is one in which the client resists the force and there is no change in lower extremity or trunk position. A failed test is one in which the client cannot maintain the test position of the lower extremity or stabilize the trunk, or if there is pain during the test.

LATERAL TRUNK FLEXION

Prime muscles being tested: quadratus lumborum, lumbar erector spinae, oblique abdominals.

Synergists: thoracic erector spinae, trunk stabilizers.

Procedure: The client lies supine on the table with the legs together and the knees straight. The tester stands on the opposite side that is being tested and positions the clients legs so that the lumbar spine is in 20 degrees of lateral flexion. The client grasps the edges of the table to stabilize the upper aspect of the trunk. The tester grasps underneath the client's ankles with the forearm perpendicular to the client's legs and places the other palm over the client's ipsilateral pelvis. The client is instructed both in the direction of the applied force and as to the start of the test. The tester applies a two-second force, attempting to laterally flex the lumbar spine through the frontal plane of the body.

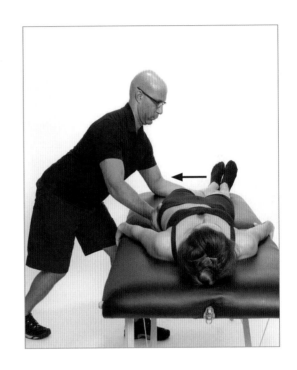

A passed test is one in which the client resists the force and there is no change in trunk position. It is a failed test if the client cannot maintain the test position or if there is pain during the test.

MUSCLE TESTING RESULTS

Assessing the results of muscle testing will aid the direction of the corrective strategy. If weakness or inhibition is noted in any of the muscle tests, begin with the corrective breathing and core activation strategy and then retest. The reason for this is simple – in the absence of proximal stability, the client will be unable to generate optimal distal force through the extremities. If this strategy improves the results of the previously weak muscle test, then proceed with an appropriate corrective exercise or conditioning program. If this strategy fails to show an improvement in the muscle tests, then a more specific activation strategy – such as the use of visualizations, isometric positioning, joint approximation, or origin-insertion palpations – will usually be required to restore stabilization to the appropriate regions. These approaches will be discussed in the corrective exercise section of the book.

Additional muscle testing can be useful in supplementing the information gained through the general FMT scan. For further information about manual muscle testing, specifically neurologically based manual muscle testing, readers are encouraged to review the work of Goodheart, Beardall, Frost, Thie, and Walther.

EVALUATING THE RESULTS OF THE ASSESSMENT

The results of the assessment will dictate the direction of the corrective exercise approach. While the goal of the assessment is to identify the biggest areas of dysfunction and improve them with some sense of accuracy, unfortunately it is not an exact science no matter what some experts may claim. Decision-making based upon the client's assessment should be systematic and performed with a reasonable degree of educated thought process. However, unlike the exactness of a field such as mathematics, the human body is highly variable, so interpreting the results of an assessment can sometimes feel as complicated as reading a language one is not familiar with. This likely explains some of the reasons why there are many clients who have failed in traditional physical therapy, chiropractic, surgical, and medication interventions despite going through a thorough assessment and an appropriate and reasonable treatment plan. The goal, however, of the evaluation process is specificity in testing and assessment of the tests, as well as in the application of the corrective exercise strategy and training program, so that there is the best chance of providing sustainable and repeatable results.

The general rule of thumb in interpreting the results of the assessment is to address the biggest problem area, that is the region with the greatest dysfunction. Since optimal breathing drives and precedes all function, this is the area that will always be addressed first if it is found to be dysfunctional. Once breathing has been normalized, if the client failed any of the functional muscles tests, these should be reassessed. Restoring optimal breathing and activation of the thoracopelvic canister will often correct proximal stabilization issues of the trunk, hip, and shoulder complex, resulting in a stronger MMT test. The next step will be to identify the region(s) with the greatest instability or asymmetry in range of motion as this is where the client is demonstrating poor motor control and/or overcompensation. Where the trainer or therapist chooses to start in the presence of multiple regions of dysfunction will be determined by their level of experience, choice of modalities (expertise in soft-tissue release, manipulation techniques, activation strategies), and clinical intuition, otherwise known as the art of the profession. There is nothing wrong with choosing one area of dysfunction and finding it does not significantly alter the client's movement and/or stabilization strategy. Make a decision, follow it through, and reassess constantly. If the dysfunctional pattern or strategy does not change in a short period of time (relative to the client and the level of function or dysfunction), then simply choose another area of dysfunction and approach that area.

CONCLUSION

A thorough assessment arms the trainer and therapist with a guide, similar to the way a road map is used to navigate one's way across a network of highways. Careful interpretation of the information gained during the assessment will help direct the trainer or therapist to the causative factors of the movement dysfunction without having to solely rely on a client's subjective complaints. While empirical evidence is the best place to start when assessing and directing a client's corrective exercise or training strategy, the trainer or therapist is encouraged to listen to their intuition as well as rely on their past clinical experiences. The last two will serve him or her well as he or she develops a strategy to marry the client's individual goals with their functional requirements.

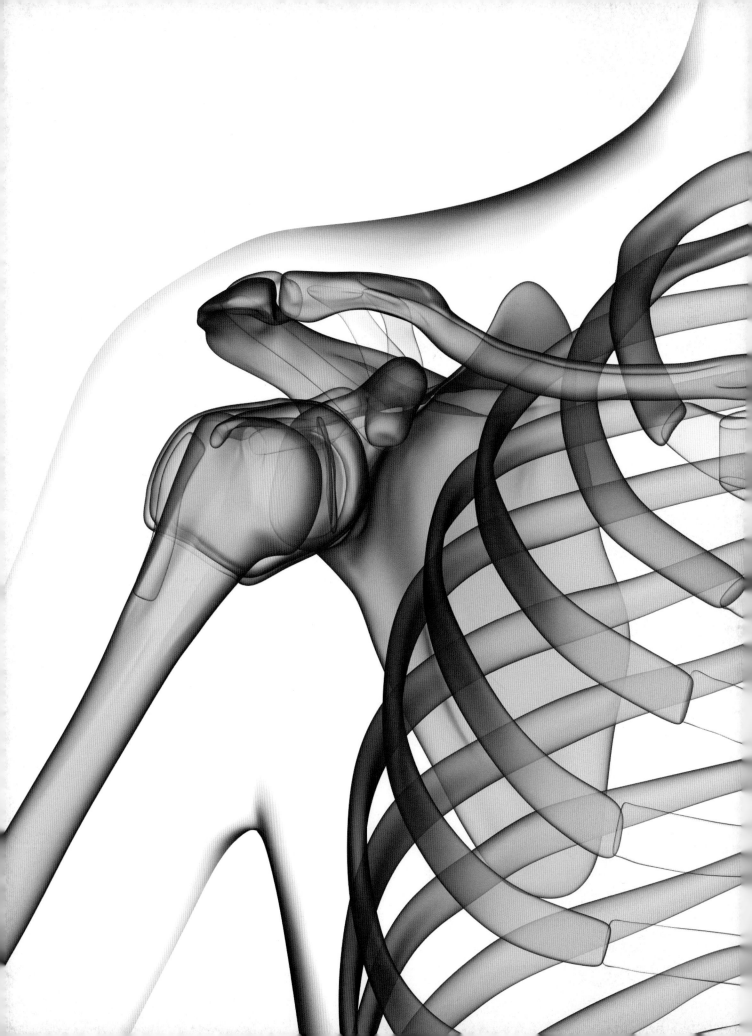

part III

Corrective Movement and Exercise Progressions: The Functional Elements

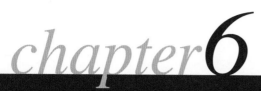

Developing the Corrective Exercise and Movement Paradigm

CHAPTER OBJECTIVES

To identify and understand the functional components of the corrective exercise and movement paradigm

To identify the key regions necessary for improving function

To develop the specific strategies for corrective exercise and fundamental movement patterns

CORRECTIVE EXERCISE

The key to improving movement patterns lies in establishing ideal alignment, activating appropriate myofascial linkages, and maintaining joint centration during functional movement patterns. These factors allow for optimal length-tension relationships between myofascial synergists, enabling the perpetuation of efficient movement patterns while reducing stress on articular structures. Recall that the most common causes of musculoskeletal pain are habitual movement patterns and clients and patients don't necessarily understand what constitutes correct movement. In other words, they only know what they know and don't know what they don't know regarding movement. The goal of corrective exercise is to help them identify their faulty patterns and to give them the best strategy for improving activation of the ideal myofascial connections while maintaining centrated joint positions and performing efficient movement patterns.

The three key areas for initial correction of faulty shoulder and hip movements are the spine, the thorax, and the foot. The reader may notice that neither the actual hip (femoroacetabular) nor the shoulder (glenohumeral) were mentioned and may wonder about their intrinsic contribution to shoulder and hip dysfunction. To answer that, it would be helpful to look at the body as a building consisting of a series of interconnected blocks, with the spine, thorax, and pelvis as the base of the building and the feet as the anchors. While this analogy may seem simplistic, the human body is at the mercy of the same gravitational pull and biomechanical forces as the building.

However, unlike the building, the human body has the ability to compensate for structural changes. A change in the foot stabilization can cause a compensatory change at the suboccipital junction as the body attempts to equal forces around the spine and maintain the eyes level with the horizon. More importantly, as this previous example of the righting reflex illustrates, the human body reacts to reflexive patterns of activation, that govern function that don't always work in a parallel or segmental manner, as compared to a static structure such as a building.

For example, during the gait cycle, the spreading of the metatarsals and stretching of the interossei muscles of the feet cause a reflexive extension of the posterior chain, which creates extension of the lower extremity and trunk during the midstance phase of gait (Michaud 1997). Trainers and therapists can enhance this reflex by focusing the clients' attention on their posture and by performing specific foot exercises in clients and patients with poor hip and thoracic extension. Conversely, clients can dampen this reflex by cramming their feet into shoes with small toe boxes, such as high heels, causing a diminished extensor reflex and potentially diminished extension of the spine and lower extremity upon lower extremity loading. This can lead to a client adopting compensatory postures and patterns of movement such as thoracolumbar junction hyperextension to help improve their stability during the midstance phase of gait.

So what does all this mean in regard to shoulder and hip correction? These examples suggest that when adopting corrective exercise strategies, the trainer and therapist must stabilize proximal neuro feedback structures, such as the feet, thorax, and spine, prior to changing the more proximal hip and shoulder structures.

The strategy adopted will include:

- stabilization of the spine to ensure ideal neurological feedback from the central nervous through the peripheral nervous system;

- stabilization of the thoracopelvic canister to ensure proper diaphragmatic breathing, development of intra-abdominal pressure and ideal extremity function;

- stabilization of the foot to ensure proper support of the lower extremity and to ensure reflexive feedback for optimal extensor chain function.

Collectively, the thorax, spine, and the feet represent three of the biggest drivers of movement dysfunction and are the more common regions of breakdown in function. Unfortunately, they also tend to be the areas on which trainers, coaches, and therapists generally spend the least amount of time, especially with clients who have specific goals such as improving athletic performance or losing weight. In these individuals, specificity of maintaining optimal curvatures and alignment, diaphragmatic breathing, and foot position take a backseat to increasing the exercise resistance, intensity, and tempo of the workout routine. When working with the general population client, the corrective approach must include the improvement of awareness both of current and ideal movement patterns, synergistic co-activation of the functional antagonists achieve ideal joint centration, and the performance of integrated movement patterns that will help the client achieve their ultimate goal.

COMMON PROBLEMS WITH THE CURRENT TRAINING PARADIGM

Before getting into the specifics about the corrective exercise training paradigm, it will be helpful to recap some of the common problems with the current training paradigm that are currently being perpetuated within the health and fitness industry. While these have been discussed earlier, there are three general problem areas: overtraining, training tonic muscles phasically, and linear training progressions.

1. **Overtraining:** Overtraining is one of the biggest problems that affects clients with movement dysfunctions who begin exercise programs. Overtraining goes hand in hand with improper rest and recuperation, as most clients who are overtrained fail to see, or their trainer/coach fails to see, the importance of this aspect of a training program. The reason for this is simple – trainers and coaches are under the impression that since athletes can perform at a high level and push their bodies very far, then so too should Mr. and Mrs. Joe Client. And if the training is not causing fatigue, sweat, or discomfort, it is deemed not a good training session. However, the trainer and/or the client fail to realize that, generally speaking, the athlete a) has superior genetics which is why they are a professional athlete in the first place and can tolerate a lot more stress and develop better compensatory strategies; b) does not live a normal life, have to go to a stressful job (although there is a great deal of stress associated with maintaining a high level of performance), work late hours, or fail get enough sleep worrying about their early morning meeting the next day; c) has daily access to professionals such as chiropractors, massage therapists, and athletic trainers to help them manage their dysfunction; d) sleeps longer every night and/or takes naps; and e) eats a healthier diet. Overtraining is one of the leading causes of dysfunction because it is precursory to pain and fatigue, which are two of the more common causes of dysfunctional movement patterns and move clients further away from developing ideal strategies.

2. **Training tonic muscles phasically:** Conventional training that focuses on improved efficiency and control of movement has been replaced with a strategy that encourages bigger, faster, and stronger. Unfortunately, while this training has produced bigger, faster, and stronger individuals, it has also ushered in an era of greater dysfunction in many of these individuals. High level training focusing on faster speed and heavier resistance preferentially recruits the phasic or two-joint muscles over the one-joint stabilizers. In the short term, the individual gets bigger and stronger; however, in the long term, the individual sacrifices joint and postural stability. This 'go hard or go home' approach turns many of the tonic muscles, especially the transversus abdominis, diaphragm, rotator cuff and other muscles of the deep stabilization system, into phasic-acting muscles. This translates into a loss of joint centration and global rigidity as the two-joint muscles increase their stabilization action and functionally lock down the body, affecting both local stabilization and respiration.

3. **Linear training progressions:** With more clients turning to the internet, magazines, and related sources for semi-personalized training programs, there is a greater propensity for these individuals to adopt high-intensity type training programs. However, all clients don't improve in a linear fashion. Work or family obligations, lack of sleep, missed workouts, current movement dysfunctions, or improper nutrition can all determine the progress that a client will make during a training program. The client may not be progressing in a linear fashion in relationship to the progression of their workout. Having these clients perpetually perform higher levels of exercise

will lead to a greater likelihood of developing movement dysfunction. Generally speaking, rather than designing training programs in a progressively more challenging manner, they should be designed in a non-linear progression, meaning that the resistance, movement progressions, and intensity should be increased relative to the client's advancing stability, strength, ability to recuperate and aptitude in performing fundamental movement patterns.

Understanding a few of the biggest problems with the current training methodologies will help lay the groundwork for the next section, which will focus on the new paradigm of training and the corrective exercise strategy.

THE TEN PARAMETERS OF THE NEW MOVEMENT PARADIGM

"... experiences where you're forced to slow down, make errors, and correct them ... end up making you swift and graceful without you realizing it." (Daniel Coyle, *The Talent Code* 2009)

What follows are the ten parameters of the new movement paradigm. However, this is not to suggest that this is novel or new but it does imply that there should be attention placed upon the included criteria when developing a corrective exercise and conditioning program.

1. **Treat every individual as an individual:** There is a trend in the training industry to place every client in a box and treat every client as if they present with the same problems. While there are many similarities in dysfunction and etiologies, each client will present with their own unique stereotypes, adaptations, and compensations for their specific movement dysfunction. Applying one method to every single client will only work with those clients who have an issue that the particular method addresses. Understanding and improving the principles of human function enables the trainer or therapist to address any client's needs and adapt their approach to help the client reach their specific functional goals.

2. **Focus on movement awareness:** Movement awareness should be the focus of the entire corrective exercise approach. Too many trainers and conditioning specialists operate under the premise that their clients are 'weak' and therefore must be strengthened. So in response to this thought process, they load their clients up, subjecting them to higher and higher loads, performing movements in progressively more challenging and less stable environments. All this does is exacerbate the movement dysfunction because the client is forced to use the strong muscle patterns he or she already knows how to access. And to make matters worse, these types of training protocols take the client further and further away from being aware of their movement because all they can focus on is their level of fatigue, muscular discomfort, and getting through the exercise. The goal of corrective exercise must be to slow the client down, to restore their consciousness of their body, and to introduce them to what correct movement looks and feels like.

3. **Educate the client on their movement strategy:** Educating the client on their movement strategy begins with developing awareness. Awareness develops the client's proprioceptive and therefore kinesthetic attention to their current movement patterns. Education helps them develop a deeper understanding of the why and how of improving these patterns. Although the client may not understand the anatomy, biomechanics, or kinesiological principles behind their movement,

education offers them the opportunity to familiarize themselves with the components of optimal function. Too often clients are talked down to and leave their decisions to the more knowledgeable medical professional. Education aids the client's training experience by respecting them as a partner in the process as well as assists their compliance to a corrective exercise strategy because they better understand the process. An educated client is the corrective exercise specialist's best client.

4. **Maximize central nervous system function and educate the brain:** Incorporate more brain activity by educating the client in both movement awareness and their movement strategies. Address the patterns that most directly affect the central nervous system, including respiration, conscious attention and body awareness, and proximal stabilization, as well as addressing central nervous system stressors, such as up-regulation of the sympathetic nervous system and fatigue.

5. **Quality over quantity:** The quality of the movement must always be stressed in corrective exercise. To reiterate, the problem with the majority of the conditioning programs that are recommended by the training 'experts' is that they are too intense and focus on the quantity of work being performed, that is the number of repetitions, amount of weight, and number of exercises performed in a given session. It is virtually impossible to focus on movement quality or awareness when fatigue and discomfort consume the central nervous system's attention. Quality of motion should always be the prerequisite to improving function. And for most general population and post-rehabilitation clients, quality will be exponentially more valuable than quantity.

6. **Movements must first be performed at a slow to moderate pace:** Improved speed of performance is the goal of many training programs, which is fine if the client is an athlete or is ready to be progressed. For the general population client and those requiring to improve their dysfunctional movement patterns, the corrective movements must be initially performed at a slow pace and then progressed to a moderate pace as the client gains competence and control of the pattern. Higher execution speeds during an exercise require that the brain pay less attention to form and more attention to the speed of the movement. Therefore, slow the client down and make them aware of how, where, and why they should be adopting a specific movement strategy.

7. **Movements must be controlled:** Improving movement patterns is all about controlling the body's motion. This comes from improving the client's awareness of a particular movement pattern, performing it at a slow to moderate pace, and teaching them how to control their body weight, ground reaction forces, and momentum.

8. **Train to the client's stabilization strength:** Most resistance training programs focus on training to the strength of the client's global movement system. This is also the problem with training to strategies that prioritize 'feeling the burn' or 'no pain, no gain' approaches. However, this is exactly what perpetuates movement dysfunction as clients will continue to strengthen what is strong, while the weak or inhibited muscles will remain just that – weak and inhibited. Generally speaking, in the presence of movement dysfunction, the stabilization system is inhibited or functionally weaker than the movement system and overloading the body results in developing more strength in the global movement system, thereby perpetuating the imbalance between the two muscle systems. Improving a client's awareness of their body will help them recognize signs of instability or when

they have lost control of proximal stabilization. Improving functional strength while decreasing the risk of injury and the perpetuation of faulty movement patterns occurs when the client is progressed appropriately, based upon their ability to stabilize proximally while moving distally.

9. **Follow the proper progressions:** In their haste to get to the 'sexy' movements or to get their clients to 'feel the burn,' it is common practice in the personal training industry to push clients too quickly, bypassing many of the fundamental patterns in the process. Unfortunately, this is often a sign of the times when 'bigger, faster, stronger' becomes the substitute for slower, more controlled, and with more awareness. As discussed previously, this strategy just layers more dysfunction on top of the client's current dysfunction. Proper progression is the best method for assuring that the client is able to optimally integrate the corrective exercise strategies into their fundamental movement patterns. The following is a list of ideal progressions during fundamental movement patterns:

- **Sagittal plane prior to coronal or frontal plane patterns:** The sagittal plane is generally the easiest for clients to control, and coronal and rotation patterns should only be attempted when they have demonstrated ability to control the plane of motion.

- **Bilateral patterns prior to unilateral patterns:** While the goal is to get clients to perform unilateral patterns as they are fundamentally more functional, unilateral patterns introduce rotary forces that need to be controlled. Bilateral patterns can help the unstable client gain confidence prior to moving them to a more unstable base (split or unilateral stance) or pattern (unilateral or alternating arm patterns).

- **Slow performance to faster performance:** Beginning clients, clients with injury, and clients experiencing instability generally have poor ability to control or stabilize their joints. They perform even simple movements at a faster pace to compensate for instability somewhere within the kinetic chain. Slow performance allows the nervous system to focus on the movement, thereby improving awareness and time to make the necessary corrections to achieve optimal and efficient movement. Training at faster speeds or with greater momentum decreases the client's ability to become aware, properly stabilize, recognize, and make adjustments because their awareness is diverted to the task at hand – the speed and execution of the movement. While proponents of the 'bigger, faster, stronger' school of thought like to point out that if one trains slow they become slow, so if one wants to get fast they must train fast; they often fail to mention that a poor movement performed fast will also advance any dysfunction at an accelerated rate. Therefore train movement efficiency prior to movement speed, adding speed when and where appropriate.

- **Stable surfaces prior to labile surfaces:** The goal is to get the client to control their body weight and momentum prior to introducing an unstable or labile surface. The advent and proliferation of labile equipment has ushered in a generation of trainers and therapists who have their clients perform increasingly challenging exercises, even when they can barely control their body on a stable surface. Progressing these clients to unstable surfaces merely perpetuates compensatory strategies, because the clients will adopt any strategy necessary to maintain stability. Training on a labile surface has also been shown to increase compressive loads on the spine, which should not be the goal when training the stiff or hypomobile client. Also, training on labile surfaces decreases force production as the body cannot generate optimal force when its attention is diverted to maintaining stability. Progress clients from bilateral to split stance, from split stance to split stance with one leg elevated and supported, and from split stance with one leg elevated and supported to unilateral stance. Once they can successfully achieve each of these progressions, progress them to labile equipment.

10. **Marry optimal movement strategies into sport- or occupation-specific movements:** Once the client demonstrates competency in the fundamental movement patterns, they can be progressed to sport- or occupation-specific movements. Just as parameters 1–9 stated, they must be able to carry the fundamentals from the corrective exercise strategies and fundamental movement patterns into their sport- or occupation-specific patterns. This progression gives the individual the best opportunity to perform at a high level while minimizing the risk of injury.

While these are the general guidelines that should be followed when improving movement, the next section will look at the seven principles and three core concepts that must be adhered to when developing a corrective exercise and functional exercise program.

THE SEVEN PRINCIPLES OF CORRECTIVE AND FUNCTIONAL EXERCISE

1. **Address the greatest area of dysfunction:** The goal of performing a proper assessment to determine a client's movement dysfunction is to drive the corrective exercise approach. Whether the client is coming in for a specific goal of losing weight, alleviating pain, or performing their sport at a higher level, improved movement efficiency should always be the goal prior to performance enhancement. If movement efficiency is achieved, the program instituted by the coach or trainer will generally lead to accomplishment of the client's goals. However, pursuing goals at the expense of improving movement efficiency will lead to problems and the likelihood that the client may not achieve their goals – or worse, achieve them and get injured in the process. Addressing the greatest area of dysfunction improves the client's tolerance to exercise by improving the proverbial 'weak link' in the kinetic chain.

Often addressing the greatest area of dysfunction will need to include down-regulation of the sympathetic nervous system. This down-regulation most often must precede other strategies, as an up-regulated system is often resistant to change. There are three main methods for down-regulating the nervous system:

   i. Diaphragmatic breathing

   ii. Slow, deep, and specific soft-tissue techniques

   iii. Visualization

   These will be discussed more thoroughly in the corrective strategy section of the book.

2. **Improve spinal posture:** Improving spinal posture generally goes with principles 1 and 3. Often the trunk and spine posture, or something related to the trunk and spine, is the region of greatest

dysfunction. Improving spinal alignment is also necessary to improve breathing patterns by placing the head, neck, trunk, and spine in a position that best enables optimal breathing patterns and activation of the local stabilizers. This can be accomplished by any combination of manipulative techniques, spinal mobility exercises, and/or postural re-education.

3. **Improve breathing patterns:** Breathing patterns must be restored and coordinated with proper activation of the deep stabilization system. This is the key to improving function of the local stabilizers while freeing up the muscles of the global system to perform movement. Improving breathing patterns will help establish and maintain optimal posture due to the diaphragm's dual postural and respiratory role. Additionally, proper diaphragm breathing mobilizes the thorax, improving the health of the discs, improves oxygenation of the body, and down-regulates the central nervous system, thereby restoring parasympathetic function.

4. **Train local co-activation and coordination with breathing patterns:** As mentioned above, once diaphragmatic breathing is restored, it must be coordinated with proper activation of the deep muscle system. The ability to coordinate respiratory and stabilization functions precedes all optimal performance, as the inability to coordinate these functions contributes to dysfunction of the entire neuromusculoskeletal system.

5. **Train proximal stabilization of the scapula and pelvis with glenohumeral and femoroacetabular dissociation:** Once the client can optimally stabilize the trunk and spine, they should be progressed to shoulder and hip dissociation at the glenohumeral and femoroacetabular joints respectively. Proximal stabilization of the scapula and pelvis will be necessary and must be maintained prior to dissociation of the hip and shoulder joints. At times, soft-tissue release will need to be performed to release the humerus from the scapula and the femur from the acetabulum, due to the up-regulation of either the local or the global stabilizers, which limits dissociation of the GH and FA joints. Once dissociation of the humerus and femoral head is established independent of the glenoid fossa and acetabulum respectively, the client is taught proper motor control of these regions.

6. **Integrate fundamental movement patterns:** Once the client learns how to stabilize proximally while performing diaphragmatic breathing and how to dissociate through the appropriate regions of the kinetic chain, they can coordinate these activities into fundamental movement patterns – squatting, lunging, pushing, pulling, rotation, and gait. They should be able to coordinate stabilization and dissociation at the appropriate levels, maintaining motor control as they progress through the patterns. Load, speed, momentum, and stability can each be challenged as the client gains more confidence and aptitude in the patterns.

7. **Progress to work or sport:** Progressing the client to occupational, recreational sport, and dynamic activities of daily living is the final step of the corrective exercise and movement progression. The specific demands of the activity – speed, loads, movements, etc. – can be challenged as the client learns how to maintain joint centration, motor control, and movement efficiency during the functional demands.

THE THREE CORE CONCEPTS OF CORRECTIVE EXERCISE

1. THE USE OF SUPINE AND PRONE POSITIONS

A common question that is asked when looking at the corrective exercise approach presented in this book is why are so many corrective patterns performed in the supine and prone positions rather than more functional, upright postures? Vaclav Vojta, a Czech pediatric neurologist, whose work with children has inspired the next generation of movement and rehabilitation specialists and whose influence can be seen throughout this book, said, "Movement is not something that spontaneously develops in the vertical posture but evolves from lying on one's belly and one's back." Many of the corrective strategies in this book are adapted and modified from Vojta's original work on reflex locomotion and Kolar's dynamic neuromuscular stabilization approach to adult rehabilitation. Both approaches were formed by working with the pediatric population and look to restore fundamental movement patterns in a manner consistent with the development milestones of the child. These patterns are thought to be engrained in the central nervous system so accessing them initially through specific supine and prone positions, specific stimulation points, and muscle activation strategies is considered to be a more ideal starting place rather than forcing the body into positions that it may not have a hard-wired familiarity with.

Additionally, many of the dysfunctional postures and patterns seen in the adult population are thought to be milder manifestations of the patterns seen in many neurological conditions such as cerebral palsy. In particular, increased tone of the flexors and internal rotators, decreased tone in the extensors and external rotators, and poor trunk stabilization and respiratory patterns are rather ubiquitous in both populations with the one big difference being that the adult orthopedic client generally has greater adaptability and better compensatory strategies. Prone and supine positions can help clients and patients gain improved activation of the deep stabilizers and joint centration by eliminating some of the resultant compensatory effects that have developed by habituation and compensation.

Furthermore, while many clients can perform rather impressive feats of strength or rather high level recreational and occupational tasks, they often carry out these activities with substitution patterns rather than optimal motor patterns. The supine and prone positions enable the client to work in positions that they can ideally control with less likelihood of substitution or compensation patterns. These positions also help the clinician or trainer provide kinesthetic feedback for the client as to the position of the their head, neck, trunk, and pelvis, which is commonly deficient or lacking when the client is in the upright position. It is also easier for the clinician or trainer to assess client activation strategies while in the prone and supine positions as well. The goal, however, is always to progress the client to the upright position and integrate this function as they gain functional control of the lower level positions.

2. DECREASE SYMPATHETIC TONE

Decreasing sympathetic tone is one of the most important components of reprogramming the central nervous system and restoring more optimal movement patterns. It is difficult and virtually impossible at times to reprogram the nervous system and institute more ideal motor patterns when the nervous system is up-regulated and overactive. Pain, fatigue, and stress all tend to stimulate sympathetic nervous system activity to a greater degree than the parasympathetic system. There are several very effective methods for dampening sympathetic nervous system activity and up-regulating parasympathetic activity prior to instituting corrective exercise.

- **Deep diaphragmatic breathing** will stimulate the parasympathetic nervous system and decrease sympathetic tone (Rattray 2000, Umphred 2007). Diaphragmatic breathing is one strategy that will be introduced in the corrective exercise section and which must be incorporated into every stage of the functional exercise continuum.

- **Visualization and imagery** of peaceful scenarios and/or quieting the mind are also beneficial and can be used in conjunction with diaphragmatic breathing to decrease tension and quiet the nervous system.

- **Light touch** (Umphred 2007) and stimulation of the Ruffini organs and interstitial receptors have been shown to decrease sympathetic tone (Lindsay 2008). Myofascial release, including holding techniques as well as general shaking and rocking techniques, is an invaluable strategy for decreasing a client's current gripping or bracing compensatory strategies.

3. IMPROVE BODY AWARENESS

It is common, even for client's who routinely exercise, to lack body awareness. While body awareness is a common part of practices such as Tai Chi, Qi Gong, Feldenkrais, and yoga, current training methodologies that stress harder, faster, or stronger approaches often move the individual away from developing body awareness. Pain and fatigue diminish a client's sensation and awareness of their body because the discomfort of the activity prioritizes the brain's attention. This disconnect between an individual's awareness of their body and what is actually happening within their body is further deepened by the use of painkillers that diminish the presence of pain, as well as from the constant stimuli of personal music devices, computers, and television. With advancing technology, greater reliance on dietary stimulants (caffeine, nicotine, etc.), and less attention on both the amount and the type of physical activity that enhances body awareness, clients have become increasingly disconnected from their body. Awareness is one of the key components of the corrective exercise approach and this practice must be a deliberate portion of all exercise sessions. In his book *The Talent Code*, Daniel Coyle lists 'learn to feel it' as one of the three rules of deep practice. By learning to 'feel it', clients can get to a deeper connection with their body, are better able to recognize current patterns, and can more readily institute changes necessary to optimize performance. Improving a client's awareness will be enhanced with the use of specific visualization and imagery techniques as well as visual, verbal, and kinesthetic cuing.

THE LEARNING COMPONENT OF CORRECTIVE EXERCISE

The learning component of developing optimal movement patterns is often overlooked in corrective exercise. Improving motor skill, or the ability of the client to perform highly efficient movement, must be the end goal of any rehabilitative, corrective, or training approach. However, it is important to understand that skill and ability are two fundamentally different individual traits. Ability is the genetic potential of an individual and is unchanged by training or conditioning. Skill is something that is developed by practice, and a client can develop skill regardless of their ability. Regardless of the client's ability, the goal of corrective exercise is always to help increase the client's skill set. An important component of developing skill is improving the client's ability to learn the ideal patterns of stabilization and movement. All individuals will learn at a different level and each skill has its own unique challenges, hence the concept of the 'learning curve.' Each individual will move through specific, distinct stages during the learning process, although the steps are often overlapping. These stages are specific sequential steps in the learning process of any new skill and are broken into the verbal-cognitive, motor, and autonomous processes (Schmidt and Wrisberg 2008).

In the verbal-cognitive stage, the individual is introduced to and develops a general understanding about an unfamiliar task. Significant time is spent giving analogies, developing basic skills, demonstrating (visual), and talking to the client (verbal) and having them think (cognitive) about the task as well as providing them kinesthetic (tactile) feedback about their actions and results. Movement patterns in this stage will be quite uncoordinated and at times can look generally 'sloppy.' The time spent in this phase tends to go quickly and there are generally large jumps in skill level.

The second step is the motor stage. During this stage the individual has mastered the basics nuances of the movement, is able to identify their mistakes, and can more consistently produce their desired actions. They begin to demonstrate refinement of skill and their movements become smoother and more efficient. This stage can last from months to years, or considerably longer, depending on the complexity of the task as well as the client's investment in improving.

The final step is the autonomous phase, where the individual has mastered the movement or activity with a proficiency that requires little conscious thought process. This is the phase of movement sophistication where the individual is able to both identify and correct their movement faults, as well as perform for longer uninterrupted periods of time.

The goal of corrective exercise is to move the client into the final phase so they can be progressed to their functional or task-specific goals. These steps will generally go rather quickly if working with someone with greater ability and internal capacity to learn new skills. The goal is not to see how quickly the client can be moved through the phases but rather to provide the individual with a high level of quality teaching so they can progress at their own optimal pace.

SPECIFICITY OF LEARNING

Specificity of learning relates to those tasks that most resemble the environment and movement patterns the individual will be performing. While some of the initial corrective patterns may not seem to look like the final product of sport or life, they are component pieces or chunks. 'Chunking' is a method that encourages improved neuromotor learning, by breaking up larger tasks into smaller ones and mastering each component before integrating them back into the final movement piece.

For example, a runner presents with knee discomfort that occurs after three miles. During a running assessment, the trainer or therapist may note increased thoracolumbar extension, a positive Trendelenburg's gait on the side of the knee pain, and decreased rotation of the trunk. Rather than having this client try to focus on all those different components, the trainer or therapist may chunk up the running pattern into the following pieces:

- The client works in the supine position on breathing and core activation to help improve the position and stabilization of their thorax.

- They then work on seated trunk rotations, maintaining alignment of their trunk.

- They progress to transitioning between a split stance squat position to a single leg stance to help them develop the neuromotor control of single leg stance that is required for running.

- Finally, they work on integrating these component pieces into their running mechanics.

PRACTICE

A final component of learning that will be utilized in the corrective exercise strategy is practice. Blocked practice, or practice where the client works on the same skill repeatedly, produces immediate benefits in performance. For example, a client performs several sets of squats in a row and gets markedly better with each set. However, random practice, where different sets of skills are practiced in a randomized fashion are performed, has been shown to produce superior learning (Schmidt and Wrisberg 2008). In this example, the client may work on a set of breathing and activation, followed by a set of bridges, and finally do a set of squats, focusing on their stabilization prior to moving back to a set of breathing and activation. The client is performing similar patterns of stabilization but there are several different variables that they have to deal with in each pattern. This will be the method by which many of the patterns are performed in the corrective exercise strategy. Regardless of the type of practice that is utilized, superior learning and improvements in talent have been demonstrated with deep practice or where there is focused exercise (Coyle). The three rules of deep practice as defined by Coyle are to break the movement or exercise into chunks, repeat it frequently, and learn to feel it or experience it at a deep or visceral level. These steps are repeated until the client learns the task.

While the goal for most clients is not to win a gold medal in the performance of fundamental movement patterns, or even to compete at a professional sporting event, they do want to live life and participate in their recreational activities at a high level of function and not be limited by pain. Understanding and applying the principles of learning can help these clients buy into the corrective exercise paradigm and realize the amount of work and concentration it takes to develop improved levels of skill. It also helps to educate the client to the fact that it is required that they perform some homework to help reinforce and 'groove' the corrections that they learned during the rehabilitation or corrective exercise session.

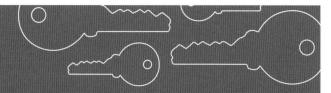

Key To Success
Developing Skill –
Does Practice Really Make Perfect?

From early childhood parents, teachers, and coaches have espoused the idea that practice makes perfect. But does this idea really help improve skill? This idea has been challenged by current research in the area of myelin, the protective coating that surrounds nerves and increases conduction velocity.

"Skill is myelin insulation that wraps neural circuits and that grows according to certain signals." And the more one struggles, the greater their ability to develop these neural connections. "... in order to get your skill circuit to fire optimally, you must by definition fire the circuit suboptimally, you must make mistakes and pay attention to those mistakes; you must slowly teach your circuit." "The truth is, practice makes myelin, and myelin makes perfect." (Coyle 2009)

KEY: There are three key concepts that come out of Coyle's book that will be instituted into the corrective exercise paradigm to improve movement patterns: 1) the client should be allowed to make mistakes; 2) the client must be made aware of their movement patterns and be given a strategy so they can identify and correct them; and 3) the training should be focused and concentrated in order to optimally develop these myelin connections.

MUSCLE ACTIVATION STRATEGIES

Improving movement patterns requires a properly functioning and integrated system. One of the biggest causes of dysfunctional movement, and a challenge during corrective exercise, is muscle inhibition. In the presence of muscle inhibition, the body will substitute by overactivating muscle synergists for a particular dysfunctional muscle. For example, the latissimus dorsi can substitute for inhibition of the lower trapezius in the action of scapular depression. While the latissimus dorsi can perform this action, it also tends to pull the scapula into downward rotation and slight protraction in direct opposition to the upward rotation and posterior tilting function of the lower trapezius. This change in muscle synergies will affect the client's ability to functionally stabilize their scapulothoracic joint during functional movement patterns.

Another common example that was addressed in an earlier section is inhibition of the gluteus maximus, which tends to lead to overactivation of the synergistic hip extensors, primarily the hamstring complex. While functionally this will enable the client to accomplish their short-term task of climbing the stairs or performing squats in their exercise class, the long-term effects of this substitution pattern are what will contribute to this client's joint dysfunction. The insertion of the gluteus maximus is located closer to the axis of rotation and therefore is more effective at maintaining an ideal axis of rotation of the femoroacetabular joint. Because its axis is not near the axis of rotation, activation of the hamstrings will drive the femoral head forward as it extends the hip. Performing corrective exercises that don't improve the inhibited local stabilizers will perpetuate rather than improve these patterns. Likewise, any inhibited muscle is not likely to respond favorably to corrective exercise without being activated prior to its inclusion into functional movement patterns. Inclusion of an inhibited muscle will only strengthen the strong synergists and thus perpetuate the movement dysfunction. This is the reason for performing a thorough assessment including functional muscle testing and having a strategy for improving muscle activation of any inhibited muscles that are discovered. It is also the reason that isolation movements are often used prior to integrating an inhibited muscle back into a functional movement pattern.

While there are many general strategies for restoring balance between muscle synergists, four specific strategies will be utilized throughout this book to facilitate or activate inhibited muscles. They are visualization, isometric contractions, palpations, and breathing, which are designated by the acronym VIP+B™; these strategies will be discussed below.

VISUALIZATION

"The use of mental imagery is useful for both spine position and muscle activation awareness." (Stuart McGill, *Ultimate Back Fitness and Performance* 2004)

While the use of visualization is widespread in the practice of meditation, yoga, and massage, the application of visualization techniques, otherwise known as guided or mental imagery, is gaining popularity outside these arenas for improving muscle activation. In fact, the use of visualization is present in many movement fields – including dance, Feldenkrais, Alexander technique, Pilates, and Gyrotonics, just to name a few – in enabling its practitioners to more fully express movements within their body. Focused visualization strategies are common among athletes before a performance and in between practices to not only maintain but additionally hone their skills. Mabel Todd, developer of the approach that would become known as 'ideokinesis', used imagery and conscious thought patterns as ways to improve posture and habitual movement patterns dating back to the early 1900s.

Advances in technology have been able to demonstrate increased brain activity on MRIs taken of clients performing visualization techniques. For example, simply thinking about a body part has been shown to activate the somatosensory portion of the cortex, while visualizing the performance of a specific activity will activate the motor cortex of the brain (Umphred 2007). These techniques have shown anecdotal clinical applications of being able to activate or awaken dormant movement patterns that have been inhibited by habituation and in new skill acquisition. Visualization can be a part of this process by encouraging the client to visualize an image of what the ideal movement pattern looks and feels like and then attempting to replicate that image and feeling.

Specific visualization and imagery techniques are a necessary part of developing the kinesthetic awareness and 'feeling' associated with a particular movement pattern. For example, a client presents with a butt-gripping strategy and poor ability to dissociate their pelvis from their hips during a squat pattern, even though they have adequate hip flexion range of motion. To get a client to decrease their learned gripping strategy, they can be asked to relax their posterior hips and visualize the hip as a ball sinking back in the socket as they relax and spread their ischial tuberosities.

Visualization as a means of improving activation strategies can be enhanced through the use of different types of verbal cuing to achieve a desired response. Linda-Joy Lee is a big proponent of using cuing phrases such as 'imagine,' 'connect,' 'activate,' or 'lengthen,' which tend to facilitate use of the deep stabilization system, and suggests that terms such as 'do it,' 'squeeze,' and 'stand up tall' correlate to increasing global muscle activity. Using cues to activate the deep stabilizers is a powerful way to improve their function during corrective exercise and their integration into fundamental movement patterns.

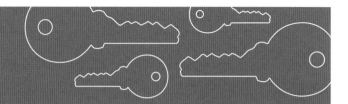

Key To Success
Visualization and Verbal Cuing

Visualization and verbal cuing virtually go hand in hand and can be used to elicit specific responses within the body. For example, if an individual was lying relaxed and breathing deeply, and being walked through a relaxation exercise where they were thinking about lying on a beach, listening to crashing waves, and basking in the sun, they would likely find that their respiratory rate decreases and sense an overall drop of tension in their body. Now imagine that once this individual was relaxed, someone burst in and started shouting, 'come on', 'get up', or 'let's do this', their respiratory rate would instantly increase and their overall state would move from relaxed to tensed. This same concept can be used to activate different muscle systems within the body, depending on the client's needs and learning style, and the response the therapist or trainer is trying to elicit.

KEY: To preferentially activate the deep stabilization system, use verbal cues such as 'think about', 'connect', 'lengthen', 'feel', and 'imagine that' and combine them with an appropriate movement visualization. To bias the global movement system, utilize 'doing' commands such as 'squeeze', 'pack', 'harder', and 'more', to attain an overall global stabilization or movement response.

ISOMETRIC POSITIONS

Isometric contractions first gained popularity from the early muscle-building pioneer Charles Atlas, who promised legions of underweight men that if they performed isometric contractions, they would soon develop the muscle mass necessary to thwart their adversarial bullies. Isometric contractions have historically been used in early rehabilitation programs where pain, inflammation, joint instability, and/ or poor proprioception limit the effectiveness of isotonic types of exercise. Submaximal contraction can be utilized during a rehabilitative or corrective exercise strategy, even beyond the initial stages of the program, to improve both strength and joint stability (Bandy and Sanders 2001). Another benefit of isometric contractions is the carry-over effect. An increase in strength across 30 degrees has been demonstrated from the position in which the isometric contraction is performed, suggesting that isometrics can be useful in improving strength and stability through a range of motion, even when pain or joint limitation prohibits full range of motion (Bandy and Sanders 2001). Additionally, isometric contractions tend to have a greater response to increasing resistance than isotonic contractions (Umphred 2007).

Anecdotally, submaximal isometric contractions are used to improve muscle inhibition and joint centration by placing the client in a position that both optimally centrates the joint and approximates the origin and insertion of a specific inhibited muscle or chain of muscles. The client is then asked to perform a submaximal contraction (approximately 10%–25% of their maximum contraction) for 5–10 seconds as the trainer or therapist resists the client's force. They hold this isometric position for 3–5 repetitions. They can gradually increase the resistance within their tolerance and ability to maintain a centrated joint position up to about 50% of their maximum resistance. Maintaining a relatively low intensity (between 10% and 50% of the client's maximum contraction) seems to clinically promote better activation of the local joint stabilizers than when using intensities that more closely approximate the client's maximum contraction. Once they can maintain the centrated joint position with 50% of their maximum contraction, they can be progressed to functional integration of these regions into fundamental movement patterns.

Isometric contractions can serve as effective take-home exercises for the client in between sessions and/or as a muscle activation strategy prior to corrective or higher level exercise. Examples of specific positions to activate the deep stabilization system and integrated global movement system are included in the corrective exercise strategy section of this book.

PALPATION

"The discovery of the physiological basis of connective tissue therapy stems from the discovery of the presence of mechanoreceptors, intrafascial smooth muscle cells, and autonomic nerves dispersed throughout the network of fascial tissue." (Lindsay 2008)

The role of soft-tissue therapy as a viable treatment of muscle inhibition is well known and documented. As early as 1964 George Goodheart, the founder of Applied Kinesiology, discovered that specific, firm, cross-friction stimulation over the origin and insertion of previously weak muscle caused immediate increases in strength of that muscle (Walther 2000, Frost 2002). This 'origin-insertion' technique' became one of the first techniques used in Applied Kinesiology. Additional origin-insertion techniques used in Applied Kinesiology include direct stimulation of either the muscle spindles or the Golgi tendon organs. Applying a steady pressure directly to the muscle spindle cells (located within the muscle belly) and pulling them towards the muscles attachments will strengthen a muscle. Similarly, direct pressure over the Golgi tendon organs (located within the musculotendinous junction) and pulling them towards the muscle belly will also strengthen a previously weak muscle (Walther 2000, Leaf 1995, Thie 2005). It is beyond the scope of this book to demonstrate these specific techniques and there are many great resources available to the trainer and therapist that adequately cover this topic.

There are three additional plausible mechanisms as to why these origin-insertion and other soft-tissue stimulation techniques work in activating inhibited muscles:

1. It has been proposed that the vibratory stimulation of the mechanoreceptors facilitates the alpha motor neurons that are responsible for increasing tone within the muscle (Frost 2002).

2. Origin-insertion palpation likely causes stimulation of the Golgi tendon organs that are located within the musculotendinous junction, thereby decreasing their inhibitory tone on the muscle (Frost 2002, Rattray and Ludwig 2000).

3. Goodheart noticed small nodules within the weak muscle, which disappeared when rubbed firmly, causing the formerly weak muscle to test strong. These nodules are thought to be the result of traumas that create micro-avulsions or regions where the muscle pulls away from its periosteal attachment (Frost 2002). Stimulation of these nodules potentially improves microcirculation and promotes the healing cascade of the muscle.

Two additional benefits of the origin-insertion technique are that slow, deep, lateral stimulation of the fascial interstitial fibers has been shown to stimulate the mechanoreceptors within the fascial system, functioning to both reset the muscle tone and increase local blood flow, thereby improving the fluidity and flexibility of the fascia (Lindsay 2008). Soft-tissue and joint manipulation techniques, especially slower, deeper methods, affect the myofascial component and can be effective at reversing chronic soft-tissue contractions (Schleip et al 2006). This stimulation functionally elongates the musculofascial fibers by resetting them to their original length, potentially restoring the contractile strength of that particular muscle.

Other palpatory techniques – including rapid tapping, scratching, or brushing methods – can increase stimulation of the muscle spindles and promote muscle facilitation (Page et al 2010). Massage techniques such as heavy tapotement have also been demonstrated to stimulate the stretch reflex and increase the tone of a muscle (Ratray and Ludwig 2000). These palpatory kinesthetic cues can also serve an important role in drawing a client's attention to an inhibited muscle and improve their conscious awareness of an area of the body where there is diminished proprioception.

Interestingly, the use of ice was able to facilitate an inhibited vastus medialis in subjects with an effused joint, whereas the use of electrical muscle stimulation did not elicit similar changes (Hopkins et al 2002).

BREATHING

"If breathing is not normalized, no other movement pattern can be."
(Karl Lewit, as printed in Liebenson 2008)

Breath work, more specifically the coordinated activity of diaphragmatic breathing with intrinsic muscle activation of the trunk and spine, has shown consistent anecdotal evidence of improving shoulder and hip range of motion as well as trunk, shoulder, and hip strength. It is likely that because of the acute improvements in range of motion and strength, the use of the diaphragm helps to normalize respiratory activity, thereby improving the overall stabilization strength of the entire system (Hodges et al 2004). Additionally, it likely improves the alignment and joint centration to allow better muscle synergy and activation patterns. Better oxygenation, down-regulation of the parasympathetic nervous system (Rattray and Ludwig 2000, Umphred 2008), and up-regulation of the parasympathetic nervous system with restoration of deep diaphragmatic breathing likely decreases overactivity of the accessory muscles of respiration while allowing the improved synchronization between the stabilizers and the prime movers of the entire NMS system.

Regardless of the reason for this improvement it is key to establish ideal respiratory patterns prior to instituting any other corrective strategy. In the absence of ideal respiratory patterns, the motor system will be forced to choose between respiration and stabilization, with preferential selection of the former (Hodges et al 2004). This decreases the stability of the system, requiring overactivation of the global trunk, shoulder and hip muscles to increase their contribution to stabilization. While effective in the short term, this strategy is a common cause of global rigidity and perpetuation of faulty stabilization and movement patterns. The specific patterns for improving respiration will be discussed in the corrective exercise section.

STRETCHING

The exclusion of specific stretching techniques in this book is not intended to imply that clients should not stretch or that stretching cannot be performed in isolated situations. The point of the book is to identify the causes of movement dysfunction, which includes habituation, joint laxity, impaired proprioception, and alterations in motor control. Tightness is merely a neurological response to these factors and stretching does little to change or improve the causes of movement dysfunction. Weakness, or more specifically muscle inhibition, and resultant synergistic substitution is at the root of most movement dysfunction and losses of range of motion.

"Because weakness is the underlying cause of loss of alignment and joint range … techniques of lengthening muscle and tissue tightness must be balanced with re-education. Isolated stretching does not result in a lasting improvement in range and may decrease functional ability if not combined with activities designed to increase control." (Umphred 2007)

One additional reason why stretching is not included is that most clients don't do it properly, rather they don't make it specific enough to be helpful in changing dysfunctional movement patterns. Generally, the muscles that clients complain are 'tight' are those that are up-regulated in response to instability and are therefore less resistant to stretching.

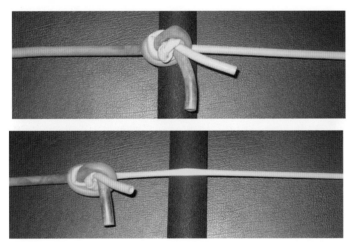

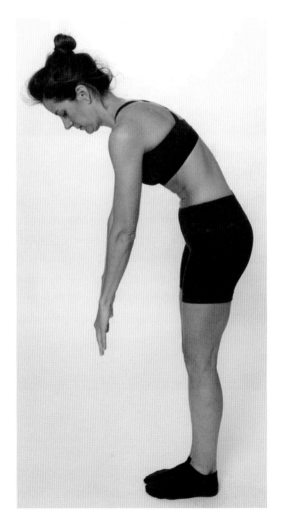

Notice in the images above how the stiffer elastic tubing is more resistant to stretching (lengthening) than the lighter, more elastic tubing. This is similar to what happens in the client with 'tight' hamstrings when these muscles are stretched. As the client attempts to stretch her hamstrings (the stiffer elastic band), the low back (the lighter band) will stretch first and further than the hamstrings. This destabilizes the low back even more and perpetuates the tension in the hamstrings. If stretching is to be used as part of a corrective strategy or conditioning program, it must be followed up with an activation strategy to diminish the potential for inhibition.

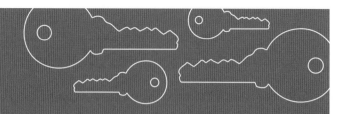

Key To Success
Manual Muscle Testing (MMT) and Flexion Intolerance

While its accuracy and clincial relevance often comes into question, MMT has been used for decades in Applied Kinesiology and Clinical Kinesiology (Walther 2000, Buhler 2004, Leaf 1995, Beardall 1982, Thie 2005) as well as other systems to test an individual's 'tolerance' to a specific substance (supplement, medication, food, or noxious stimulus) or other stimulus such as a particular exercise or movement. In corrective exercise, MMT can be used to determine a client's response or tolerance to a specific exercise or activity. For example, if MMT is performed prior to stretching and the client is found to be strong (activated), clients with lumbar instability will generally test weak (inhibited) post-stretching or after performing a flexion-biased pattern such as a crunch or sit-up.

These clients are referred as flexion-intolerant and is often the reason that sitting for long hours or performing flexion-biased exercises (e.g. stationary bike, seated resistance exercises, abdominal exercises) increases their back discomfort and creates inhibitory effects down the lower extremity.

KEY: To determine your client's response and tolerance to a particular activity, exercise, or movement, do a MMT on them prior to and after the activity. If the MMT remained strong, the activity can be considered to be tolerated by the client's NMS. If a previously strong test goes weak – or they lose range of motion – the activity was not tolerated and must be modified or eliminated from their program, because further exposure to the activity will continue to stress their system.

SUMMARY

The use of specific activation techniques is a powerful strategy for improving muscle inhibition and coordination within the neuromuscular system while restoring function. Although there are many techniques that can be employed, particularly visualization, isometric positions, palpations, and breathing are powerful techniques that directly affect the central nervous system through their stimulation of various central and peripheral receptors. The incorporation of these techniques provides the trainer or therapist with multiple tools for addressing muscle inhibition and movement pattern dysfunctions, while additionally providing a practical strategy for improving function.

Key To Success

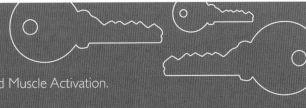

Applying the VIP+B™ Strategy

See Video: Using the VIP+B™ Strategy for Improved Muscle Activation.
www.fitnesseducationseminars.com/osar-book

While each individual component of the VIP+B™ corrective paradigm can be used independently, the maximum effect in improving muscle activation and therefore functional movement patterns requires a combined approach using components of several of the strategies. These will be based upon the therapist's or trainer's skill set and comfort level, as well as the client's needs. For example, a client complains they have trouble walking up stairs. While performing a step-up pattern, the client demonstrates pelvic unleveling (positive Trendelenburg's test), an overly adducted hip position and valgus knee position. The trainer or therapist notices the following during the client's assessement: poor respiratory patterns favoring the accessory muscles of respiration, decreased internal hip rotation and poor dissociation of the femoropelvic joint on the dysfunctional side, and poor muscle strength in the hip abductor functional muscle test. Here is how the trainer or therapist might utilize the VIP+B™ corrective paradigm to help improve this client's pattern:

1. **Breathing:** Instruct the client how to develop optimal breathing by placing their hands on the lateral and posterior aspects of the thoracic cage (kinesthetic cue). The trainer or therapist verbally cues the client by instructing them to 'breathe down and back' into their thorax. The trainer or therapist can also demonstrate the ideal breathing pattern on themselves to provide the client with a visual cue.

2. **Palpation:** The therapist can perform an origin-insertion approximation technique or slow, deliberate, cross friction palpatory stimulation over the osseous attachments of the hip abductors (tensor fasciae latae, gluteus medius, and gluteus maximus) to activate the inhibited hip abductor muscles and investing fascia.

3. **Isometric positioning:** The client is instructed to perform isometric contractions to activate the deep stabilizers of the hip joint, primarily the hip abductors (gluteus medius and minimus) and rotators (psoas major, gemelli, and obturator) in the side lying position (see corrective exercise section). The client performs 5 repetitions of holds for 5–10 seconds with approximately 25% of their maximum strength.

4. **Integration:** The client is then asked to integrate breathing and a centrated joint positon into their step-up pattern, performing it with the addition of the following verbal cues:

   • 'Activate the foot tripod and align the lower extremity.'
   • 'Achieve a squared pelvis position and maintain a long spine.'
   • 'Step up onto the step being sure to lift from the lower, inner portion of the gluteal complex.'

With the client's permission, the therapist or trainer can gently poke or scratch the posterior aspect of the hips to facilitate the lift by using the gluteal complex over the hip flexors and knee extenders. The therapist can also position their hands over the pelvis to help the client feel what it is like to maintain the squared pelvis and lower extremity alignment during the process.

KEY: Utilizing a multi-sensorial approach, the VIP+B™ strategy gives the client the best chance of activating a more optimal stabilization and movement strategy while improving their performance during fundamental movement patterns.

THE COMPONENTS OF IMPROVING FUNCTION

Several keys to improving function will be discussed throughout the corrective exercise phases and carried into the functional movement progressions. These are the long spine, the squared pelvis, the foot tripod, diaphragmatic breathing, and the neutral hand-wrist. Additionally, the concept of ipsilateral and contralateral support will be discussed. Descriptions of each of the keys are given below.

THE LONG SPINE

Achieving neutral posture of the head, thorax, and pelvis is key to improving movement efficiency in both the hip and shoulder complexes and decreasing areas of postural overload. The long spine refers to maintaining neutral alignment of the head, cervical spine, thorax, and lumbopelvic complex. When asked to stand up tall, many clients mistakenly raise the sternum, hyperextending at both the thoracolumbar and occipitocervical junctions. This postural strategy overloads these areas, making the client's movements inefficient, potentially leading to common patterns of overload and overuse injuries as well as making movement of the extremities less efficient.

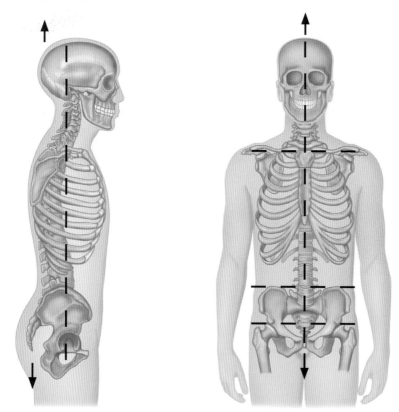

Achieving the long spine should not include a lot of effort on the client's part and they should not be given the common cues to 'lift the chin' or 'tuck the pelvis' as these cues can perpetuate faulty movement patterns. Rather, the client should be verbally cued to visualize a string pulling their head towards the ceiling and their sacrum towards the floor to help achieve the long spine posture (see images above).

Achieving the long spine position is an important key to improving movement patterns and must be relatively maintained regardless of the client's position.

Ideal alignment of the head, thorax, spine, and pelvis are shown in the table below.

Region	Ideal Alignment
Head	Eyes are level with the horizon, occiput is in cephalic-oriented position and chin is in caudal-oriented position
Thorax	Sternum is in vertical alignment with pubic symphysis, lower anterior aspects of ribs are in a caudal position and posterior aspects of ribs are in superior position
Spine	Neutral curves – gentle lordosis in cervical and lumbar regions and gentle kyphosis in thoracic region
Pelvis	Anterior superior iliac spine is in vertical alignment with pubic symphysis

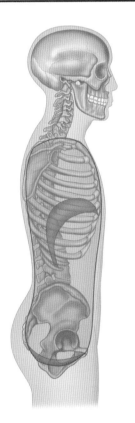
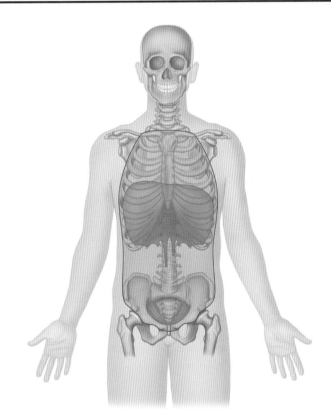

Another related concept to the long spine that will be discussed throughout this book is the thoracopelvic canister (TPC, above). The thoracopelvic canister comprises the thorax and pelvis, including the thoracic and lumbar spine and ribs. The thoracopelvic canister can be cued similarly by having the client maintain the long spine posture with the anterior aspect of the rib cage positioned in a slightly caudal position and the sternal aspect being lightly lifted towards the ceiling. Functional control of the thoracopelvic canister will be discussed overleaf.

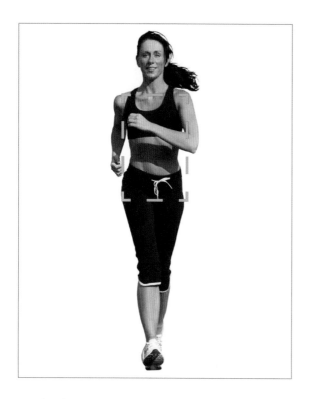 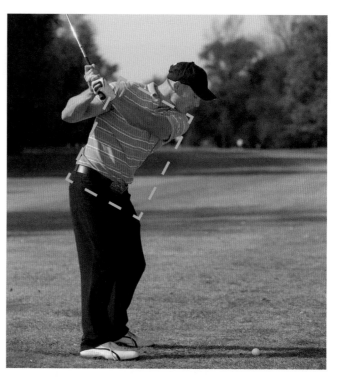

Notice how the athletes maintain a long spine and control of the thoracopelvic canister whether running or swinging a golf club.

FUNCTIONAL CONTROL OF THE THORACOPELVIC CANISTER

Functional control of the thoracopelvic canister (TPC) is achieved by the deep stabilization system. Most important in this control are the transversus abdominis (TrA), which supports the front and sides, the quadratus lumborum, which controls the posterior aspect, and the psoas major and multifidi, which control the anterior and posterior aspects of the spine respectively, in addition to the diaphragm and pelvic floor. These structures are fascially bound superiorly through the thoracolumbar fascia and inferiorly through the pelvic floor fascia. Collectively they function to provide a stable base of support for the kinetic chain and act as a relay station between the upper and lower extremities in addition to their role in visceral support.

The diaphragm deserves special mention in TPC stabilization because of its dual role in respiration and stabilization. The diaphragm is key to maintaining optimal stability of the thoracopelvic canister as well as improving intra-abdominal pressure. Fascially attaching to the quadratus lumborum, psoas, and TrA, the diaphragm forms the roof of the TPC. Because of its unique attachments, the interlinking fascial attachments of the diaphragm act to stabilize the thoracolumbar junction – the important region where the thoracic spine meets the lumbar spine. In the absence of optimal TPC stabilization, many of the faulty stabilization and resultant movement pattern dysfunction will be noted. The characteristic lumbar hyperlordosis more commonly occurs at the thoracolumbar junction than at the lumbosacral junction, as these individuals use a posterior extensor stabilization strategy rather than a circumferential-type stabilization strategy. Individuals with a flexion-dominant strategy will rely too much on their trunk flexors and anterior myofascial and ligamentous structures for stability.

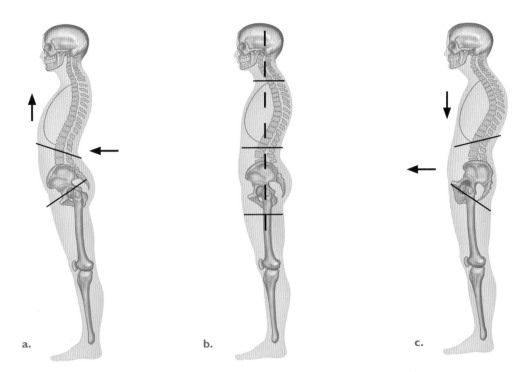

a. Extension dominance: The individual demonstrates overactivation of the extensor muscles, resulting in thoracolumbar hyperextension and stretching of the anterior abdominal wall. This individual will have an accessory dominant breathing strategy, increased thoracolumbar erector tone, and poor TPC stabilization. This posture is generally the result of extension-dominant stabilization strategies during exercise patterns, and cuing that encourages the individual to 'lift the chest' and 'squeeze the shoulder blades down and back.'

b. Neutral posture: Note the parallel alignment of the thoracic inlet, diaphragm and pelvic floor.

c. Flexion dominance: The individual demonstrates overactivation of the trunk flexors and hip extensors. This individual will also demonstrate accessory dominant respiratory patterns, increased abdominal (oblique and rectus) tone, overstretched thoracolumbar erectors, and poor TPC stabilization. This posture generally results from an over-reliance on flexion-biased exercises and cues that encourage the individual to 'squeeze' or 'tuck in the butt' and 'flatten the low back to the floor during supine exercise patterns.'

Studies have demonstrated that fatigue of the respiratory muscles can result in decreased tolerance to imposed stresses on the body (Eliasz 2004). While obesity and the lack of physical activity have been cited as causative factors in the development of low back pain, dysfunctional breathing and alterations in continence strategies (suggesting pelvic floor dysfunction) have been shown to have a greater role in the development of pain than the individual's weight or exercise habits (Hodges et al 2001). Clients and patients with chronic low back pain also demonstrate increased postural sway as compared to individuals with acute induced back pain during forced respiration. Changes in central nervous system responses, alterations in breathing strategies, and the preferential prioritization of breathing over stabilization are several plausible explanations for increased postural sway in the individuals with chronic low back pain (Hodges et al).

STABILIZATION OF THE THORACOLUMBAR JUNCTION

One important key in the stabilization of the thoracopelvic canister is the thoracolumbar junction. Several key muscles responsible for stabilization of the trunk and spine take their origin or insertion at the thoracolumbar region. These include the psoas major and minor, transversus abdominis, quadratus lumborum, and diaphragm and are bound with the thoracolumbar fascia, which suggests their role in stabilization of this key region of the spine. Notice how the child lifts her pelvis to stabilize at the thoracolumbar junction (image below left). This is an important developmental point in that she is able to coordinate trunk stabilization with diaphragmatic respiration, and is key to improving function in fundamental movement patterns such as the squat (image below right).

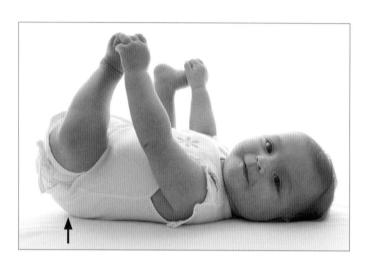 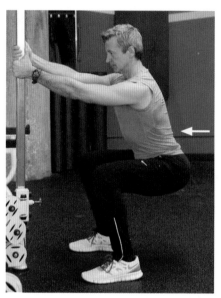

Loss of thoracolumbar stabilization results in many of the common postural and movement dysfunctions observed in the assessment process, including:

• hyperextension of the thoracolumbar region;

• hypertonicity of the erector spinae over the thoracolumbar region that contributes to thoracic rigidity;

• compensatory flexion of the lower lumbar spine.

These compensations for the loss of thoracolumbar stabilization compromise the stability of the thoracopelvic canister and contribute to dysfunctional movement strategies.

The primary corrective exercise strategy for improving dysfunctions of the hip and shoulder as well as the trunk and spine involves optimally stabilizing the TPC, especially at the thoracolumbar junction. The goal of the corrective movement strategy is to improve stabilization in this key region and ensure that the client can maintain control of the entire thoracopelvic canister throughout their fundamental movement patterns.

There are three primary mechanisms for achieving thoracopelvic stabilization: intra-abdominal pressure, the hydraulic amplifier, and the fascial chains. These mechanisms will be discussed next.

1. INTRA-ABDOMINAL PRESSURE

Intra-abdominal pressure (IAP) is perhaps the most important of the three strategies for achieving a long spine, although its usefulness in contributing to force production and stabilization of the spine has been the source of debate.

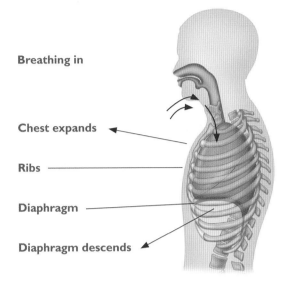

Breathing in

Chest expands

Ribs

Diaphragm

Diaphragm descends

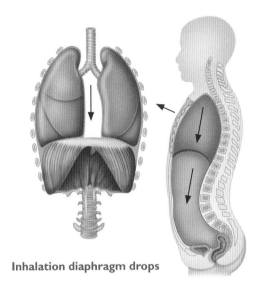

Inhalation diaphragm drops

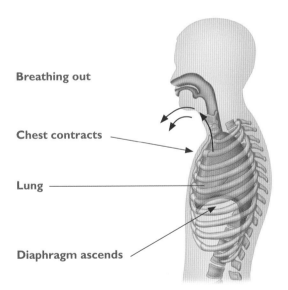

Breathing out

Chest contracts

Lung

Diaphragm ascends

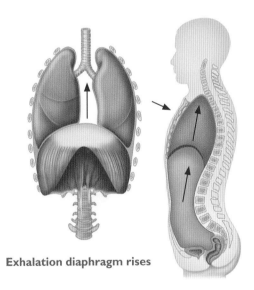

Exhalation diaphragm rises

As the diaphragm descends during inspiration, it pushes the abdominal visceral inferiorly, creating negative internal pressures, causing air to be drawn into the lungs. The intercostal muscles contract to resist the inward forces of this pressure change, while the abdominal muscles, in particular the transversus abdominis, contract to support the positive pressure in the abdominal cavity and the descent of the viscera. The muscles of the pelvic floor are co-activated during this process to help maintain continence and support the abdominal and pelvic viscera. This process increases the IAP, which functionally stiffens and elongates the spine. IAP can be thought of in terms of internal pressure creating outward stabilization, or the image of blowing up a sturdy balloon inside a box, thereby increasing internal stability of the box. Developing optimal IAP also requires optimal abdominal wall and erector spinae muscle function to resist the thoracic and abdominal expansion that results from the increase in IAP. It has been suggested that IAP is greatest with inhalation and breath-holding during a lifting task (Hagins); therefore greater strength and trunk stability is achieved with breath-holding. While this specific strategy will not be a part of the corrective exercise strategy, improving activation of the abdominal wall while generating increases in IAP will benefit clients as they return to higher level training.

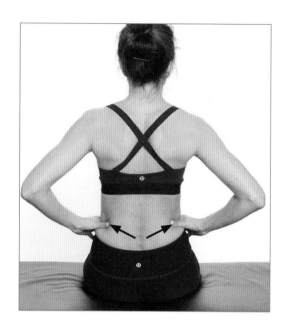

The client ensures three-dimensional activation of her core by lightly pushing out towards her fingers and maintains this tension as she continues to breathe low and wide with her diaphragm.

2. HYDRAULIC AMPLIFIER

The hydraulic amplifier effect occurs with the contraction of muscles within their fascial envelopes. All muscles are invested inside fascia and as they contract, push out into the fascia, creating a stiffening around the joint. In the spine, contraction of the lumbar erector spinae and multifidus within the thoracolumbar fascia creates an extension force, assisting extension of the spine. When the lumbosacral multifidus contracts it broadens posteriorly into the lumbodorsal fascia (image below).

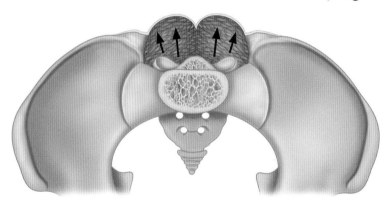

As the multifidii contract, it pushes into the thoracolumbar fascia and along with contraction of the transversus abdominis provides intersegmental stability (image above).

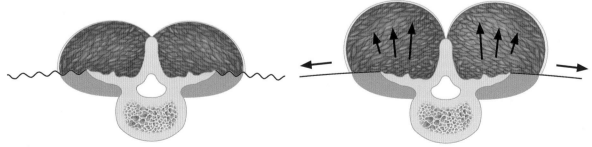

The relaxed multifidi muscle in transverse section (left image). Co-contraction of the transversus abdominis and multifidi creates a stiffening tension on the thoracolumbar fascia thereby providing intersegmental stability (right image).

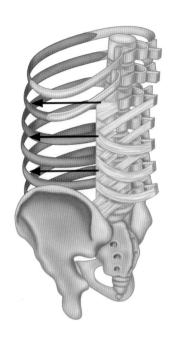 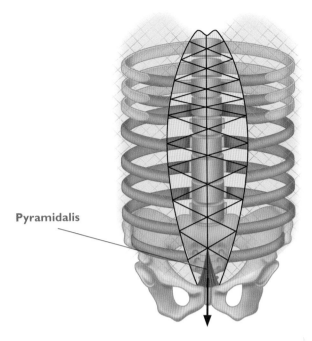

Pyramidalis

This effect is aided by contraction of the transversus abdominis, which pulls the thoracolumbar fascia tight around the contracting erector spinae and multifidi, thereby creating a stable column (image above left). Note how contraction of the pyramidalis tenses the linea alba (central tendon), creating a stable base for contraction of the transversus abdominis (image above right, anterior view). As the transversus abdominis contracts, it tenses the thoracolumbar fascia, which allows the multifidi and lumbar erector spinae to contract against it and aid spinal elongation and stiffness (image above left, posterolateral view).

Tensor fasciae latae

Iliotibial band

Vastus lateralis

Vastus medialis

In the lower extremity, contraction of the vastus lateralis against the iliotibial band helps to transform the lower kinetic chain into a stable column to help support the upper body and resist ground reaction forces during unilateral stance.

3. FASCIAL CHAINS

As mentioned earlier, all muscles are invested within fascia, which interlinks muscles to form myofascial chains surrounding the thorax and extremities. Muscles taper into tendons, which fascially blend into a bony attachment. Adjoining muscles will take their attachments on the other side of the bone, making a fascial interlink with the first. Essentially, these chains are formed as series of muscle-tendon-fascia-bone-ligament-fascia-tendon-muscle linkages.

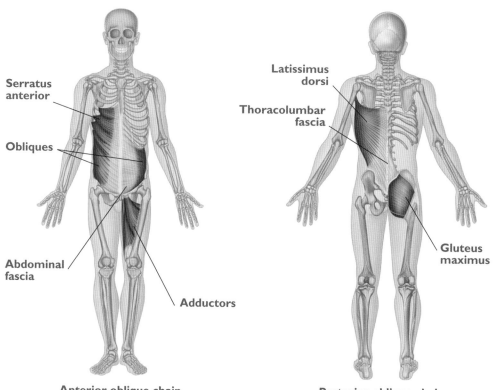

Serratus anterior

Obliques

Abdominal fascia

Adductors

Latissimus dorsi

Thoracolumbar fascia

Gluteus maximus

Anterior oblique chain.

Posterior oblique chain.

While muscles and fascia form numerous myofascial chains throughout the body, there are two distinct chains that connect the upper and lower extremities with the trunk and spine. These are referred to as the anterior and posterior oblique chains. The anterior oblique chain is formed from the left splenii, right rhomboids, right serratus anterior, right external obliques, abdominal fascia, left internal obliques, and left adductor complex. The posterior oblique chain is formed from the latissimus dorsi, thoracolumbar fascia, contralateral gluteus maximus, iliotibial band, and peroneus longus. Each chain has a corresponding partner chain on the opposite side of the body. They each cross the midline, connecting the contralateral upper and lower extremities, and function to accelerate and decelerate rotation of the trunk and extremities. The left anterior oblique chain works with the contralateral posterior oblique chain to improve the force production and reduction abilities of the trunk and extremities. Additionally, because the chains cross the midline of the body connecting contralateral limbs, they provide a criss-cross or 'X'-type of stabilization to the trunk and spine. One additional chain that plays an important role at the heel strike and loading phases of gait is the longitudinal chain. This chain, through the sacroiliac and sacrotuberous ligaments, fascially conjoins the contralateral erector spinae with the ipsilateral long head of the biceps femoris, and fibularis peroneus longus, which prepares the body for loading by stabilizing the lower extremity and functionally locking the sacroiliac joint.

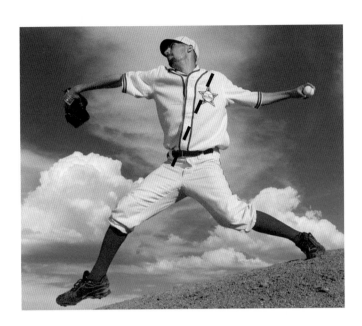 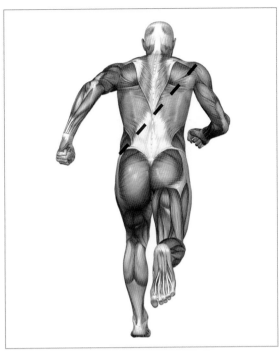

Needing to maximally accelerate their shoulder, the athlete in the left image loads their anterior oblique chain. With activities requiring increased speed, individuals will pre-load their posterior oblique chain to extend their contralateral shoulder and hip during the propulsion phase of the running cycle.

TRAINING THE CHAINS UTILIZING IPSILATERAL AND CONTRALATERAL STABILIZATION

Earlier in this book the concept of early child development was briefly touched upon. One of the key concepts is that in early development, the extremities are used as stable points and the spine rotates around the fixed limb, which may call into question some of the commonly accepted beliefs of functional anatomy. Also presented was the idea that many patterns that clients are asked to perform actually contribute to movement dysfunction by creating stiffness of the thorax and hypermobility at the scapulothoracic and lumbopelvic articulations. In particular, bilateral patterns such as barbell or dumbbell versions of the bench press, rows, pull-downs, and overhead presses, squats, and deadlifts contribute to dysfunction because the trunk and spine are called on to be a stable base and the extremities are moved around the fixed base.

Unilateral and alternating patterns help free up the thorax and aid driving motion through the spine, taking advantage of Serge Grecovetsky's concept of the spinal engine. In these patterns, the free arm will be used to stabilize one side of the thorax, while the trunk and spine will drive motion of the free arm. The resisted arm will complete the motion by either pushing or pulling the resistance.

Cables and resistive tubing are generally the preferred method of resistance as they allow the client to be upright and motion can be driven in an infinite number of directions. The cables enhance the functional carry-over of these patterns and can make the patterns somewhat sport or occupation specific. However, dumbbells and kettlebells can be used for bent-over rows, overhead presses, and chest presses. The form of resistance is not important but rather the concepts of the patterns.

Generally speaking, the anterior oblique chain is trained with pushing patterns, while the posterior oblique chain is trained with pulling patterns. However, a more realistic view is that the right anterior oblique chain functions with the left posterior oblique chain and vice versa, so training one of the chains is likely also working its synergistic partner. Listed below are the parameters for the proper execution of movement patterns, involving the anterior and posterior oblique chains.

Regions	Description
Thoracopelvic canister	Client must be able to maintain alignment, activation, and diaphragmatic breathing through the pattern. They must rotate their trunk on a vertical axis that extends through their spine.
Legs	Split stance, with neutral alignment of the hip, knee, ankle, and foot. The majority of the weight is on the client's front leg (approximately 70%), with the remainder on the back leg. The heel is raised on the back leg.
Lead hip	Internal hip rotation can be driven by having the client hold the cable in the same hand as the forward hip during pulling patterns. During pushing patterns, internal hip rotation is driven by holding the cable in the contralateral hand of the forward leg.
Pushing patterns – anterior oblique chain	The free arm stabilizes the trunk as the resistance is pushed away from the body either horizontally or vertically.
Pulling patterns – posterior oblique chain	The free arm stabilizes the trunk as the resistance is pulled towards the body either horizontally or vertically.

In ipsilateral support (left image) the lead leg and ipsilateral arm will be used as the fixed points, while in contralateral support (image far right) the lead leg and contralateral arm will be used as the fixed points. The decision to use one over the other is based on the desired training goals and needs of the client. Each pattern will be used at different times to elicit specific results throughout the corrective exercise and functional progressions.

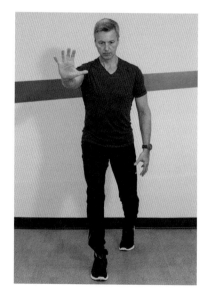 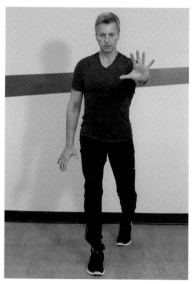

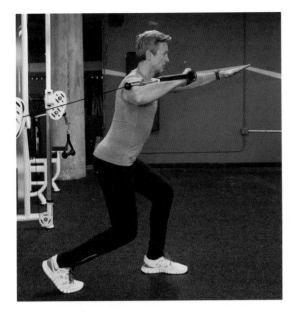 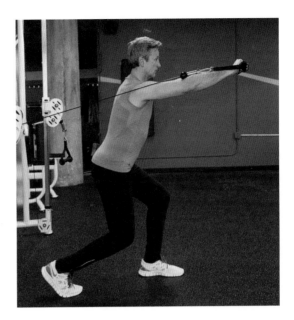

Training the anterior oblique chain: cable chest press – ipsilateral support (see images above). The client maintains a stable base in the left upper and lower extremities and allows the trunk and spine to drive the motion.

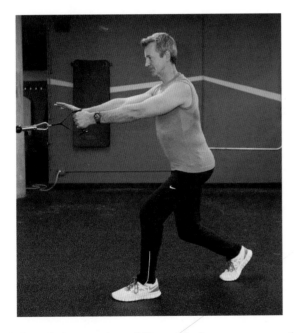 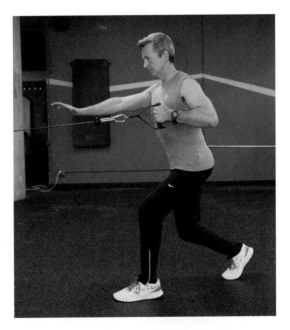

Training the posterior oblique chain: one arm cable row – contralateral support (see images above). Contralateral support can help drive internal hip rotation of the lead hip as the trunk and spine are rotated over the stationary limb.

See Video: Utilizing Stabilization Strategies for Improved Performance, www.fitnesseducationseminars.com/osar-book

THE SQUARED PELVIS

The squared pelvis comes from the idea of the client being able to 'square' their pelvic pyramid over the femoral heads and maintain this alignment during functional movement patterns. Thinking of the pelvis and hips as a pyramid, the base must be squared in relation to the lower extremity during lower extremity patterns. While in real life and sport this position is rarely achieved, the goal of squaring the pelvis is to activate the deep hip stabilizers while maintaining a stable base for the spine, an optimal axis of rotation for the hip, and ideal lower extremity mechanics. The visual cue of standing on a clock is useful, where the client is facing 6:00 and the pelvis remains squared with the hips at the 3:00 and 9:00 positions. This position should be maintained whether performing a movement pattern in a bilateral, split, or unilateral stance.

The pelvis is a functional pyramid supported by the lower extremities. It functions to support the weight of the trunk, spine, and upper extremities, as well as absorb and dissipate ground reaction forces from the lower extremities. Achieving optimal alignment and stabilization of the thoracopelvic canister is a prerequisite of the squared pelvis. The ability to stabilize the thorax over the pelvis and the pelvis under the thorax is key to improving function of the lower extremity. Alterations in thoracopelvic stabilization result in alterations in lower extremity stabilization.

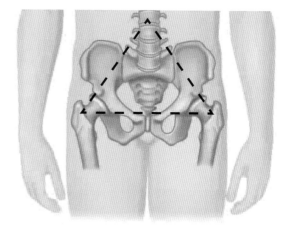

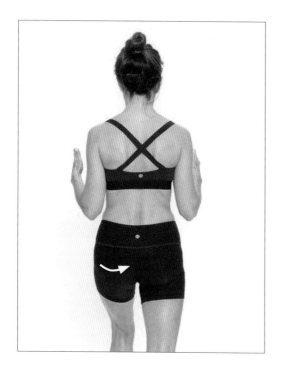

The deep rotators of the hip and the coccygeal fibers of the gluteus maximus are responsible for assisting leveling of the pelvis. Directly, they help draw the femur posteriorly within the acetabulum and, fascially, help pull the pelvis up over the femur (arrow). This position is key to optimal alignment and performance of all lower extremity patterns.

THE FOOT TRIPOD

The foot essentially functions as a tripod, balancing delicately on the heads of the first and fifth metatarsals and the calcaneus. This position helps create the positive support reflex, which turns the lower extremity into a rigid lever for support during lower extremity movement patterns. While functional training purists and biomechanists may argue the point that the tripod is not biomechanically correct during functional movement patterns, the goal of the foot tripod is to help improve a client's awareness of their foot position as well as improve the functional control of the arches of the foot. Even the client with a 'flat' foot should strive to achieve the tripod, albeit a lower tripod position with the goal not being to necessarily restore the arches but rather to activate the intrinsic muscles required to help stabilize the foot architecture.

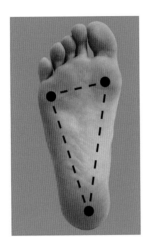 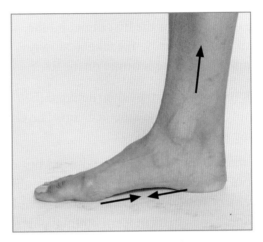

The client is instructed to maintain the tripod and visualize a tension wire from just behind their big toe to the medial aspect of their heel (horizontal arrow). During lower extremity patterning such as squats and lunges, they visualize about initiating the lift from the apex of their medial arch (vertical arrow). This is a powerful cue to help the client connect their foot to their lower extremity and to functionally 'lighten' the load through their transverse and medial arches.

The foot tripod should be maintained during all lower extremity patterns. Generally cuing should be performed with the naked foot so that the trainer or therapist can evaluate the competence of the foot architecture and musculature and so that the client can see and feel what their foot is doing and utilize these mechanics even when wearing shoes.

See Video: Establishing the Foot Tripod and Medial Stabilization Chain,
www.fitnesseducationseminars.com/osar-book

For clients who experience difficulty in getting into or maintaining this position, begin seated and then progress to a parallel stance before progressing to the split stance position. The client always begins in a squared pelvis and long spine position. For the advanced client who can begin in a split stance position, follow the steps below to activate and connect the foot tripod to the lower kinetic chain.

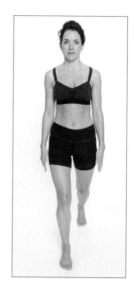 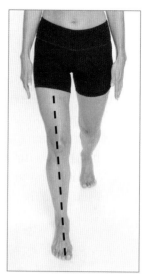

- The client starts by placing the big toe and medial aspect of their foot onto the floor.

- Maintaining the connection of the first digit and the medial aspect of the calcaneus, the client slowly rolls their foot until the fifth toe is firmly on the floor.

- Maintaining this foot position, they then activate their deep external hip rotators to externally rotate the lower extremity and align the kinetic chain. The client rotates the hip only as far as they are able while maintaining the foot tripod.

Activation of the medial foot stabilizers and deep hip rotators helps maintain optimal alignment of the entire lower kinetic chain. The client should be able to maintain this alignment throughout the fundamental movement patterns. Once the client is able to maintain this activation sequence, they begin with small squats to help them learn optimal control of this alignment through the pattern. They then progress to deeper patterns and more unstable patterns such as the split squat position as described above. Follow the proper progressions, stopping the pattern once the client is unable to stabilize any segment of the kinetic chain.

There are two dysfunctional stabilization patterns that are common with poor connection through the medial stabilization chain (medial column of foot, adductors, and sacral and coccygeal divisions of the gluteus maximus). The first is in clients with poor internal hip rotation secondary to overactivity

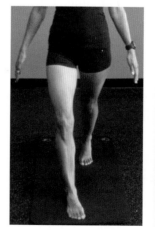 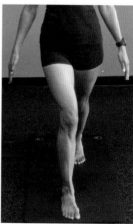

of the posterior hip complex, restriction in the posterior joint capsule, and/or a combination of a genu varus knee position and a supinated, high arch foot (image below left). The client is unable to load through the medial aspect of their leg and foot. The second pattern is when there is poor control of hip rotation, which leads to increases in internal rotation and adduction of the knee (image far right). This is a common dysfunctional pattern, which increases medial stress on the knee and is a contributor to injuries of the medial collateral ligament, medial meniscus, and anterior cruciate ligaments during functional activities. These patterns must be corrected prior to functional loading or the client is at risk of developing repetitive movement dysfunctions and/or soft-tissue injury.

DIAPHRAGMATIC BREATHING AND CORE ACTIVATION

Respiration is the single most important function of the neuromusculofascial system. While dysfunction of the diaphragm in postural stabilization has been noted in several studies (Hodges et al 2001), poor respiratory habits have also been linked to global issues including anxiety, hypertension, headaches, irritable bowel disease, and dizziness (Lum 1987). Therefore, it is imperative to improve respiration and include it in the correction strategy of common dysfunctional movement patterns of the hip and shoulder.

While factors such as smoking are obvious contributors to changes in respiratory patterns, there are several causative factors that lie beneath the radar including:

- asthma;

- chronic stress and/or pain;

- exercise that is too intense for the client's current level of conditioning;

- chronic allergies;

- chronic overuse of stimulants such as caffeine and over-the-counter diet products and energy drinks that stimulate the sympathetic nervous system;

- chronic inflammation of the respiratory tract such as sinusitis;

- disease processes such as chronic obstructive pulmonary disease.

However, the challenge for the trainer and therapist is in convincing their clients of the importance of proper breathing in the restoration of normal function and the development of efficient movement patterns. Unfortunately, while many clients rarely come in with the chief complaint of breathing difficulties, they often present with clinical signs of poor breathing stereotype. The following is a short list of common signs of respiratory distress. Like most movement dysfunctions, they are far easier to recognize in the later stages of the disease process than in the earlier stages.

- **Forward head posture:** The accessory muscles of respiration (primarily the scalenes and sternocleidomastoid) become overactive as they work to elevate the thorax, resulting in shortness and stiffness of these muscles. This in turn pulls the head forward and into suboccipital extension, potentially increasing the likelihood of headaches and temporomandibular issues.

- **Anterior tilt of the scapula:** The scapula gets pulled over the thorax by the overactive pectoralis minor (another accessory muscle of respiration), resulting in the winged, anteriorly tilted scapula posture.

- **Rib cage flare**: The intercostal space and the angle of the ribs increase, producing a wide position of the rib cage. This position is also exaggerated by stiffness in the lateral and posterior aspects of the thorax, resulting in the client's inability to efficiently perform lateral and posterior excursion of the diaphragm. This rib cage posture also leads to overstretching of the anterior abdominal wall and an inspiratory position of the diaphragm, and is a common cause of abdominal hernias and diastasis recti.

- **Stiffness of the thorax:** The thorax becomes stiff as the client increases the use of the accessory muscles, loses the stabilization function of the diaphragm, and subsequently overuses the large thoracic muscles for additional trunk stability.

- **Respiratory rate:** The client will generally breathe shallower and more rapidly when using a poor breathing strategy. As a result, the respiratory and cardiac rates increase as the body attempts to improve oxygenation to the body. This can lead to several global symptoms, including anxiety, hypertension, and dizziness, as well as contributes to overloading the accessory muscle system. The client may appear to 'sigh' a lot in an attempt to expel the air from their lungs.

- **Additional signs:** These can include hypertrophy of the scalene, sternocleidomastoid and pectoralis minor muscles, as well as increased skin pigmentation (usually a deep reddish color), most obvious in the face and neck.

There are several reasons to include breathing in improving function of the hip and shoulder. Diaphragmatic breathing:

1. helps restore alignment of the axial skeleton (trunk and spine), which in turn will help align the appendicular skeleton (limbs);

2. decreases accessory muscle activity, which will diminish some of the global rigidity especially in the muscles directly connecting the shoulders and hips to the neck and trunk;

3. activates the parasympathetic nervous system and down-regulates the sympathetic nervous system, improving overall sense of well-being as well as making it easier for the client to adopt new movement strategies;

4. improves oxygenation of the body, which can decrease pain and sensitivity;

5. improves a client's awareness of their body.

Key To Success
Coordination of Respiration

The key to improving stabilization function of the trunk and spine lies in the ability to maintain activation of the deep stabilization system while diaphragmatically breathing. Clients with spine and trunk instability generally have a poor ability to coordinate diaphragmatic breathing and tend to develop restrictions of the hip and shoulder complexes.

KEY: Improving diaphragmatic breathing and co-activation of the deep stabilization system is an important first-level correction for improving function of the hip and shoulder complexes.

The stabilization approach that follows is modified and adapted from Pavel Kolar's dynamic neuromuscular stabilization and Shirley Sahrmann's lower abdominal progression series. The visualization and alignment cues are modified and adapted from Linda-Joy Lee (2008).

PHASE I: DIAPHRAGMATIC BREATHING

The client lies supine with her legs elevated on a ball or bench, so that her hips and knees are at 90 degree flexion and her arms resting at her sides. If the head and neck are in excessive extension, a pillow is placed under the head to position the head and neck in a more neutral alignment. The goal of this posture is to relax the neuromusculoskeletal system as well as align the diaphragm with the pelvic floor.

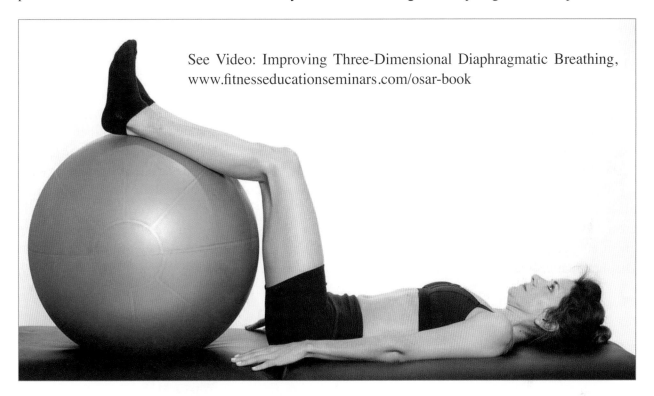

See Video: Improving Three-Dimensional Diaphragmatic Breathing, www.fitnesseducationseminars.com/osar-book

Next the client is asked to breathe laterally and posteriorly into her rib cage. While the rib cage should elevate superiorly and the abdomen should rise, the large majority of the motion should come from lateral and posterior excursion of the diaphragm. Hence, it should appear as if the thoracopelvic canister is a giant balloon and enlarges with inhalation and deflates slightly with exhalation. The ideal duration of the expiratory phase should be approximately one and a half times the inspiratory rate. When retraining clients with poor breathing stereotypes, it is helpful to have them pause for a second at the end of the exhalation prior to taking another breath in, as well as at the end of the inspiration before exhaling. This helps slow the client's rate of breathing while allowing them to take full advantage of the lung volume as well as the inspiratory reflex that comes at the end of a full expiration. The client repeats for several breaths before returning to their normal respiratory pattern. With clients who have an excessively stiff thorax, one breath cycle using the above strategy may be all they are able to handle before they have to rest.

The trainer or therapist can facilitate posterior and lateral diaphragmatic excursion by kinesthetically cuing the client. The trainer or therapist places their hands over the posterior aspect of the thorax and provides a gentle squeeze medially while cuing the client to 'breathe into my hands.' The trainer can facilitate a more caudal rib cage position and expiration by placing their hands over the anterior portion of the thorax and gently gliding the thorax inferiorly during the expiratory phase.

PHASE II: CORE ACTIVATION

Next the client must be instructed on how to optimally activate their deep stabilization system. Research has consistently demonstrated deficiencies in the ability to activate the deep stabilization system in individuals with chronic low back pain (Hodges et al 2004). While some question the validity of isolated training of the deep stabilization system (McGill 2007) there is sufficient research (Hodges et al 2004, Lee 2008, Lee 2004) and clinical evidence that supports this approach. Unfortunately, for clients with the chronic low back pain, bracing strategies are generally their default stabilization strategies, and evidence suggests those individuals may have too much activation of the global system. Therefore a lighter, submaximal effort is utilized, and verbal cues such as 'tighten your stomach as if you are going to be punched' should not be used with these clients.

The client is asked to take a deep breath in and let all the air out. The trainer or therapist then attempts to gently push their index fingers into the client's abdomen just inside the anterior superior iliac spines. It should feel as if the client pushes slightly out into the therapist's hands as she activates her deep abdominal wall. The trainer or therapist can repeat this procedure to ensure lateral wall activation by placing their fingers into the client's lateral abdominal wall and pressing between the client's iliac crest and last rib. The therapist should feel their fingers push slightly out of the abdominal wall as the client activates the deep stabilizers. See Video: Establishing Core Activation with Coordination of Diaphragmatic Breathing, www.fitnesseducationseminars.com/osar-book

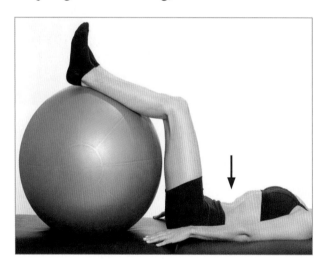 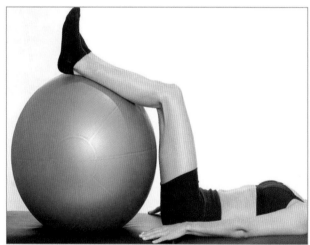

The client attempts to activate her deep stabilizers by performing an abdominal 'draw-in' maneuver (left image). She overactivates her abdominal wall, which leads to lumbar spine flexion, functionally limiting the stabilization effect of the deep system with this type of strategy. The client achieves a much better activation by the trainer providing them with the cue of 'don't let me push my fingers into your abdomen' (right image). It is important to note that the client is not 'braced' when using this strategy but is able to maintain some activation of the transversus abdominis and other deep stabilizers as she performs diaphragmatic breathing.

Once the client is able to activate and sustain an isometric contraction for 6 seconds, they coordinate the activation with diaphragmatic breathing. The client begins with one breath cycle, working up to maintaining this coordination for an entire 1-minute cycle.

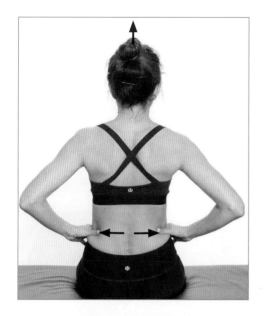

The client must be given homework to change their daily strategy and to 'groove' the pattern and engrain it in their nervous system. During the day, they sit tall in the chair, placing their thumbs above the iliac crest and their fingers inside the anterior superior iliac spines to ensure lateral and posterior diaphragmatic excursion (image left). The client activates their core and performs several diaphragmatic breaths while visualizing being long through the spine. They perform this exercise 6–10 times per day to help alleviate tension and to ensure that they are using a proper breathing-activation strategy throughout the day. The above strategy is then incorporated into trunk stabilization patterns such as the modified dead bug progression. There should be no change in alignment, breathing, or activation strategy throughout any of these progressions.

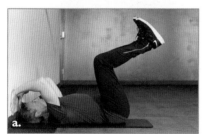
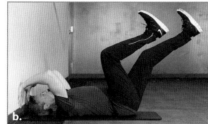
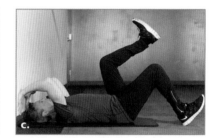
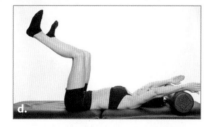
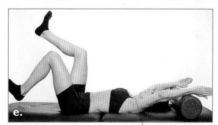

a. **Modified dead bug isometric:** The client lies in neutral spine posture, places his palms against the wall, and activates his serratus anterior, scapulae depressors, and core. He holds this position as he performs 10 reps of 10 deep breaths.

b. **Modified dead bug heel slide:** The client maintains activation from a) and slides one leg away from the starting position, alternating each side and working up to 3 sets of 10 repetitions per leg.

c. **Modified dead bug with heel drop:** The client maintains activation from a) and drops one heel towards the floor, alternating each side.

d. **Modified dead bug with extension bias:** This pattern is great for teaching overhead athletes spinal stabilization with shoulder dissociation. The client lies in neutral spine posture and activates her serratus anterior, scapulae depressors, and core. She maintains pressure into the foam roll and performs 10 repetitions of 5 deep breaths, working up to 10 repetitions of 10 deep breaths.

e. **Modified dead bug with extension bias and heel drop:** The client maintains her activation strategy from d) and performs alternating heel drops.

The most advanced progression is the pelvic lift. The client grasps a supported step or machine and maintains the activation strategy from above. He initiates lift from the abdominal wall and intra-abdominal pressure to raise his pelvis vertically towards the ceiling. He performs 5 sets of 2–3 repetitions, building up to sets of 5–10 repetitions.

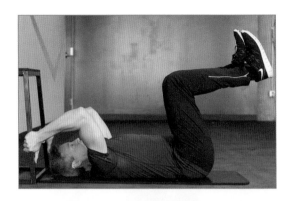

Most clients substitute by posteriorly tilting the pelvis or by performing lumbar flexion – these are incorrect substitutions. The action must be a pure vertical lift to optimally train the high level coordination between intra-abdominal pressure and co-activation of the TPC musculature.

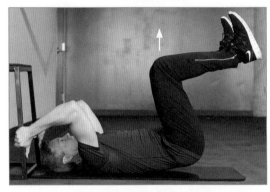

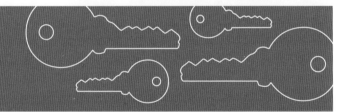

Key To Success
Bracing Vs Activation Strategies

There has been much debate about which is the superior strategy for stabilizing the spine – bracing or hollowing. McGill (2004) has presented the argument that the transversus abdominus and multifidus – in effect the muscles of the local system – can not effectively stabilize the lumbo-pelvic region. Research by Hodges and others (Lee, Hides, Richardson, Jull, et. al.) has demonstrated atrophy and timing delays in the activation of the deep (local) muscle system of the lumbo-pelvic, thorax, and neck region. Their research does not suggest the deep muscle system functions alone in stabilizing the spine, rather that bracing alone does not ensure optimal intersegmental control. Furthermore, studies on individuals with chronic low back pain have demonstrated these individuals tend to use a constant co-activation or bracing strategy (Radebold et. al. 2000) so additional bracing will unlikely improve performance and may actually contribute further to the problem. Therefore, it is necessary to adopt different stabilization strategies given the tasks at hand, as well as teach clients with lumbar instability the technique of isolated activation of the deep stabilization system prior to integrating it back into functional movement patterns.

KEY: The key to improving functional spine stabilization strategies is to increase the client's options rather than provide them with only one option. Improve the client's ability to breathe and maintain co-activation of the deep stabilization system. Use a lighter activation strategy when performing low levels of activity and a bracing-type strategy (i.e. McGill approach) when higher loads are applied to the spine.

THE NEUTRAL HAND AND WRIST

Just as proper foot position is essential to function of the lower extremity, proper hand and wrist alignment enables irradiation to spread through the entire upper extremity and shoulder complex. Similarly, poor hand and wrist stability compromises stability in the entire upper extremity.

In neutral alignment and while loading the upper arm, pressure should be distributed on the tips of the fingers, the metacarpal heads, and equally between the thenar and hypothenar regions of the hand. An equally supported arch should form between the ulnar and radial aspects of the hand.

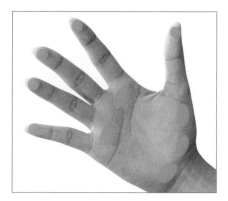

Note the ideal alignment when the hand is loaded – the hand, wrist, elbow, and shoulder are stable (image below left). Also note the increased load-bearing on the hypothenar aspect of the hand and subsequent ulnar deviation of the wrist (image below right). This is a destabilized position of the hand and wrist and must be avoided in all corrective and fundamental movement patterns.

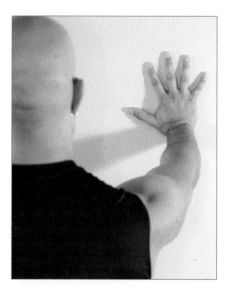 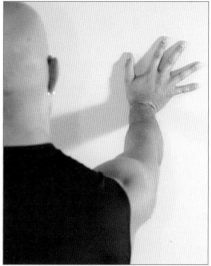

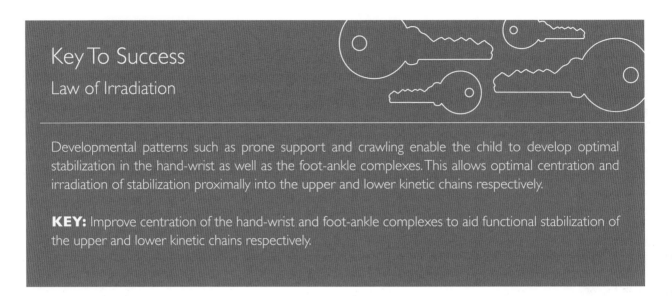

Key To Success
Law of Irradiation

Developmental patterns such as prone support and crawling enable the child to develop optimal stabilization in the hand-wrist as well as the foot-ankle complexes. This allows optimal centration and irradiation of stabilization proximally into the upper and lower kinetic chains respectively.

KEY: Improve centration of the hand-wrist and foot-ankle complexes to aid functional stabilization of the upper and lower kinetic chains respectively.

SUMMARY

The coordination of neutral alignment of all joints, between breathing and stabilization of the thoracopelvic canister, and maintaining this in functional positions of lying, sitting, kneeling, and standing must be included in the first steps of corrective exercise. This activity ensures proximal stability of the spine and trunk with optimal alignment and forces around the proximal structures. Once the client can maintain coordinated activity of diaphragmatic breathing and core activation in these positions, they are ready to progress to functional movement patterns.

chapter 7

Corrective Patterns for the Shoulder and Hip Complexes

CHAPTER OBJECTIVES

To identify and understand the functional components of the corrective exercise and movement paradigm

To identify the key regions necessary for improving function

To develop the specific strategies for corrective exercise and fundamental movement patterns

SHOULDER COMPLEX

DYSFUNCTIONS IN UPPER EXTREMITY PATTERNS

Identifying dysfunctional movement patterns is the first step in the corrective strategy because if dysfunction is not identified, the client will perpetuate their habitual patterns. Therefore, the fitness professional and therapist must become adept at recognizing the signs of dysfunctional patterns which can be identified both visually and through palpation. The fitness professional or therapist will want to observe the client's ability to proximally stabilize while performing diaphragmatic breathing while being able to dissociate the extremities as they perform their patterns. The following section will look at common dysfunctions in the shoulder and upper extremity while the next section will look at similar dysfunction as they relate to the hip and lower extremity. Also, the reader is encouraged to revisit the assessment chapter in Part II for additional observations.

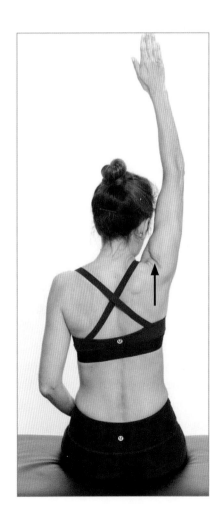

THE DOWNWARD ROTATION SYNDROME AND ANTERIOR HUMERAL GLIDE SYNDROME

The lack of optimal scapular stabilization leads to compensatory patterns during overhead motion. There are several common movement dysfunctions that can be noted as the client to the right raises her arm overhead:

- **Non-optimal scapulothoracic stabilization:** The scapula is moving up over the thorax rather than around it (arrow).

- **Excessive levator scapula activity:** At the superior angle insertion of the levator scapula there is increased tone (arrow) and the neck is pulled into right rotation by the levator scapula.

- **Non-optimal cervical and thoracic spine stabilization:** The cervical spine moves into excessive right lateral flexion and the trunk moves into left lateral flexion due to poor stabilization at the left cervical and right thoracolumbar regions respectively.

In clients with a downward rotation syndrome, the levator scapula and rhomboids assume the primary role of scapular stabilization. During many common exercises such as triceps cable push-downs, the levator scapula will become prominent because there is inadequate inferior stabilization of the scapula by the serratus anterior and lower trapezius. The 'levator scapula sign' (arrow) will be present as the client loads their shoulder (images below. The levator scapula sign is common in many patterns where there is poor scapular stabilization. The therapist or trainer can palpate hypertonicity in the lateral aspect of the neck during many common exercises as increased, indicating overactivity of the levator scapula. The levator scapulae should be relatively quiet and there should not be palpable overactivity during functional movement patterns.

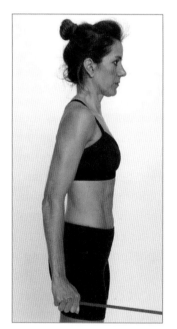
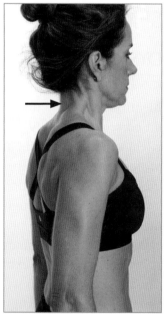

The anterior humeral glide syndrome (Sahrmann 2002) is a common result of scapulohumeral muscle imbalances and is commonly observed as the shoulder moves into extension. A divot will be noted at the posterior aspect of the joint due to the loss of joint centration (right arrow), and the head of the humerus can be observed (left arrow) or palpated as it translates forward, moving on the fossa (image below right). This occurs most often as the arm moves into extension during patterns such as the concentric phase of pulling patterns (e.g. cable rows) and during the eccentric phase of pushing patterns (e.g. cable chest presses). In the anterior humeral glide syndrome, more than one-third of the humeral head will be palpated in front of the acromion process, and the posterior aspect of the humeral head will be palpated forward of the posterior aspect of the acromion process.

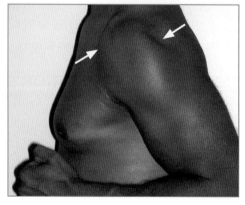

There are three main causes of anterior humeral glide syndrome:

1. **Short posterior joint capsule:** To remain centrated in the glenoid fossa, there must be proper extensibility of the joint capsule. Shortness in the posterior joint capsule does not allow the humerus to move posteriorly in the glenoid fossa, causing an anterior shift in position during extension of the shoulder.

2. **Short posterior rotators:** As mentioned above, the humeral head must remain centrated in the glenoid fossa. Shortness of the posterior rotators, infraspinatus, teres minor, and/or posterior deltoid causes a shift in the axis similar to the short posterior joint capsule.

3. **Muscle imbalances:** Recall, the function of the subscapularis is to draw the humeral head back in the socket. Weakness or inhibition of the subscapularis and pectoralis major and/or dominance of the latissimus dorsi and teres major as internal rotators will drive the head of the humerus forward.

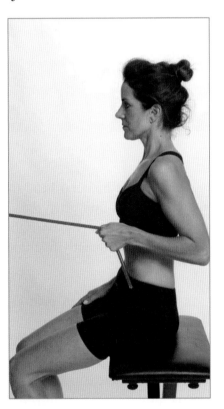 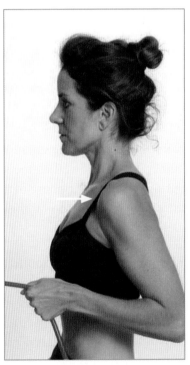

Note the anterior shoulder position which also tends to cause slight elevation of the scapula. Also notice the ulnar deviated position of the wrist – the wrist should remain neutral while performing pushing and pulling patterns.

It is important to observe and correct this position during functional movement patterns because every repetition that the individual is allowed to perform incorrectly brings them one step further in establishing a permanent movement dysfunction. While the short posterior joint capsule is usually a soft-tissue restriction secondary to repetitive injury, the short posterior rotators are usually a result of poor motor patterning or up-regulation secondary to poor motor control of the GH joint by the scapulohumeral muscles. Mobilization of the posterior capsule, release of the posterior rotators, and activation of the subscapularis, in addition to movement retraining, will help reverse this problem. It is helpful to palpate the head of the humerus during corrective exercise and functional patterns to help monitor and cue proper humeral head positioning.

During ideal patterning, the humeral head remains centrated in the glenoid fossa. There should be no anterior migration of the humeral head and no gapping or divots observed in the posterior aspect of the shoulder. Poor patterning is common with biceps curls and many pushing patterns in the presence of poor ST and/or GH stabilization, and the humeral head is consequently driven forward during the eccentric phase of the exercise. If posterior humeral glide is restricted, the humeral head needs to be reseated to help the individual achieve more optimal mechanics. Humeral head centration will be present next.

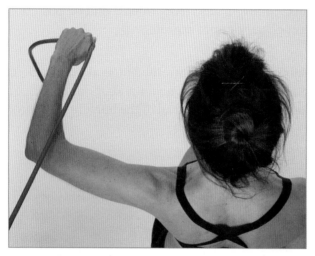 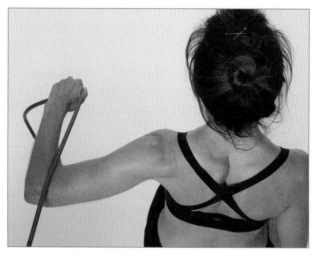

Optimal.   Non-optimal.

Note the optimal alignment of the scapula and humeral head (above left), and poor control of the humeral head as well as the scapulothoracic position when the shoulder is allowed to overly adduct during the eccentric phase of a cable chest push pattern (above right). This can also result from allowing the elbow to come too far posteriorly which subsequently fulcrums the humeral head anteriorly on the glenoid fossa.

The lack of optimal stabilization is often the cause of pain at the compensatory joint segments. Hypermobile segments are created that tend to be where the client will experience pain. The nervous system responds by compensating with areas of hypertonic muscles that are the corresponding locations of myofascial trigger points. As mentioned earlier, this example also illustrates why myofascial approaches that focus on trigger point release often fail to produce long-term results because the primary problem is a stabilization issue and the trigger points are the compensatory issue.

The key to improving shoulder motion function lies in retraining the motor system in three key areas:

1. Stabilize the cervical spine and thorax.

2. Improve stabilization in addition to posterior tilting and upward rotation of the scapula.

3. Integrate steps 1 and 2 into functional movement patterns.

HUMERAL HEAD CENTRATION

RESEATING THE HUMERAL HEAD:
RELEASING POSTERIOR CAPSULE AND EXTERNAL ROTATOR RESTRICTIONS

To reseat the humeral head, perform the posterior capsule and external rotator muscle release. The client lies supine with the arm abducted to around 90 degrees and the therapist standing at the side of the table facing the patient's head. The therapist gently yet firmly grasps the head of the humerus – the fingers wrap around the posterior aspect of the humeral head and the pisiform aspect of the palm is placed over the anterior aspect of the humeral head. Their opposite hand grasps the client's arm, providing a gentle traction to the arm. The therapist instructs the client to take a deep breath in and perform a submaximal isometric contraction of their arm into horizontal adduction against the therapist's resistance for a five-second count. The client then exhales as the therapist simultaneously tractions the arm and, pushing anterior to posterior on the humeral head, glides the humeral head posteriorly in the glenoid fossa (down-facing vertical arrow). This process is repeated 3–5 times until the posterior structures release. Since the posterior capsule restriction is generally due to shortness and stiffness resulting from chronic irritation, it generally requires slightly greater pressure and longer holds. This technique also works well to release a stiff pectoralis minor by simply shifting the hand position and placing the pisiform just above the coracoid process of the scapula and repeating the similar motions. Generally with these releases, the lighter the pressure, the more the client will relax and release the restrictions. Stiffness of the external rotators is a motor control issue and responds much more rapidly and easily to this type of down-regulating technique. Perform ST stabilization and GH integration immediately following this release.

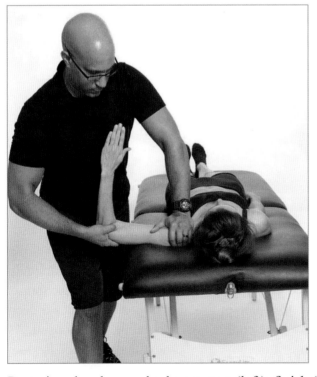 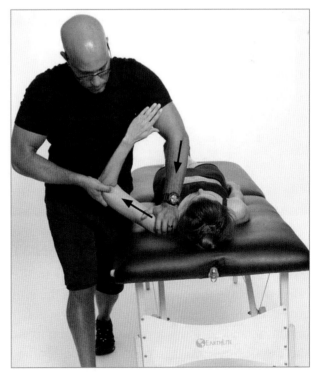

Posterior glenohumeral release: start (left); finish (right).

EVALUATION OF GLENOHUMERAL FLEXION

As mentioned earlier, GH dissociation can also be limited by musculofascial restrictions in the latissimus dorsi so it is important to evaluate shoulder flexion in the unstable shoulder.

ASSESSING THE LENGTH OF THE LATISSIMUS DORSI AND THORACOLUMBAR FASCIA

The client lies supine with her arms straight and by her sides. The client is instructed to keep her arm straight and raise it overhead (sagittal plane flexion). Assess both the range of motion (ROM) as well as the client's ability to maintain her spine on the table and the thorax in an inferior position. Common compensations include thoracolumbar hyperextension and an inability to keep the arms straight and in the sagittal plane. See Video: Establishing Proper Scapular Mechanics, www.osarconsulting.com

Latissimus dorsi length assessment: poor performance (top, note the increase in thoracolumbar extension); ideal performance (below). Note the decrease in shoulder range of motion as the client stabilizes her thoracolumbar junction.

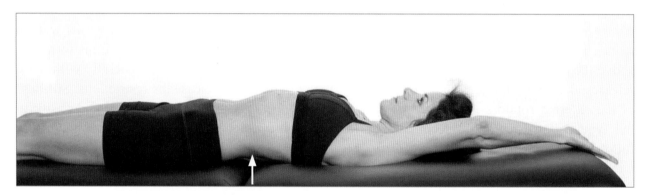

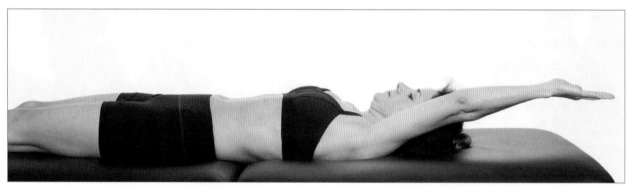

RELEASING THE LATISSIMUS DORSI AND THORACOLUMBAR FASCIA

Using a neuromuscular approach similar to the strategies mentioned above can also be extremely effective. Have the client lie supine with the arm flexed as far as she is able while keeping the thorax connected to the pelvis. The client activates her core to maintain this thorax position, takes a deep breath in, and performs a five-second submaximal isometric contraction into the therapist's hand. As she exhales, release the contraction and let the client's arm move to the next end range of flexion. Repeat this process 3–5 times as additional ROM is gained. Follow up this release with activation of the ST stabilizers and integrate immediately into functional movement patterns.

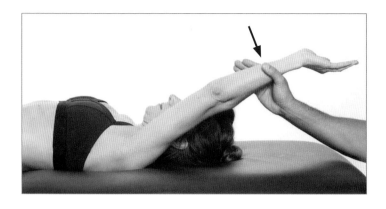

Latissimus dorsi release: the client performs an isometric contraction into the therapist's/trainer's resistance. The resistance is released and the client lowers her arm to the new end range, progressing as far as she can without compromising her TPC stability.

Foam rolling the latissimus dorsi attachments at the posterior scapulohumeral and thoracolumbar regions can be effective at lengthening these structures. Foam roll release of the latissimus dorsi and teres major attachments (below left) and thoracic spine (below right).

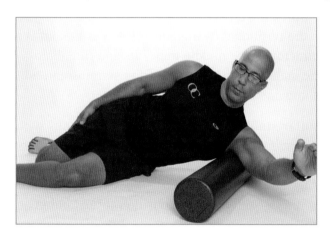 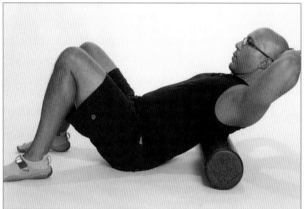

IMAGERY AND CUING FOR IMPROVED SHOULDER FUNCTION

Verbal cuing can have a rather dramatic effect on ideal motor recruitment. The client in image below left was cued to 'squeeze the shoulder blades down and back,' which has resulted in over-adduction, depression, and slight downward rotation of the scapulae. Also notice the slope of the shoulder, indicating overlengthening of the upper trapezius (below left). By cuing the individual to 'relax and wrap the shoulder blades around the thorax,' the scapular position improves (below right).

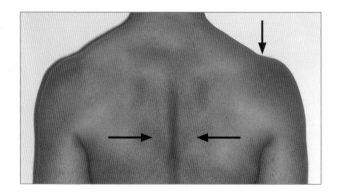 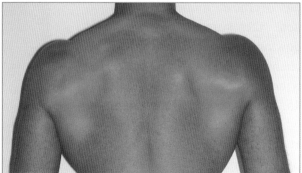

SCAPULAR STABILIZATION – YS, TS, AND WS

Many rehabilitation and corrective exercise articles, books, and on-line resources covering shoulder stabilization contain some version of the Ys, Ts, Ws, and wall angel exercises. These exercises are given to help clients and patients combat the all-too-familiar forward and internally rotated shoulder position. Specifically, Ys, Ts, and Ws are aimed at addressing elevation and protraction of the scapula by having the client or patient perform a combination of scapular adduction and depression. Unfortunately, these exercises fail to address the fundamental issue with the unstable shoulder: scapular dyskinesis. There are two primary issues with scapular dyskinesis that will be discussed below: inadequate scapulothoracic integrity; and poor timing and sequencing between the scapular stabilizers.

1. **Inadequate scapulothoracic integrity:** Poor activation of the scapular stabilizers, primarily the serratus anterior and lower trapezius, in addition to overactivity of the scapula protractors, primarily the pectoralis minor, results in the scapula favoring an anterior tilted position. Termed scapular winging, this is when the inferior angle and lower medial border of the scapula move away from the thorax. This is the position from which the client then performs all their resisted exercises, which tends to perpetuate and worsen the positional dysfunction. The Ys, Ts, and Ws focus primarily on the scapular adductors and retractors – the middle trapezius and rhomboids – and have very negligible effect on improving the stabilization function of the serratus anterior, upper and lower trapezius or improving scapulothoracic integrity.

2. **Poor timing and sequencing between the scapular stabilizers:** One of the biggest faults with scapular dyskinesis is improper timing and sequencing of the scapular stabilizers that favors downward rotation. Often this is seen during the eccentric phase of an overhead motion. The client can often lift their arm overhead with rather good mechanics but as they lower it to the starting position, the scapula seems to 'crash', or returns to the starting position faster, and in an uncontrolled fashion, than the arm. The scapula will often wing more significantly, and even move into downward rotation, before it returns to its resting position. This is an eccentric motor control issue so no amount of Ys, Ts, and Ws will correct this dysfunction as these exercises focus only on the concentric function of the scapular adductors and retractors. The client's scapular motion must be in view to witness these aforementioned mechanics or the trainer or therapist must palpate lightly through their shirt, being careful not to disrupt their normal patterning.

Notice how this client's right scapula is fairly well controlled in the overhead motion (left). Then note the scapular winging and downward rotation (arrow) as the client lowers their arm (right). This winging generally occurs around 45 degrees of shoulder elevation, where the scapular stabilizers are at their most disadvantaged point (longest length-tension).

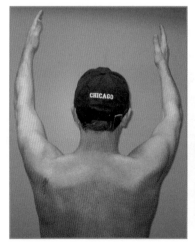 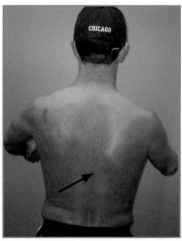

So is there a place for Ys, Ts, and Ws in corrective exercise? These exercises do serve one benefit in corrective exercise and rehabilitation: to train movement awareness of the scapula. In the early phases of rehabilitation or corrective exercise, many clients and patients have very poor scapular awareness. During this phase, Ys, Ts, and Ws can be an effective way to help bring a client's or patient's awareness to their scapulae prior to having them perform more dynamic exercise. However, as stated above, they should only be used on a short-term basis, because the problem these clients have is with eccentric and stabilization control of the scapula, and rarely will concentric exercises such as Ys, Ts, and Ws improve a motor control problem. Ys (left), Ts (middle), and Ws (right). Note the scapular adduction and lack of ST control in this client while performing the patterns.

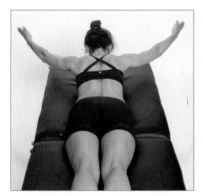 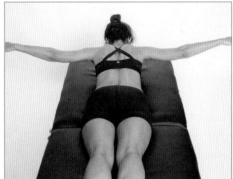 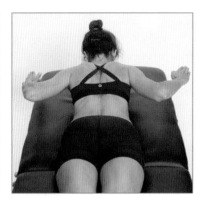

WALL ANGEL

The wall angel is another common scapular stabilization exercise. There are three main problems with this exercise and are discussed below.

1. This exercise creates problems for the client with scapular dyskinesis because the focus of the wall angel is on scapular adduction. Clients experiencing scapular dyskinesis have issues with scapular stabilization, more specifically with scapulae abduction and upward rotation (wrapping the scapulae around the thorax) during overhead motion. The wall angel does not improve this function and can actually add to the lack of optimal abduction of the scapulae during overhead movement.

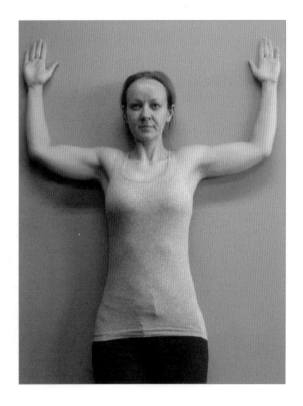

2. The second problem with the wall angel is in clients with poor thoracic stabilization. Often clients will make up for poor thoracic extension by overextending at the thoracolumbar junction (a). This will compromise thoracolumbar stabilization and will not improve scapular function once the client moves away from the wall.

3. The third problem with the wall angel is the disruption of the GH axis of rotation that occurs as the client tries to get the arms against the wall. Clients with a stiff posterior joint capsule or tightness in the external rotators will drive the head of the humerus forward in the socket as they attempt to put their arms against the wall. Clients with poor range of motion in external rotation and/or lacking strength in their scapular stabilizers and external rotators of the GH joint will be unable to get the back of the forearm flush with the wall.

Like the Ys, Ts, and Ws, the wall angel can be beneficial for the client who needs scapular adduction or the kinesthetic postural response provided by the wall. However, ensure that the client can both stabilize the thoracolumbar junction as well as obtain ideal scapular and humeral positions before recommending this exercise.

With soft-tissue release of her latissimus dorsi and thoracolumbar junction, as well as education on TPC stabilization, the client is able to perform a more precise wall angel (b).

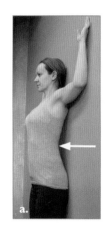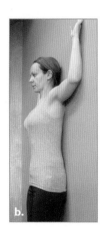

EXERCISE PERFORMANCE

To optimally use the wall to improve spinal and scapular stability, the client stands with their back to the wall. They activate the serratus anterior by reaching their arms long (horizontal arrows in image below). They activate the core stabilizers to maintain a long spine and their back flush to the wall without excessive neck flexion or posterior tilting of the pelvis – the goal should be to get long in the spine. The client reaches their arms to the ceiling in an arcing motion, which helps maintain a stabilized scapular position, and returns to the starting position, reversing the arcing motion. This pattern will generally not be used with individuals with significant postural alterations as they will be unable to achieve the optimal positioning without significant compensations.

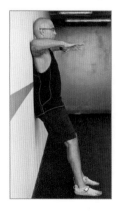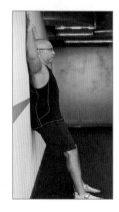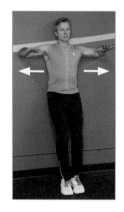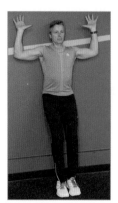

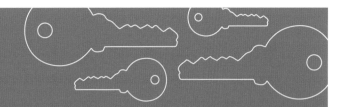

Key To Performance

Wall Angel

- The client maintains a long spine position and core activation throughout the pattern.

- They reach their arms long, maintaining serratus anterior activation throughout the pattern.

- The arms are moved in an arcing-type pattern – the scapula should not elevate during the pattern.

CLIENT SENSATION: The client should feel the tension in the serratus anterior and lower thoracic stabilizers and not experience any neck and upper back tension.

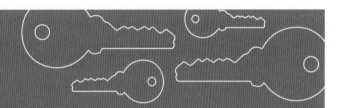

Key To Success

Scapular Dyskinesis: Ys, Ts, and Ws and Wall Angels

Scapular dyskinesis is most accurately described as a motor control issue where there is generally over-activation of the downward rotators and anterior tilters of the scapula. Additionally, improving the stabilization and eccentric function of the upward rotators and posterior tilters of the scapula are key to improving motor control during movement of the shoulder complex. Y's, T's, and W's and wall angels will not improve scapular dyskinesis because the issue is a motor control issue, not an inability to adduct or retract the scapula.

KEY: Work first on improving isometric control and then on eccentric control before proceeding to concentric exercises such as Ys, Ts, and Ws and wall angels for clients and patients with scapular dyskinesis.

PRONE THORACIC EXTENSION

Prone thoracic extensions (PTEs) help to improve most dysfunctional postures – including increased or decreased thoracic kyphosis, lumbar hypo- or hyperlordosis, and pelvic anterior or posterior tilts – because it addresses the fundamental problem of these postural alterations: altered stabilization strategies of the head, neck, and thoracopelvic canister.

By addressing the three key areas of stabilization – the deep neck flexors, the thoracopelvic canister (TPC), and the deep spinal extensors – PTE becomes one of the most effective corrective exercises as well as a necessary prerequisite to performing many of the plank and pushing progressions that will follow.

EXERCISE PERFORMANCE: PHASE I

The client lies prone with the forehead resting on the hands and the elbows resting on the table (below). The client gently tucks the chin and remains with the chin tucked throughout the pattern. Their pubic bone should rest gently on the table and they should visualize the 'long spine.' The scapulae are gently pulled down and around the thorax; essentially they are moving inferiorly and into upward rotation. The client can be cued to gently push the elbows into the table if they are having difficulty determining how to position their scapula. They are then instructed to breathe into the abdomen and low back.

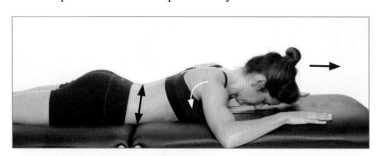

This position is maintained through three breath cycles, working up to maintaining the position and breathing pattern continuously for five minutes.

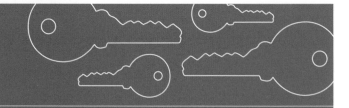

Key To Performance
Prone Thoracic Extension: Phase I

- The client's chin remains tucked and they visualize someone pulling them superiorly from the occiput and inferiorly from the coccyx (horizontal arrows).

- They activate the serratus anterior and lower trapezius to move their scapulae slightly inferior and towards the mid-axillary line of the thorax.

- The client is cued to diaphragmatically breathe from the anterior abdominal wall through to the lumbar spine (vertical arrow).

CLIENT SENSATION: The client should feel as if they are getting longer and that their erector spinae muscle group is relaxed.

EXERCISE PERFORMANCE: PHASE II

Phase II begins the abdominal-breathing co-activation sequence. The client maintains the same position and imagery as in phase I. She activates her abdominal wall and continue diaphragmatic breathing. Begin with one coordinated co-activation breath cycle, working up to ten breath cycles.

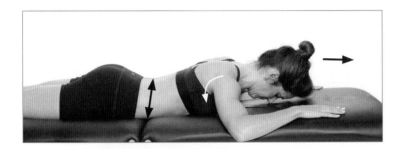

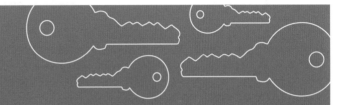

Key To Performance
Prone Thoracic Extension: Phase II

Similar to phase I with the added component of abdominal wall co-activation. The client should be able to maintain this activation throughout the entire breath cycle.

CLIENT SENSATION: As in phase I, the client should feel as if they are getting longer and that their erector spinae muscle group remains relaxed.

EXERCISE PERFORMANCE: PHASE III

Phase III adds in the thoracic extension component to the above sequence. Maintaining phase II co-activation of the abdominal wall with diaphragmatic breathing, the client inhales and begins to slowly lift the thorax and head towards the ceiling. It should be a combined lift with spinal elongation so there should be minimal activity in the lumbar or thoracic erectors. This lift is accomplished through a combination of intra-abdominal pressure and hydraulic amplifier-type activation of the deep thoracic extensors (multifidi and semispinalis thoracis). The client maintains this position for a two-second count and then slowly returns to the starting position on the exhalation.

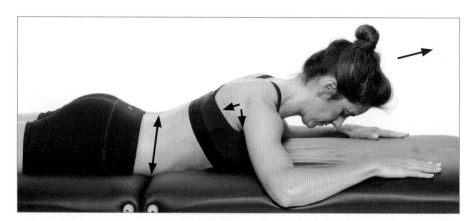

Prone thoracic extension:
Phase III – side view.

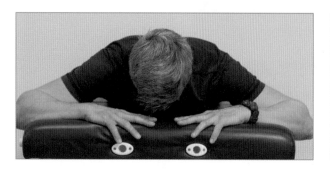
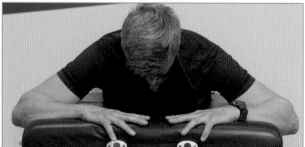

Prone thoracic extension: Phase III – axial view.

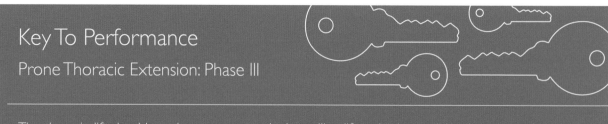

Key To Performance
Prone Thoracic Extension: Phase III

The thoracic lift should not be an up towards the ceiling lift as in the traditional 'superman' exercise, but rather an elongation lift, almost as if blowing up a long balloon. Because the goal of this exercise is activation of the deep spinal stabilizers as well as spinal elongation, palpate your client's erector spinae to ensure that there is no excessive activity. If there is excessive erector activity, have the client relax, reset the position, and repeat with decreased emphasis on the lift and an increased focus on elongating the spine.

Many clients with downward rotation syndrome and overactivation of the levator scapula will struggle with getting the proper activation of the serratus anterior and lower trapezius. If the client has this problem, try the following kinesthetic cue: gently push the client's scapula into elevation and downward rotation and ask them to resist your push (see hand position below). They will then engage the kinesthetic and reflexive action of serratus anterior and lower trapezius activation to resist your tension. Perform this for several repetitions of five-second holds, increasing it to ten-second holds until the client is able to achieve this position on their own.

CLIENT SENSATION: The PTE should be relatively effortless and be a relief position for clients and patients experiencing neck and upper back tension.

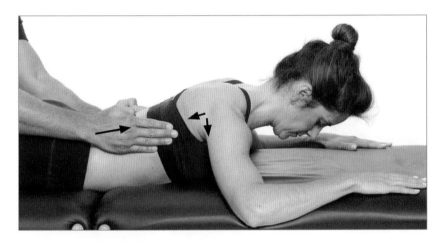

Prone thoracic extension: Phase III – kinesthetic cuing. Cue your client to depress and upwardly rotate the scapula by simultaneously pushing their scapula up towards the head and in towards the spine (longer arrow) as the client resists by pushing inferiorly and anteriorly (two smaller arrows).

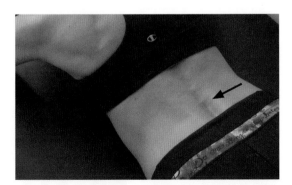 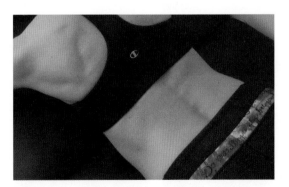

Prone thoracic extension: Phase III – verbal cuing. Notice the hypertonicity and deep valley (arrow) that is created when the client overuses their lumbar erector spinae to perform the thoracic lift (left). Then notice the decreased tonicity and smoother contour that is created once they are cued to 'activate the core and maintain a long spine' (right).

ARM SLIDE

The challenge in restoring ST stability and optimal GH motion lies in the proper positioning of the client as well as in the exercise selection. The following exercise progression is extremely effective at activating the scapular stabilizers, mainly the serratus anterior and the lower trapezius, in their most functional position – abduction, upward rotation, and posterior tilt. Moreover, these patterns aid in 'grooving' the proper plane of scapulothoracic and glenohumeral motion in addition to improving scapulohumeral dissociation. Recall that in ST dyskinesis, the lack of optimal scapulohumeral dissociation can drive ST dysfunction. The arm slide can help restore this dissociation and improve the coordination between the ST and GH articulations, achieving better serratus anterior and lower trapezius activation. Latissimus dorsi shortness often limits the range of overhead motion and this progression is an effective way to actively lengthen this muscle. Attention must be paid to the nuances of this exercise, as this is a deceptively challenging exercise.

EXERCISE PERFORMANCE: PHASE IA, IB, AND IC

The client begins by facing the wall approximately one step away from it. The arms should be placed with the upper arms parallel to the floor, the medial aspect of the hands in contact with the wall, and the arms slightly wider than shoulder width. The wall aids in supporting some of the weight of the limb as the individual is developing motor control and GH coordination. The client lightly pushes the ulnar aspect of their hand into the wall, activating the serratus anterior, and takes a step towards the wall, simultaneously sliding the arms up the wall in a slight 'Y' angle. The scapulae should be controlled, both during the lifting and lowering of the arms, through activation of the serratus anterior and lower trapezius. Once the client develops proficiency, progress them to a narrower pattern and then perform the unilateral pattern with concurrent thoracic rotation.

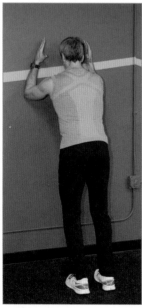 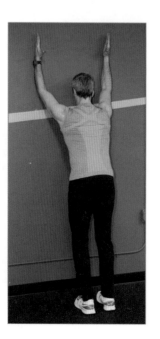 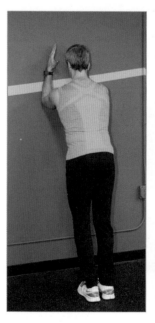 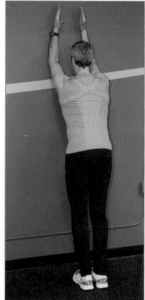

Wall arm slide:
Phase Ia – Y-pattern.

Wall arm slide:
Phase Ib – with narrow arm position.

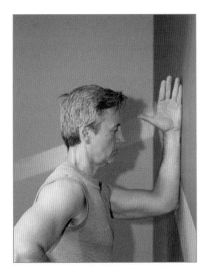 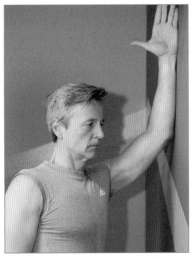

Wall arm slide:
Phase Ic – with thoracic rotation.

EXERCISE PERFORMANCE: PHASE II

Phase II begins with the client lying supine, their hand placed next to the head. The elbow must remain close to the head and pointed towards the ceiling. They activate the core to stabilize the rib cage in an inferior position. The client maintains this position throughout the pattern. They slide their arm along the table or floor as far as they can while maintaining the rib cage and arm positions. They then pull the arm back to the starting position. Begin with ten repetitions, progressing to twenty repetitions as the client gains control.

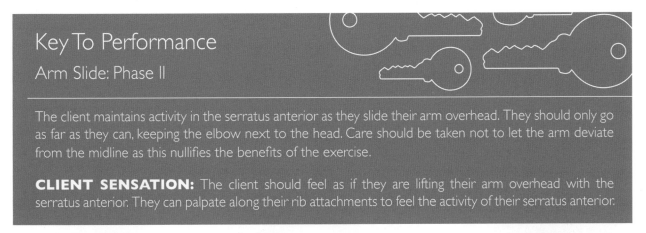

Key To Performance
Arm Slide: Phase II

The client maintains activity in the serratus anterior as they slide their arm overhead. They should only go as far as they can, keeping the elbow next to the head. Care should be taken not to let the arm deviate from the midline as this nullifies the benefits of the exercise.

CLIENT SENSATION: The client should feel as if they are lifting their arm overhead with the serratus anterior. They can palpate along their rib attachments to feel the activity of their serratus anterior.

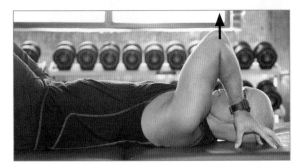 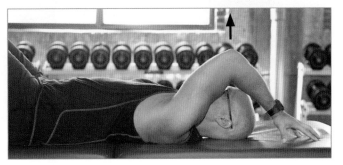

Arm slide: Phase II – supine.

EXERCISE PERFORMANCE: PHASE III

Phase III begins with the client standing with their back against a wall. The spine should remain in a neutral position with the rib cage in an inferior position against the wall. The arm placement is the same as in the lying version. The client activates their core to stabilize the rib cage in an inferior position. They maintain this position throughout the pattern. The client slides their arm along the wall as far as they can while maintaining the rib cage and arm positions. They then pull the arm back to the starting position. Begin with ten repetitions, progressing to twenty repetitions as the client gains control.

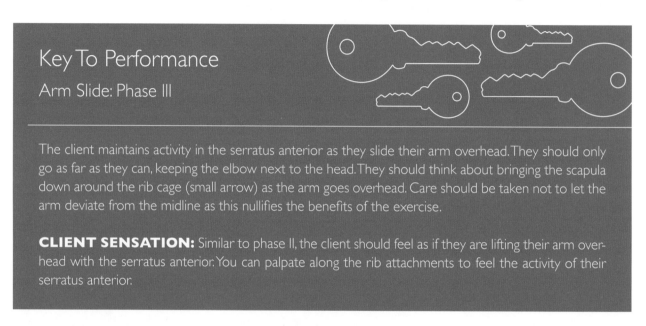

Key To Performance
Arm Slide: Phase III

The client maintains activity in the serratus anterior as they slide their arm overhead. They should only go as far as they can, keeping the elbow next to the head. They should think about bringing the scapula down around the rib cage (small arrow) as the arm goes overhead. Care should be taken not to let the arm deviate from the midline as this nullifies the benefits of the exercise.

CLIENT SENSATION: Similar to phase II, the client should feel as if they are lifting their arm overhead with the serratus anterior. You can palpate along the rib attachments to feel the activity of their serratus anterior.

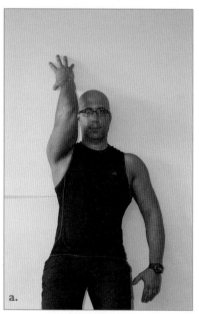
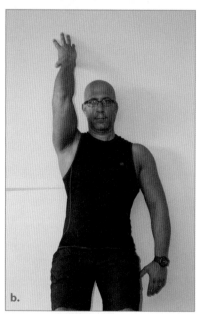
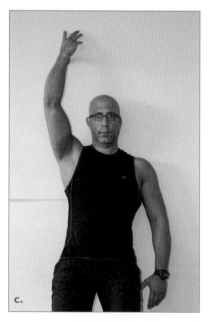

Arm slide: Phase III – wall (a–b). Note poor dissociation in the GH joint and loss of sagittal plane motion when the client tries to exceed his available range of motion (c).

WALL PLANK: PHASE I

Often categorized as a core exercise, the plank series is to the upper body what the squat progression is to the lower body. It is one of the most effective upper body exercises as it trains the entire anterior flexor chain in addition to the scapular stabilizers. Unfortunately, these also tend to be among the most poorly performed exercises by the majority of clients and patients. Precision in performance is key and several progressions for utilizing the plank patterns are outlined next.

Due to low level loading, the wall plank is one of the most effective ways to train, cue, and restore scapular stabilization. Additional benefits include:

1. It teaches neutral spine posture from the head to the feet.

2. It is an easy way to begin teaching core activation and diaphragmatic breathing in the upright position.

3. Because of the flexed arm position, it is an excellent way to restore upward rotation and posterior tilting of the scapulae.

EXERCISE PERFORMANCE

The goal of this exercise is scapular stabilization so the focus is on maintaining a stable position of the stationary arm. The client begins with arms at a comfortable level of flexion – generally with the upper arms approximately parallel to the floor – with the goal of obtaining upward scapular rotation and stabilization. They step approximately 6–12 inches from the wall, placing the forearms and hands flat against it. The client maintains a long spine, core activation, and diaphragmatic breathing. Using the serratus anterior, they push their trunk away from the wall. Maintaining serratus anterior activation, the client reaches one arm up the wall and returns it to the starting position. The stationary arm is the working arm, not the moving arm. There should be no shifting of the neck or thorax throughout the pattern.

Phase II of the wall plank adds a rotational component to the shoulder, which makes it an effective closed-chain rotator cuff exercise. To ensure serratus anterior activation, the client makes sure to push away from the wall throughout the patterns.

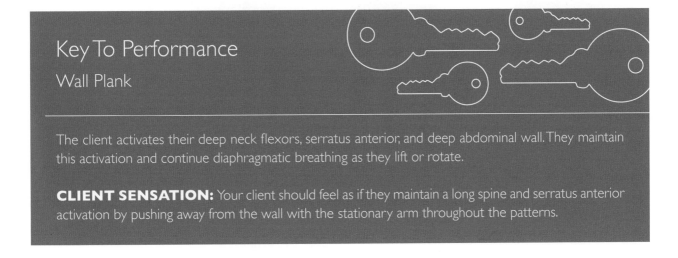

Key To Performance
Wall Plank

The client activates their deep neck flexors, serratus anterior, and deep abdominal wall. They maintain this activation and continue diaphragmatic breathing as they lift or rotate.

CLIENT SENSATION: Your client should feel as if they maintain a long spine and serratus anterior activation by pushing away from the wall with the stationary arm throughout the patterns.

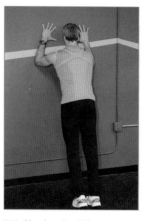 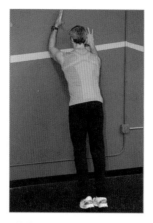 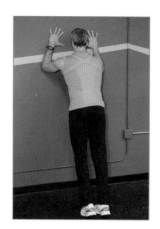 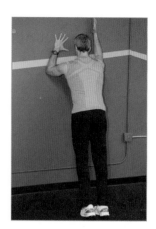

Wall plank: Phase I – arm slide.

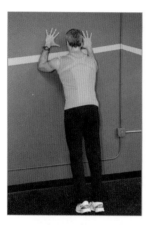 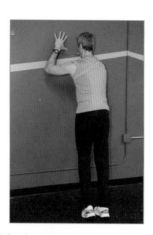 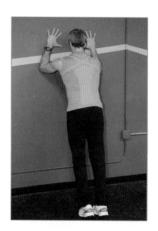 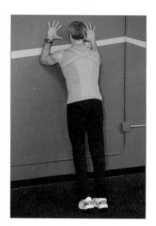

Wall plank: Phase II – with shoulder rotation (elbow support).

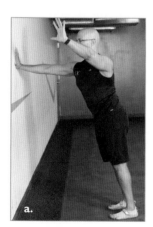 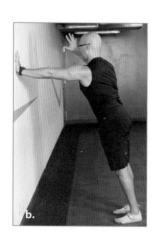 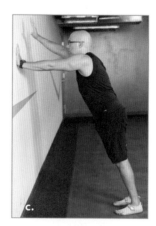

Wall plank: Phase II – with shoulder rotation (hand support) (a–c).

It is important to observe the client for signs of scapular instability throughout the plank series. Note how the client has lost scapular control and the superior, medial border of the right scapula has elevated rather than abducted around the thorax (c). This posture will only get worse once the arm is loaded so it is important to establish scapular stability prior to adding resistance or progressing to a lower plank position.

HIP COMPLEX

DYSFUNCTIONS IN LOWER EXTREMITY PATTERNS

As discussed previously, identifying dysfunctional movement patterns is the first step in the corrective strategy because if dysfunction is not identified, the client will perpetuate their habitual patterns. Therefore, the fitness professional and therapist must become adept at recognizing the signs of dysfunctional patterns which can be identified both visually and through palpation. The fitness professional or therapist will want to observe the client's ability to proximally stabilize while performing diaphragmatic breathing while being able to dissociate the extremities as they perform their patterns. Also refer back to the earlier sections on assessment and hip function, for additional signs of movement dysfunction.

RESEATING THE FEMORAL HEAD

The following technique is extremely effective for improving hip mobility that results from a tight posterior hip capsule restriction or an overactive posterior musculature including the deep external rotators (gemelli and obturators) or superficial fibers of the gluteus maximus. If used with relaxation techniques, this procedure is also effective for relaxing an overactive rectus femoris and tensor fasciae latae. Additionally, it improves hip centration (centers the femoral head in the socket).

Key To Performance
Reseating the Femoral Head

Begin with the client in a supine position with the therapist standing on the affected side. The therapist places their superior hand around the lateral aspect of the client's iliac crest with their fingers monitoring the posterior aspect of the hip, and their inferior hand cupped around the client's knee (1).

Beginning with a gentle compression with the inferior hand, the therapist moves the client's hip into flexion, adduction and internal rotation until a tautness (inability to easily move the joint) is felt (2).

The therapist holds resistance at that point and the client pushes (with approximately 25% of their strength) into the therapist's resistance for approximately 5 seconds (3).

As the client relaxes, the cue to 'relax the hip' or to 'let the hip sink gently back into the socket' is given as the therapist moves the hip to the next barrier or to the point at which the joint cannot be easily moved (4).

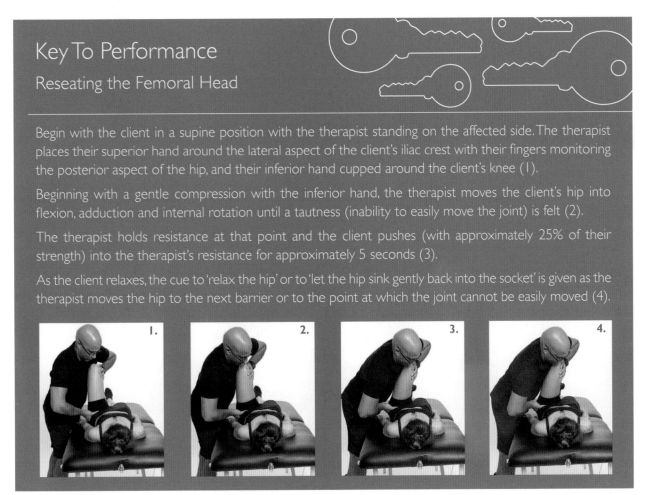

This cycle is repeated 3–5 times or until no further motion at the hip joint is possible. Additionally, with the superior hand, the examiner can palpate a taut area, either in the posterior hip region or over the anterior aspect of the hip, and instructs the client to relax underneath the examiner's fingers by using the cue 'allow the muscles to melt or relax under my fingers.'

This release is followed up with quadruped weight shifts, hip rotations, or some other integrative pattern to allow the client to utilize their newly acquired range of motion.

Please note: If the client experiences hip impingement during this technique, the trainer can bring the hip into more abduction and external rotation during this correction. If this does not change the pattern, specific release techniques for the posterior hip capsule or hip distraction may have to be performed prior to reseating the femoral head.

CLIENT SENSATION: The client should feel as if their hip is more relaxed and there is less restriction to motion.

Clients who are unable to get direct soft-tissue work or require on-going intervention can be given home exercise techniques such as using a foam roll or tennis ball over the posterior hip structures. This strategy works well prior to using a relaxation technique for those clients with overactivity in their posterior hip musculature. Clients without knee problems can perform a pigeon stretch following the soft-tissue release to help relax the posterior hip capsule, which will make it easier for the client to sit back through their hips during the quadruped, hip hinge, and squat patterns. The client must be able to sit back through the hip

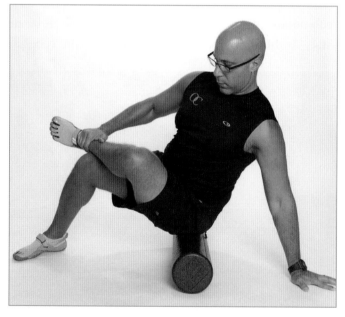

and maintain a squared pelvis during this stretch, otherwise the sacroiliac and lumbosacral joints may be compromised as they become the compensatory regions of mobility. They must follow this release technique with a connection strategy to help engrain and pattern in the newly acquire motion.

HIP DISSOCIATION PATTERNS

As discussed earlier, a common cause of hip restriction is stiffness or tightness in the posterior hip capsule. Stretching of the posterior hip joint structures is rarely effective on its own when there is a restriction in the joint capsule. Hip dissociation is one key to improving functional movement because the inability to dissociate at key joints will lead to dysfunctional movement. While poor dissociation is often a sign of more proximal problems, how and where to move often needs to be brought to the individual's conscious attention. The hip dissociation patterns, including the lying hip rotation, quadruped weight shift, and standing hip hinge, are excellent patterns to teach hip dissociation while actively mobilizing the hip joint and teaching the client to relax the deep hip rotators. Additionally, the quadruped aids in the teaching of neutral scapulae and spinal postures in a low load position. It is an excellent exercise to give to individuals who have just had their hips released from overactive muscular contractions or capsular restrictions.

LYING HIP DISSOCIATION

Hip rotation in the supine position is a low level position to help a client understand how to rotate the hip independent of the pelvis, which is required for normal gait, rotation sports, and essentially every upright fundamental movement.

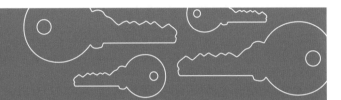

Key To Performance
Lying Hip Dissociation

- The client lies on their back with the knees and hips bent so the feet are flat on the table.
- The core is activated and maintained during the pattern.
- They rotate one hip, dropping the leg away from the midline.
- They then rotate the leg back to the starting position and repeat on the other side.

CLIENT SENSATION: The client should feel as if they are maintaining core activation and a stable pelvis/spine position throughout the pattern.

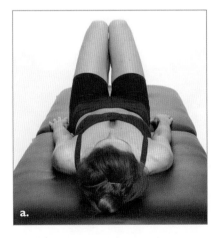
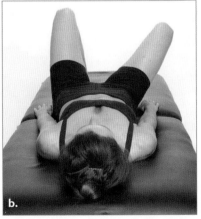
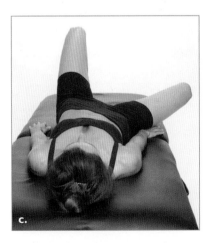

Lying hip dissociation (a–b). Poor hip dissociation: notice how the client's pelvis rotates as they rotate their right hip, because they are unable to optimally dissociate the hip (c). They should be cued to hold their pelvis and spine in neutral positions and repeat the movement. If this strategy fails to improve the pattern, there may be myofascial, capsular, and/or joint restriction that need to be released prior to performing hip dissociation.

QUADRUPED WEIGHT SHIFT

While this pattern may seem simplistic and relatively low level, it is interesting to note that many clients, including high level athletes, have trouble just maintaining a stable quadruped posture. The following key points must be considered to ensure both ideal posture and optimal stabilization of the scapula, spine, and TPC.

- The hands are placed on the floor approximately shoulder width apart and slightly forward of perpendicular.

- The hips are slightly wider than hip width, with the knees under the hips.

- The scapulae stabilizers are activated to wrap the scapula around the thorax.

- The spine is in neutral posture – a stick placed upon the client's spine can help by kinesthetically cuing them to maintain the long spine posture.

- The cue to imagine a string pulling their head superiorly and their tailbone inferiorly is helpful for maintaining the long spine posture.

- The client diaphragmatically breathes while in this position, without changing the spinal position.

- Once they can perform the pattern for 30 seconds in this position without any compromise, they can progress to the quadruped weight shift.

Key To Performance
Quadruped Weight Shift

- The client begins in a quadruped position: the arms and hips are at right angles to the body with the hands slightly wider than the shoulders and the knees slightly wider than the hips.

- Instruct the individual to relax the abdomen in order to relax the lumbar spine into a lordosis while pushing the upper back gently towards the ceiling to restore the thoracic kyphosis. The scapulae are wrapped around the thorax to activate the serratus anterior.

- The client activates their core by gently visualizing a tension wire from the lower abdomen (white arrow) to the low back (or any unstable segment in the spine) – there should be no alteration in spinal position.

- Visualizing a wire attached to the top of their head and one attached to their tailbone, the client imagines the wire on the top of the head and the one on the tailbone being pulled in opposite directions, gently elongating their spine.

- They push through the arms and glide back through the hips while the trainer/therapist monitors and cues them to relax through the posterior hips and maintain a long spine.

- The client continues sliding back as long as they can maintain a neutral spine and there are no deviations (lateral shifts of the pelvis or spine or flexion of the lumbar spine).

- They return to the starting position and as they improve range of motion and 'let go' through the hips they can shift further posteriorly, increasing the range of motion.

- Diaphragmatic breathing should be maintained as they move through the pattern.

- Verbal cues such as 'spread through the sit bones (ischial tuberosities),' 'relax through the back of the hips,' and 'let the hip sink back into the socket' are effective ways to enhance mobilization of the joint capsule.

CLIENT SENSATION: The client should feel as if their hips are completely relaxed with their scapulae stabilized and they more easily achieve a long spine posture.

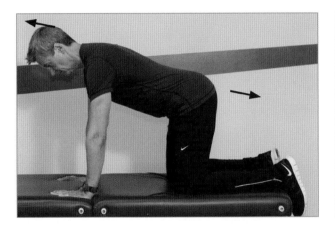 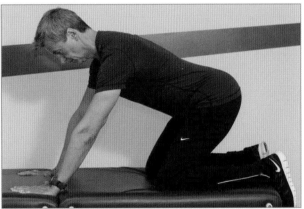

Quadruped weight shift: monitor the individual and ensure that they move only within their ability to stabilize while dissociating through their shoulders and hips. Be sure to assess for neutral spine and scapulae as well as core activation throughout the movement.

HIP HINGE

The hip hinge is a dissociation pattern designed to teach dissociation of the hips from the pelvis. This pattern is key in 'sparing' the spine from the deleterious effects of spinal flexion for those clients with lumbar flexion instabilities. Additionally, it teaches the client to use the posterior hip complex rather than the back and is the preliminary pattern that can be used to 'groove' the squat or deadlifts pattern. The goal is to perform 'pure' hip motion without concurrent spinal motion.

The client begins with her feet approximately hip width apart. She achieves a long spine posture with core activation. The movement begins by the client flexing her hips and pushing them posteriorly. The client thinks of maintaining a long spine posture by visualizing a string pulling her tailbone back (horizontal arrow) and pulling her neck long (oblique arrow). She reaches as far forward as she can without losing spinal neutral and then uses her posterior hip complex to pull herself back to the starting position. Once she can perform fifteen perfect repetitions with no pain, she can be loaded with a light medicine ball or dumbbells. If the client can use more than 25% of her body weight with no pain or loss of control, she can progress to the modified straight leg deadlifts pattern.

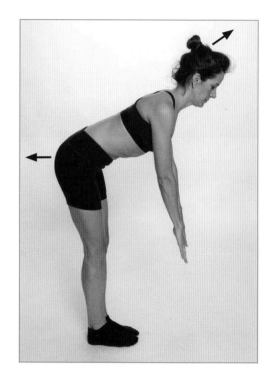

The client demonstrates a poor hip hinge pattern and does not anteriorly rotate her pelvis as she bends forward. She flexes through her lower spine (arrow) and extends her upper spine, thereby overloading the discs and soft tissue structures in both regions.

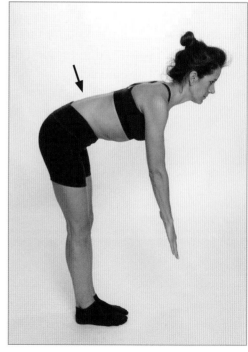

OPEN CLAM SHELL

In both the rehabilitation and training settings, the clam exercise remains king as a common pattern for improving gluteus medius function. Clam shells are performed as a functional warm-up as well as a means of activating the gluteus medius in the hope that it will improve pelvic/hip stability in the upright position. Unfortunately, this rarely occurs as this pattern does little to improve hip centration or coordinate the other hip muscles that help maintain stability in unilateral stance. This does not mean that there is no place for the open clam shell exercise. This pattern is effective for improving dissociation awareness of the hip as well as for improving hip rotation in clients who are in the early phases of rehabilitation.

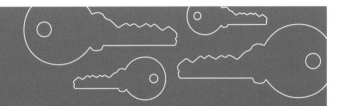

Key To Performance
Open Clam Shell

- The client lies on their side in a neutral spine position with the legs stacked – the hips are flexed to 45 degrees and the knees are flexed to 90 degrees.

- The core is activated and maintained during the pattern.

- They lift their top knee off the bottom knee, raising it as high as they are able without changing their pelvic position.

- This position is held for 1–3 seconds before returning slowly to the starting position.

- Resistance can be applied by the trainer or therapist over the top knee or by wrapping a theraband over the knees, but making sure that there is no breakdown in form.

CLIENT SENSATION: The client should feel as if the posterior aspect of the top hip is activating and that they are maintaining core activation and a stable pelvis/spine position throughout the pattern.

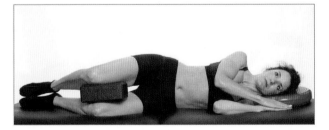 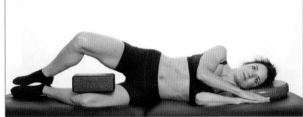

Open clam shell.

REVERSE CLAM SHELL

Any client participating in a rotary sport such as tennis, golf, or throwing requires significant internal rotation of their lead hip during the follow-through portion of the exercise. Loss of internal rotation leads to compensatory movement dysfunction through the lumbar spine and/or knee. The reverse clam shell exercise is a direct way of restoring internal hip rotation and specifically the function of the tensor fasciae latae and anterior fibers of gluteus medius.

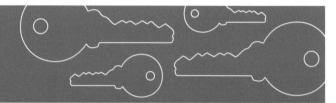

Key To Performance
Reverse Clam Shell

- The client lies on their side in a neutral spine position with the legs stacked – the hips are flexed to 45 degrees, the knees are flexed to 90 degrees, and a small ball or towel is placed between the knees.

- The core is activated and maintained during the pattern.

- They rotate their hip by lifting the top ankle/foot up towards the ceiling as high as they are able without changing their pelvic position.

- This position is held for 1–3 seconds before returning slowly to the starting position.

- Resistance can be applied by the trainer or therapist over the top knee or by wrapping a theraband over the knees, but making sure that there is no breakdown in form.

CLIENT SENSATION: The client should feel as if the anterior aspect of the top hip is activating and that they are maintaining core activation and a stable pelvis/spine position throughout the pattern.

Please note: this pattern should only be performed with clients specifically requiring internal rotation and only for specific pre-event activation. This pattern can cause increased tensor fasciae latae tension in clients who overdo this motion and in those with poor overall hip stability. Often, improving hip centration and function of the TPC will improve deficits in internal hip rotation.

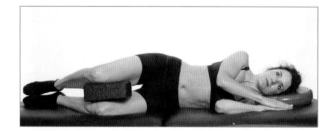
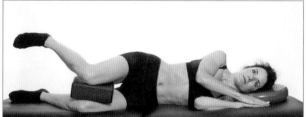

Reverse clam shell.

CLOSED CLAM SHELL

As mentioned earlier, the open clam shell pattern is rarely effective beyond the initial phases of therapy for improving stabilization in unilateral weight support as it does not improve either centration of the hip or closed-chain function of the gluteal complex. The closed clam shell exercise improves hip centration by activating the hip flexors (psoas major), hip abductors (posterior fibers of gluteus medius and minimus), and external rotators (gemelli, obturators, piriformis). Additionally, this pattern begins the progression of closed-chain hip activation, making it one of the most effective exercises for improving hip centration and stability.

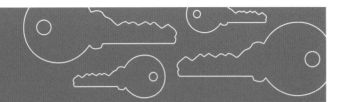

Key To Performance
Closed Clam Shell

- The client sets up in a similar position to the traditional clam shell exercise except that they move the top leg behind the bottom leg and support it on a towel or pillow.

- The bottom hip and knee are flexed to 90 degrees and the core is activated.

- They push their bottom knee into the table and rotate their foot and lower leg off the table – they must maintain constant pressure of their knee into the table.

- This position is held for 5–10 seconds before returning slowly to the starting position.

- Resistance can be applied by the trainer or therapist both at the knee (into hip extension) and on the medial aspect of the ankle (into hip internal rotation), to help facilitate proper activation.

CLIENT SENSATION: The client should feel as if the posterior aspect of the bottom hip is activating and that they are maintaining the pressure of their knee into the table with no change in pelvis/spine position as the leg is lifted.

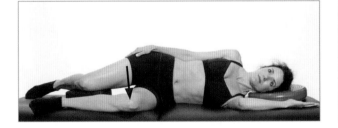
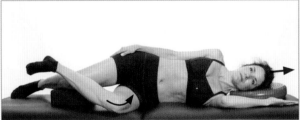

Closed clam shell. The client activates her core, pushes her knee down into the table, and raises her foot off the table.

STANDING HIP DISSOCIATION

The standing hip dissociation pattern is similar to the supine version except that the range of motion will be much less due to the weight bearing nature of the pattern. The client stands against a wall, maintaining a long spine, core activation, and their foot tripod throughout the pattern. This pattern should be slow and controlled as the internal rotation of the hips (a) can stress the medial structures of the knee if performed beyond the client's level of control. External hip rotation (b) must be initiated from the hip rotators, and rotation stops when the client can no longer maintain the big toe in contact with the floor.

Split stance femoroacetabular dissociation is an excellent way to train pelvic dissociation from the femoral head. The client must be able to maintain a neutral TPC and lower extremity symmetry during internal (c) and external (d) hip rotation.

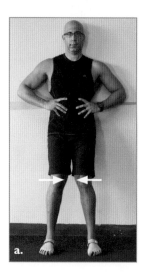
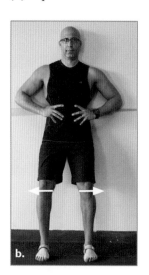
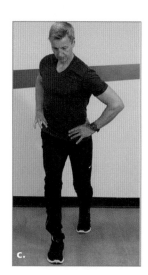
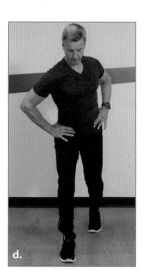

THE CRAB WALK

The crab walk is a common strengthening exercise for the gluteus medius. It is important, however, to ensure that the client maintains a stable spine and control of the lower extremity as the step is performed (a–e). This pattern can be performed by stepping forward, back, to the side, or diagonally. The goal is not to lose centration of the stationary leg or compromise TPC stability against the pull of the band.

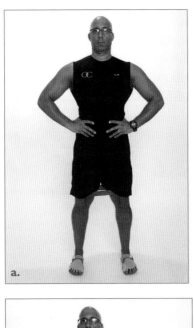
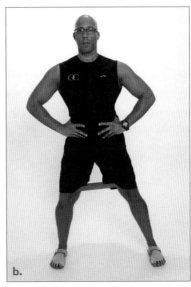
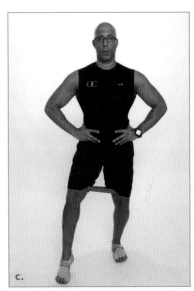
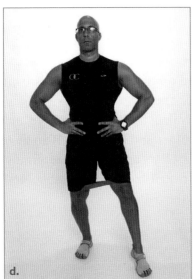
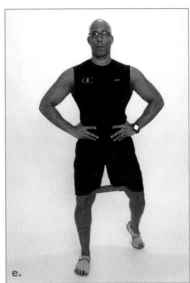
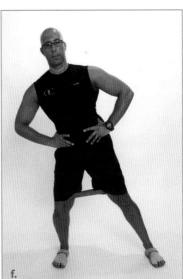

It is common for the client to laterally flex the trunk or pelvis over the leg that they are stepping towards in the presence of hip abductor weakness or poor TPC stability (f). Another common compensation is abduction or internal rotation of the leg that they are stepping away from as the band is pulled taut.

MODIFIED SIDE BRIDGE

The modified side bridge pattern is an excellent corrective exercise progression that effectively works to improve unilateral shoulder, trunk, and hip stabilization. It is designed to teach unilateral support while synergistically connecting the scapular and TPC stabilizers. Reaching of the unsupported (top) arm helps drive spinal mobility as the support (bottom) arm helps stabilize the spine in the level III pattern.

LEVEL I

The starting position can be used as an isolated stabilization exercise progression by having the client isometrically activate their scapular and trunk stabilizers. The client lies on their side with the shoulder, elbow, hip, and knee flexed to 90 degrees. They push their down-side elbow and knee into the table, activating the stabilizers and external rotators of both the shoulder and hip (see image right). This isometric position is held for 5–10 seconds and repeated 5–10 times.

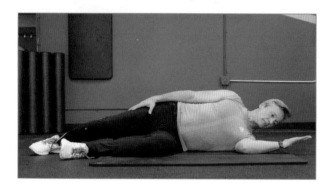

LEVEL II

Progressing to level II, the client begins in a side lying pattern propped on the elbow, which is bent to 90 degrees. Their down-side hip and knee are flexed to 45 degrees. Their top arm rests on their side and the top leg rests behind the bottom leg (image above left). The client activates their core and pushes their downside elbow into the floor to internally rotate their shoulder and lift themselves so they are supported on their forearm (image above right). This is held for 1–3 seconds before returning slowly to the starting position, controlling the descent until they are rested back on the table, and repeating 3–5 times. They maintain the long spine position throughout the pattern.

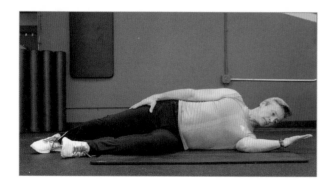
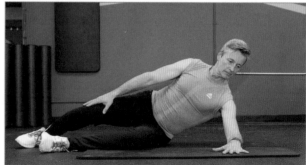

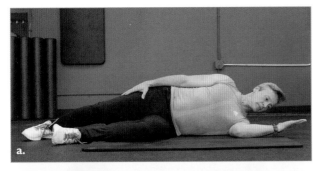
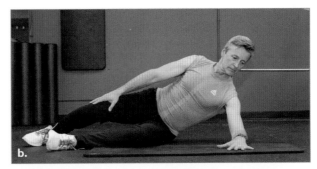
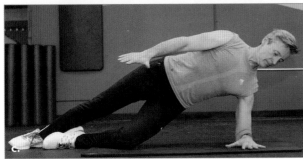
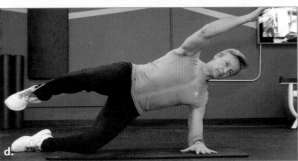

The final progression incorporates levels I – II as the client supports themselves in ipsilateral support and contralateral reaching (a–d). They hold this supported position for a 3-second count and slowly decelerate back to the starting position. It is important that the client is able to maintain ST and TPC stabilization throughout the entire pattern.

LOWER EXTREMITY STABILIZATION TECHNIQUE

Once the client establishes a centred hip position and they understand and can incorporate an ideal hip hinge strategy, increased attention can be directed to the functional integration of the lumbopelvic-hip complex and lower extremity in functional patterning. Focus can be placed on activation of the

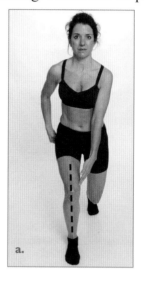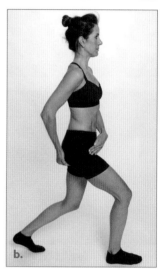

medial stabilization chain by visualizing a wire connecting the medial aspect of the foot and knee to the medial portion of the hip (dashed line), or by the client applying tactile feedback over the ipsilateral vastus medialis and ensuring that their hip does not shift laterally during the pattern (a). This connection is extremely effective for clients demonstrating a pronation syndrome (adduction and internal rotation of the hip and knee, in addition to collapse of the medial longitudinal arch of the foot), for which a connection can be visualized from the medial aspect of the arch to the ipsilateral gluteus medius or maximus.

Clients who are chronic 'butt-grippers' can be cued to improve their hip centration during functional patterns (b). They are instructed to relax through their posterior hip 'gripping', by placing one hand over the anterior hip and one hand on the posterior aspect of the hip, and thinking about relaxing through the front of the hip and sitting back through the back of the hip.

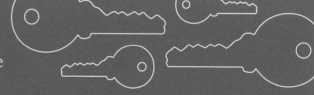

Key To Performance
Lower Extremity Stabilization Technique

- The client sets up in a split stance position with neutral spine posture, a squared pelvis, and the foot tripod.

- They visualize a connection from the arch of the foot, up the inside of the lower leg, and into the medial lower gluteus maximus or laterally into the gluteus medius.

- The client maintains this connection as they lower themselves into a squat position. Again maintaining this connection, they lift from the gluteus maximus to return to the starting position. There should be no gripping or lateral pelvic translation as the client returns to the starting position.

(Modified and adapted from specific cues as taught and demonstrated by Linda-Joy Lee in *The Pelvic Girdle, Third Edition* by Diane Lee, 2004 and Lee (2008).

CLIENT SENSATION: The client should feel as if their foot and lower extremity is more stable. They should feel activation through their vastus medialis, adductors, and lower medial gluteus maximus.

MAINTAINING LOWER EXTREMITY STABILITY

Maintaining lower extremity stability is key to performing functional movement patterns in daily life as well as in occupations and recreational activities. Once the client understands how to achieve centration of the lower extremity, a theraband can be used to challenge stability. The client maintains centration of their lower extremity against a medially (a), laterally (b), or diagonally oriented force.

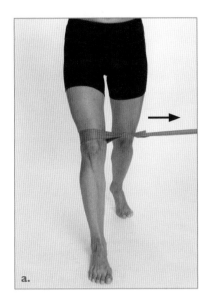 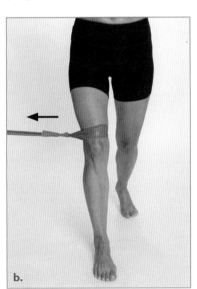

See Video: Hip Dissociation and Lower Extremity Stability During Squat and Split Squat, www.fitnesseducationseminars.com/osar-book

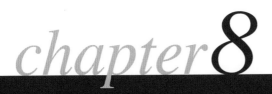

Key Patterns and Movement Progressions for the Shoulder Complex and Upper Extremity

CHAPTER OBJECTIVES

To identify the key patterns of the shoulder complex and upper extremity

To develop the specific strategies for progressing the fundamental movement patterns of the shoulder complex and upper extremity

SCAPULAR MECHANICS DURING FUNCTIONAL EXERCISE

There are many opinions and recommendations by strength, conditioning, and rehabilitation specialists regarding the ideal scapular mechanics during functional movements. Many of these concepts are based upon the movements of scapular depression and retraction to improve stabilization. Unfortunately, these instructional cues often add to shoulder dysfunction rather than help, as they do not improve the most common causes of scapular dyskinesis – mainly stabilization and upward rotation.

Optimal scapular mechanics during functional exercise is described below in relation to common functional vertical and horizontal movement patterns. Regardless of the pattern performed, the scapulae must remain in contact (flush) with the thorax throughout the exercise.

See Video: Neutral Spine Posture and Corrective Exercise,
www.fitnesseducationseminars.com/osar-book

HORIZONTAL PUSHING PATTERNS

Example: dumbbell (DB) and cable chest press

- Concentric phase: the scapulae should abduct (wrap) around the thorax and end up mid-axilla in a neutral or slight upwardly rotated position.

- Eccentric phase: the scapulae should adduct around the thorax under control and end up in the neutral starting position.

VERTICAL PUSHING PATTERNS

Example: overhead shoulder press

- Concentric phase: the scapulae abduct, posteriorly tilt, and upwardly rotate around the thorax and should reach the mid-axilla.

- Eccentric phase: the scapulae should adduct, remain posteriorly tilted, and downwardly rotate to return to the neutral starting position.

HORIZONTAL PULLING PATTERNS

Example: DB and cable row

- Concentric phase: the scapulae should adduct slightly towards, but not reach, the midline – they must remain in neutral alignment.

- Eccentric phase: the scapulae should slightly abduct around the thorax and remain in contact with it, but there should not be excessive scapular abduction – they must remain in neutral alignment.

VERTICAL PULLING PATTERNS

Example: pull-up and cable pull-down

- Concentric phase: the scapulae should posteriorly tilt, adduct slightly, and be pulled into downward rotation to return to a neutral scapulae position – there should be no excessive adduction or squeezing the shoulder blades together, and the client should not be cued to 'pull down and back.'

- Eccentric phase: the scapulae should remain in posterior tilt, abduct slightly, and upwardly rotate – they should remain flat and wrap around the thorax throughout this phase.

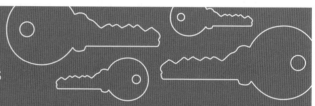

Key To Success

Push-up Plus and Other Similar Serratus Anterior Corrective Exercise Patterns

EMG studies on the push-up plus have demonstrated that it activates the serratus anterior more than other exercises that target this muscle. Unfortunately, EMG studies only show muscle activity and do not demonstrate whether or not the muscle is contracting optimally to provide the desired functional control. Clinically, most clients who demonstrate scapular dyskinesis during their general patterns will display continued dysfunction during the push-up plus exercise. Usually this pattern encourages further downward rotation and anterior tilting of the scapula, despite increased activation of the serratus anterior. Similarly, Lunden et al (2010) demonstrated that the push-up plus exercise, when performed against the wall by healthy individuals, placed the scapula in the exact position that contributes to GH impingement.

KEY: Recall that most cases of scapular dysfunction are problems with functional control and not with strength. So, while the push-up plus may strengthen the serratus anterior, it often does so at the expense of scapulothoracic stability. Ensure optimal scapulothoracic positioning and control prior to performing a push-up plus, regular push-up, or similar type of pattern.

HORIZONTAL PUSHING PATTERNS

Description: Any pattern where a resistance that is perpendicularly oriented to the position of the body and is pushed away from the body or where the horizontally oriented body is being pushed away from the fixed hands.

Example: Standing – cable or band chest press; supine – chest press using dumbbells, barbells, medicine balls, or kettle bells; prone – push-up.

PUSH-UP

The push-up (PU) is a progression from the plank and one of the great functional exercises providing a training stimulus to the entire shoulder complex, thorax, and lumbopelvic-hip complex. It can be utilized as a tool for both evaluation and training purposes. All clients can perform PUs by manipulating the angle of the body. For clients demonstrating poor scapular stability, rehabilitating an injury, or possessing lower levels of strength, the incline push-up is a great way to begin. This pattern is preferred to the modified knee version of the PU because it incorporates the entire lower kinetic chain. Through all PU progressions, adhere to the following guidelines:

- The client begins with a slightly wider than shoulder width grip on the bar or surface.
- The head, thorax and lumbar spine, and pelvis must be held in a neutral position and remain in this position throughout the entire pattern.
- The client activates their serratus anterior and core and maintains this activation.
- They slowly lower their trunk towards the bar while maintaining their posture and activation patterns – the body should remain in a straight line.
- They push away from the bar, floor, or apparatus to return to the starting position.

As mentioned earlier, the scapulae should remain stable throughout the movement, with only minor abduction (scapula moving away from the spine) during the concentric phase (pushing up) and minor adduction (scapula moving towards the spine) during the eccentric phase (lowering down). Using the visualization and verbal cue of 'push the bar or floor away from you' during both the lowering (eccentric) and raising (concentric) phases of the exercise seems to result in improved activation of the serratus anterior.

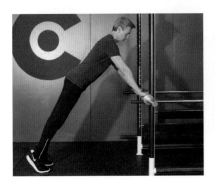 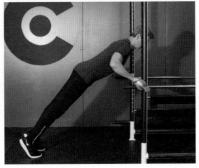

Incline push-up.

As the client progresses, simply lower the bar to increase the challenge. A Smith machine or power rack with a barbell are ideal for progressing clients to lower levels.

Progress to a floor-based PU for clients demonstrating control in the incline version. Ensure neutral spine posture as well as serratus anterior and core activation throughout the movement.

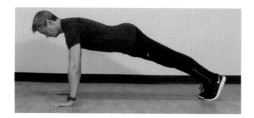 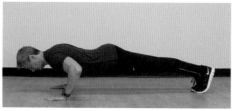

Floor-based push-up.

Performing the PU with the upper body over a stability ball adds a proprioceptive challenge to the exercise. Using balls of varying sizes and densities adds different challenges to both the stabilization and movement systems. Ensure that your client can perform the basic PU before progressing to the following versions. As strength and stability improve, increase the challenge by performing the PU over a pair of medicine balls or a stability ball.

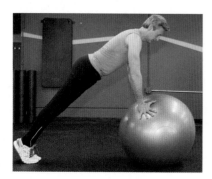 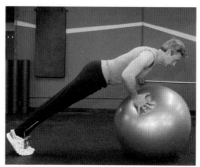

Push-up with stability ball.

Alternating limb patterns, elevating the body, or elevating the legs add increased proprioceptive and stabilization challenges to those individuals who demonstrate exceptional core stability and upper body strength.

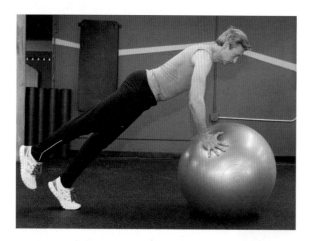 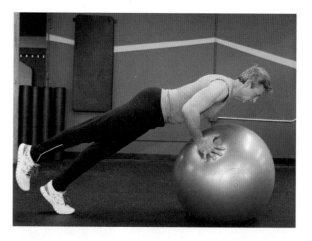

Push-up progressions on the stability ball (continued opposite).

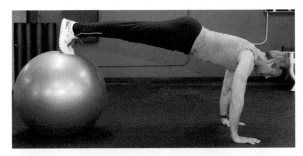

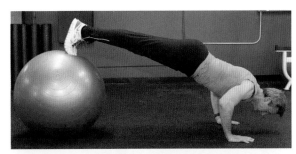

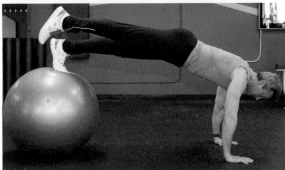

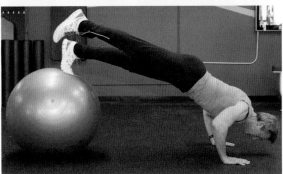

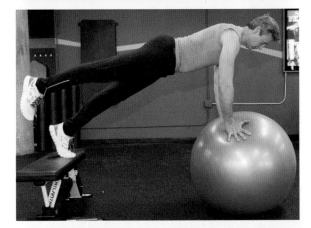

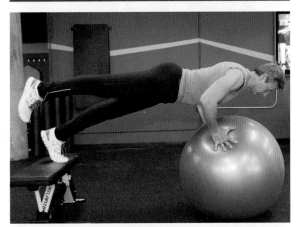

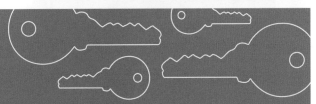

Key To Performance

Push-up Progressions

Throughout each of the progressions, the client activates their deep neck flexors, serratus anterior, and deep abdominal wall. They maintain this activation and bend the elbows as the body is lowered towards the hands and as the arms are extended to return to the starting position. Their body should remain in a straight line throughout the pattern.

CLIENT SENSATION: Your client should feel that they maintain activation and a long spine throughout the pattern. They should feel significant tension in the anterior flexor chain, including the pectoralis major, serratus anterior, abdominal wall and arms.

TRX PLANK PUSH-UP PROGRESSIONS

The TRX can be utilized to perform many plank and push-up type patterns. The individual is progressed appropriately, based on their ability to stabilize and complete the pattern without compensations.

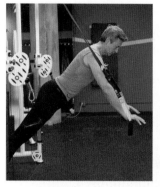 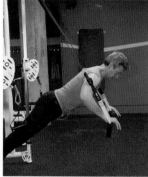 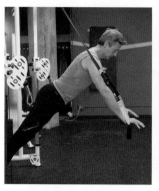 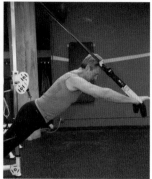

TRX push-up.   TRX plank level I.

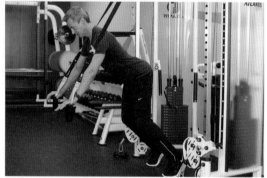 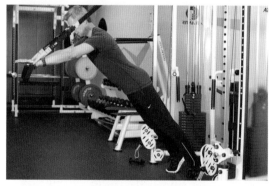

TRX plank level II.

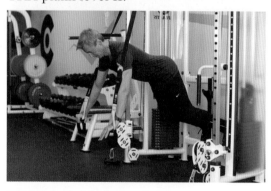 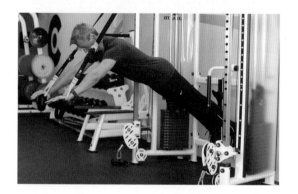

TRX plank level III.

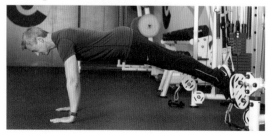 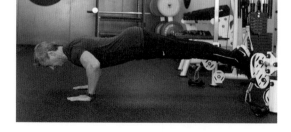

Advanced TRX push-up.

PIKE PUSH-UP

The pike push-up, also known as a V-up, over a stability ball or on a TRX is a great way to train motion of the scapula around a stable humeral head. The individual must be able to maintain scapulothoracic and thoracopelvic control throughout the pattern.

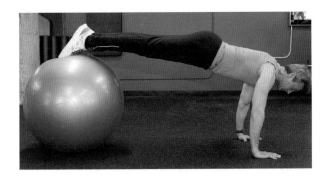
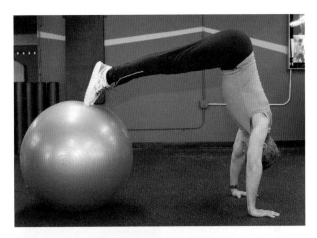
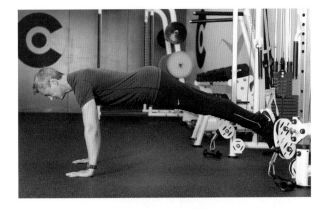
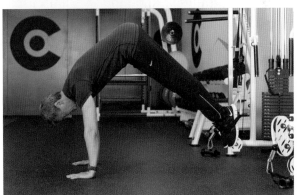

T-STABILIZATION PUSH-UP

The T-stabilization push-up (T-PU) is an excellent movement for the more advanced individual requiring strength and stability through the shoulder complex. This is an especially effective pattern for football linemen, wrestlers, and anyone needing dynamic strength and stability of the shoulder complex. It is vitally important that the client can perform the basic push-up and plank walk-out flawlessly before beginning the T-PU. (The plank walk-out is achieving the plank position and slowly walking the arms away from the start position and moving them back to the start position without losing scapular or spine control.)

EXERCISE PERFORMANCE

The client begins in a push-up position. They lower their body towards the floor and then push themselves up, rotating their torso onto one arm. At the top of the movement, the arm should be straight, the scapula should be resting flat against the thoracic cage, and the spine and pelvis should be neutral. The client should not have excessive sway during single arm support as this indicates instability in the shoulder and/or core. They hold this position for a moment, return to the starting position, and repeat the sequence on the other arm. The progression begins with a split leg position, progresses to a stacked leg position, and finally the abducted leg position.

T-PU:
split leg position.

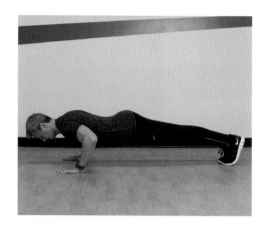
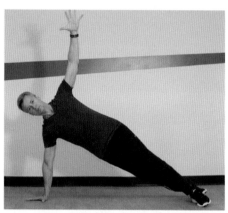

T-PU:
stacked leg position.

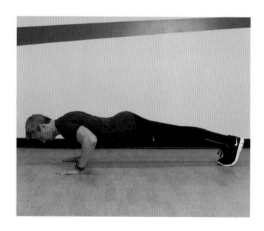
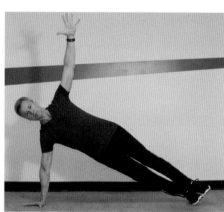

T-PU:
abducted leg position.

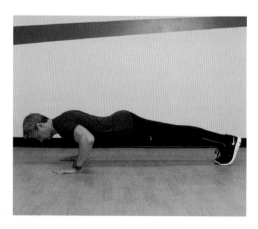
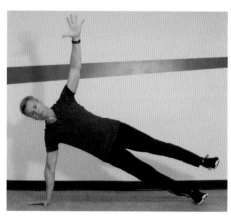

T-PUs can be loaded with light dumbbells (usually 5–20 lb) to increase the stabilization demands on both the core and the shoulder complex (a–c). Ensure a neutral spine position and monitor for the following signs of instability or weakness of the stabilization system: swaying (excessive motion) or sagging of the spine (spine goes into lateral flexion in the unilateral arm support position and can no longer be maintained in a straight line), as well as adduction, downward rotation, and/or flaring of the scapula.

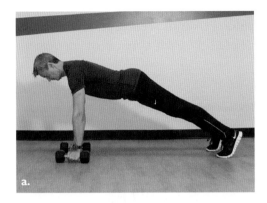
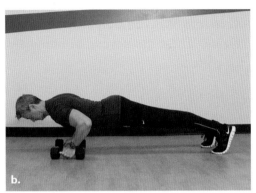

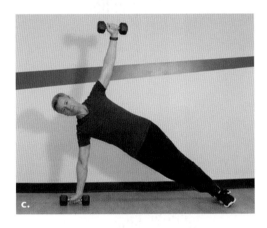

T-PU:
with dumbbells.

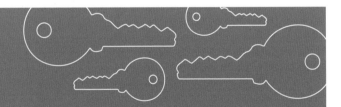

Key To Performance
T-Stabilization Push-up Progressions

Throughout each of the progressions, the client activates their deep neck flexors, serratus anterior, and deep abdominal wall. They maintain this activation, bend the elbows as they lower their body towards the hands and extend up onto one arm to return to the starting position. The body should remain in a straight line throughout the pattern and a straight support arm maintained, with no significant swaying or scapular collapse.

CLIENT SENSATION: Your client should feel that they maintain activation and a long spine throughout the pattern.

CABLE CHEST PRESS

Pushing patterns are one of the fundamental movement patterns equally targeting every stabilizer of the upper extremity and core. Cables and bands offer an additional dynamic training component, enabling the conditioning of the anterior flexor chain and allowing the lumbopelvic-hip complex to work in unison with the upper extremity in an upright versus supine posture. Performing a unilateral pattern introduces a rotary component that must be controlled by the anterior oblique chain. While there are several progressions that can be performed, the unilateral pattern with a parallel or split stance is the basic version. There are several commonalities shared by each version of movement pattern. Throughout the pattern:

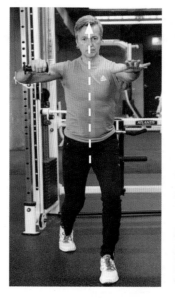 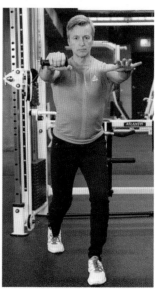

- the spine must remain in a neutral position and long;

- the core and scapular stabilizers must remain activated;

- the arm must be decelerated during the return and the elbow not allowed to extend past the shoulder in individuals with scapular or humeral instabilities;

- motion is initiated at the trunk and finished through the extremity;

- the scapula must abduct around the thorax during the concentric phase, and there should be a controlled adduction back to the starting position.

Once the basic version has been mastered, follow the proper progressions by varying the client's stance, trunk position, and torso range of motion.

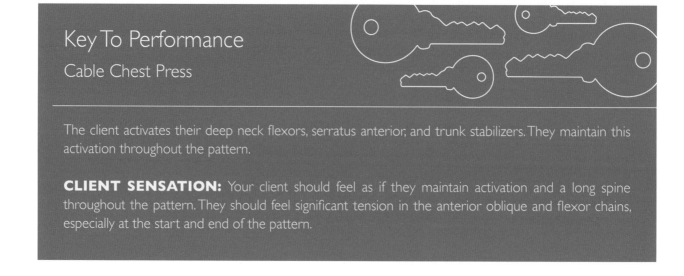

Key To Performance
Cable Chest Press

The client activates their deep neck flexors, serratus anterior, and trunk stabilizers. They maintain this activation throughout the pattern.

CLIENT SENSATION: Your client should feel as if they maintain activation and a long spine throughout the pattern. They should feel significant tension in the anterior oblique and flexor chains, especially at the start and end of the pattern.

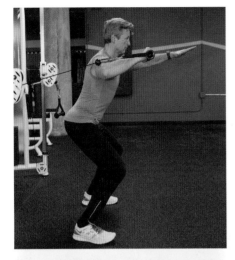
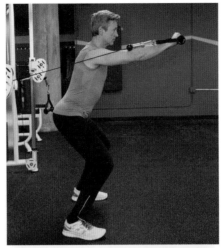

Cable chest press: parallel stance.

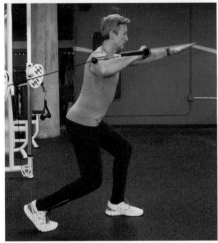
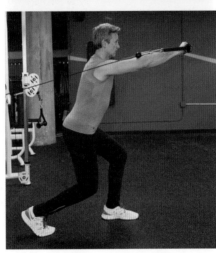

Cable chest press: split stance.

While any pattern performed in unilateral fashion introduces a rotary component, adding the trunk rotation component helps to turn this movement into a mobility pattern for the thorax. The free arm can remain fixed or can perform a pulling-type motion to aid thorax rotation. With the dynamic version, be sure the individual rotates through the front hip and pivots on the ball of the rear foot.

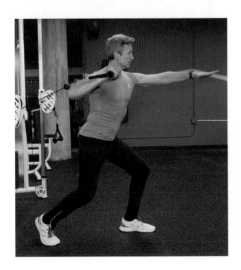
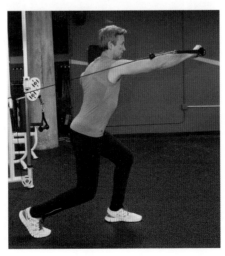

Cable chest press with rotation.

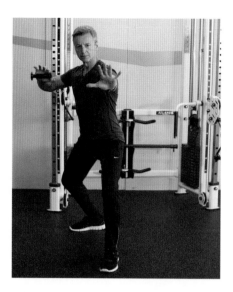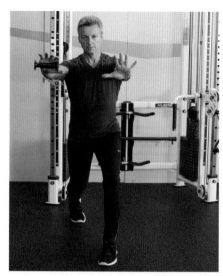

Cable chest press
with rotation: dynamic.

The alternating cable chest press with rotation is one of the most effective ways to train dynamic rotational strength and stability in the anterior oblique chain. This exercise also serves as a more functional alternative to the oblique crunch, as it works the entire abdominal wall in the more functional upright position while integrating hip and core co-activation. The static version without hip motion requires significant core control while the rotating version (with hip rotation, e–f) can be performed more rapidly to increase functional carry-over of the anterior oblique chain.

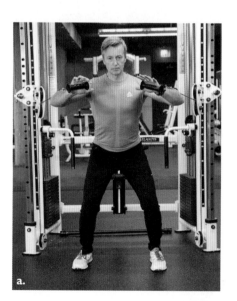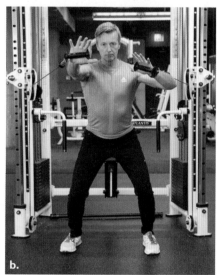

Alternating cable chest
press: static stance.

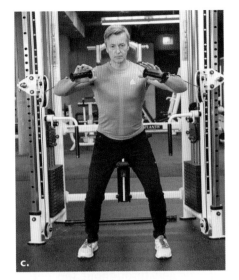

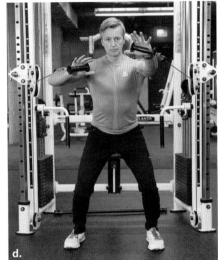

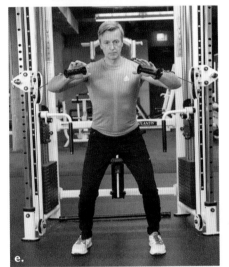

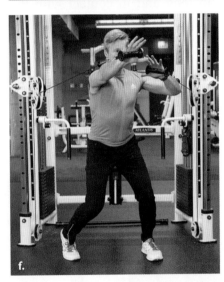

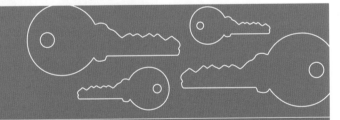

Cable chest press with hip rotation.

Key To Performance
Alternating Cable Chest Press

The client activates their deep neck flexors, serratus anterior, and trunk stabilizers. They maintain this activation and a long spine throughout the pattern. Rotation occurs around the stationary hip with a slight amount of trunk rotation.

CLIENT SENSATION: Your client should feel as if they maintain activation and are rotating on a longitudinal axis through the spine. They should feel significant tension in the anterior oblique and flexor chains, especially at the start and during the eccentric phase of the pattern.

DUMBBELL CHEST PRESS

While DB and barbell versions of the chest press are extremely popular and effective for developing upper body strength, the way many clients perform them actually adds to postural dysfunctions, such as forward head position and internal shoulder rotation, as well as ST and TL instabilities. These patterns are often cued using the powerlifting model, where the client is instructed to pull the scapula down and back and arch the back as much as possible. While this posture allows powerlifters and bodybuilders to lift more weight, unfortunately these cues perpetuate depression and downward rotation of the scapula and hyperextension of the thoracolumbar junction. Remember, the goal for the general population clients is injury reduction. The aforementioned cues increase the likelihood of injuries and, given the high incidence of shoulder injuries in clients who perform these exercises, it is better to avoid these exercises with the general and post-rehabilitation populations.

Ideally, the scapula should remain in a neutral, activated position, which is wrapped around the thorax. The entire spine should remain long and in contact with the bench surface throughout the entire duration of the exercise. If performing the chest press on a stability ball, the head and shoulders should be positioned on the ball and the spine should remain long. Utilize both alternating and unilateral patterns to reduce the potential for thoracic stiffness and to promote reciprocal motion through the trunk and upper extremities. In unilateral patterns, hold the free arm stable to stabilize one side of the thorax while the other side drives thoracic motion as it performs the press.

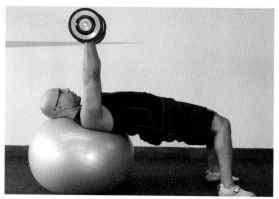
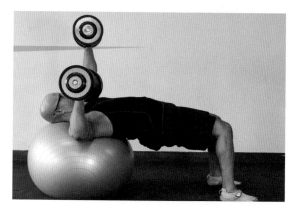

DB chest press on stability ball: alternating.

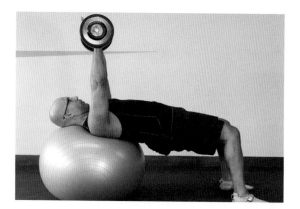
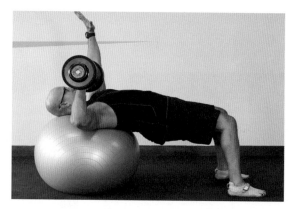

DB chest press on stability ball: unilateral.

ALTERNATING CABLE CHEST FLY

Cable flys are a common exercise, routinely performed as part of a pushing circuit. The basic version of the cable fly as performed by most individuals is essentially a non-functional movement as it is performed in a stationary position and often with little attention to what is occurring through the shoulder complex. With simple modifications such as alternating stepping leg and reaching arm, the cable fly can be an extremely effective exercise in training the entire anterior shoulder complex along with the anterior oblique chain.

There are several key points to adhere to during the alternating cable fly pattern. The client should:

- maintain neutral spinal alignment and core activation during the pattern;

- maintain a long spine and rotate on a longitudinal axis through the spine;

- stabilize the scapula throughout the pattern;

- not allow overstretching of the anterior joint capsule of the shoulder, by allowing the upper arm to decelerate only to the scapular plane (approximately 30 degrees anterior to the frontal plane).

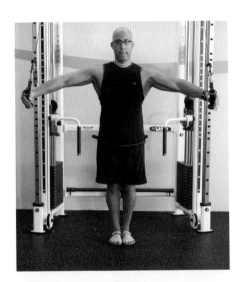
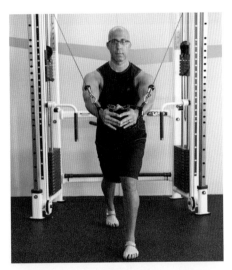
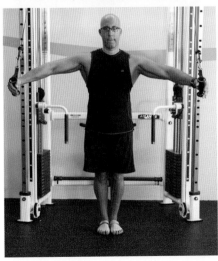
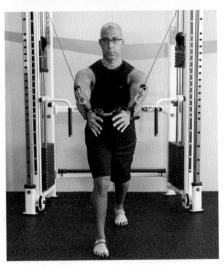

Cable chest fly
with alternating step.

EXERCISE PERFORMANCE

Facing away from a dual cable pulley machine, the client grasps the handles, with the arms in the scapular plane. After activating the core and shoulder stabilizers, the client steps out on one side, pulling the cable in the opposite arm towards the midline of the body. They return to the starting position under control.

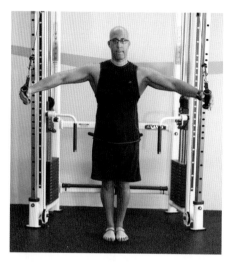
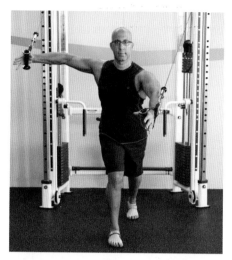
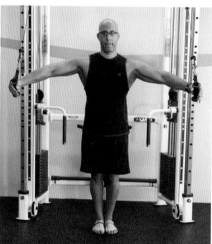
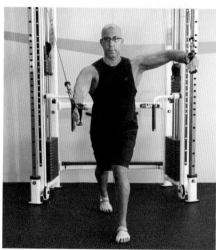

Alternating cable chest fly with contralateral step-out.

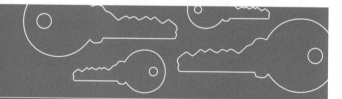

Key To Performance
Alternating Cable Chest Fly

The client activates their deep neck flexors, serratus anterior, and trunk stabilizers. They maintain this activation and a long spine throughout the pattern, and reach long through the forward arm. The trunk and torso should face forward during bilateral patterns and rotate during unilateral and alternating patterns.

CLIENT SENSATION: Your client should feel as if they maintain activation and are rotating on a longitudinal axis through the spine. They should feel significant tension in the anterior flexor chain at the start of the pattern and in the anterior oblique chain especially at the end of the pattern.

VERTICAL PUSHING PATTERNS

Description: Any pattern where resistance is pushed overhead against the pull of gravity.

Example: Overhead press using dumbbells, barbells, medicine balls, or kettlebells.

Overhead dumbbell pressing is another fundamental movement pattern that is much more than merely a shoulder exercise. It is an excellent movement for developing strength and stability in the entire shoulder complex, thorax, and lumbopelvic-hip regions. Regardless of the goal, by varying arm position, angle of push, and load levels, almost anyone can perform the overhead press. However, it is important to establish proper cervical spine, thorax, and ST stabilization prior to loading the upper extremity, otherwise the client will compensate.

Traditionally, overhead presses have been performed while sitting and stabilized against a bench. While there is nothing wrong with doing presses in this fashion, there are far greater benefits to be gained performing them while sitting on a stability ball. There is the increased demand on the core to stabilize the trunk while sitting on a stability ball, as compared to performing them while seated with the back stabilized or using a machine. However for most clients, standing will be the preferred pattern since so many of them sit for most of their day.

For most clients, DBs are used instead of barbells for a variety of reasons, including:

- DBs allow the client to move through their range of motion. Barbells require the client to lean back to clear the bar from hitting their chin; often the client compensates by extending through their thoracolumbar junction, rather than getting spinal extension through their entire spine.

- DBs enable the client to work the shoulders through multiple planes of motion.

- DBs allow the client to perform alternating and unilateral patterning, which better addresses unilateral instabilities or weaknesses.

The ideal position of overhead pressing is where the scapula is in upward rotation, with the glenoid fossa facing upward and the humerus is on the vertical axis with the body. A common cue to achieve this position is 'pack the shoulder joint by pulling the scapula down and back.' Unfortunately, in the client with an unstable shoulder joint, poor upward rotation of the scapula, or limited GH range of motion, this cue will generally result in the client pulling the ST joint into a depressed and downwardly rotated position. A better cue is to have the client imagine wrapping the scapula around the thorax and maintaining this position as the humerus moves in the glenoid fossa. This guarantees constant serratus anterior activity and ensures that the scapula remains in a relative upwardly rotated position.

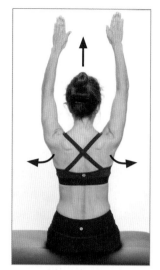 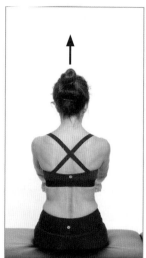

The client is instructed to maintain a long spine (vertical arrow), wrap (curved arrow) the scapula around the thorax, and to maintain this activation as they lower their arm. This ensures that the serratus anterior remains active as the arm is lowered. They must be able to perform this action without weight in the arm before adding a load.

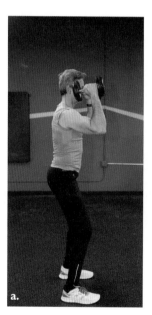 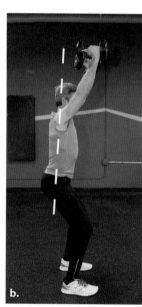 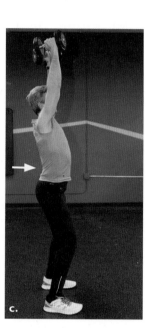

During the overhead press, the spine must remain neutral (vertical line) as the arms are pushed overhead. The serratus anterior remains active and the scapulae are wrapped around the thorax (arrow) as the arms are lifted only to the level at which the spine remains neutral (a, b).

Author's note: The question is often raised as to why the arms are held out in front of the body rather than directly overhead. The arms are raised only to the point where the client can maintain their thoracopelvic canister (TPC). For this particular client in the image to the right, to get the arms completely overhead would require him to hyperextend through his thoracolumbar junction, thereby comprising his TPC stability (c). He will use lighter weight to help spare his spine from the deleterious effects of trying to achieve a purely vertical overhead position of the weights.

SEATED AND STANDING OVERHEAD DUMBBELL PRESS

Seated and standing overhead DB presses are a great alternative to traditional bench-supported overhead DB presses as they have a greater stabilization requirement than their supported and machine counterparts. The client must maintain a long spine and activation of their TPC throughout the pattern.

Performing a standing overhead DB press provides even greater benefits than the seated version. These benefits include:

- increased demands on the core – the standing overhead press increases the demands on the core stabilizers of the thorax as the arms are extended overhead;

- integration of the entire kinetic chain – the standing press integrates the shoulder complex, thorax, hips, and lower extremities, simulating many activities of daily living;

- ability to perform transverse plane patterns – encourages integration of hip rotation and spinal stability;

- decreased stress on the lumbar spine – less pressure is placed upon the spine when standing as compared to sitting;

- can be performed in bilateral, alternating, and unilateral patterns, respectively adding progressively increased stability demands on the core.

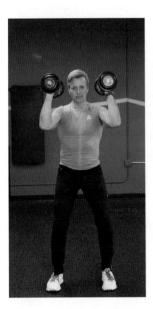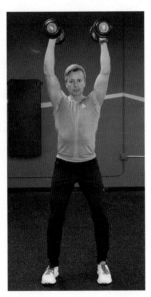

Overhead DB press: sagittal plane – front view.

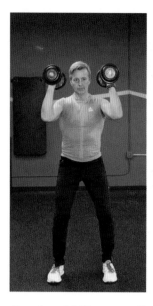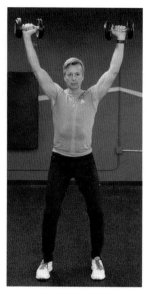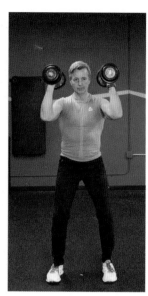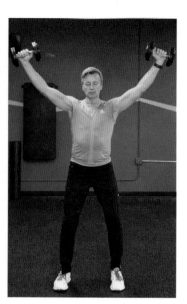

Overhead DB press: frontal plane – V-press (far left & left); Y-press (right & far right).

Key To Performance
Shoulder Press

The client activates their deep neck flexors, serratus anterior, and trunk stabilizers. They maintain this activation and a long spine throughout the pattern.

CLIENT SENSATION: Your client should feel as if they maintain activation as they press overhead. They should feel significant tension in the trunk and shoulder stabilizers throughout the pattern.

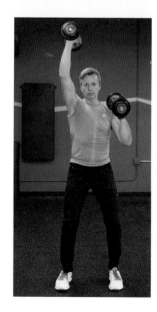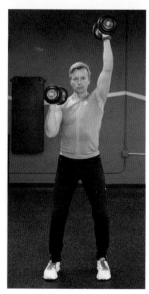

Author's Note: For clients with shoulder stability issues, stick with sagittal and frontal plane patterns. V and Y presses should only be performed by individuals with advanced levels of shoulder stability.

Alternating overhead DB press: sagittal plane.

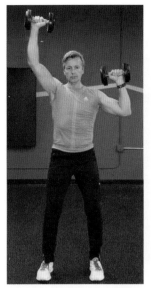
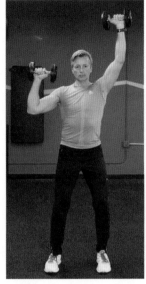
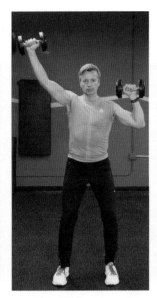
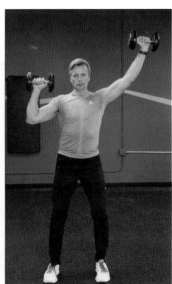

Alternating overhead DB press:
frontal plane – V press.

Alternating overhead DB press:
frontal plane – Y press.

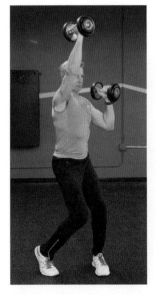
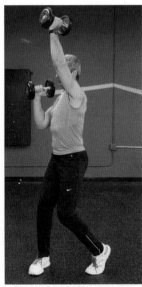
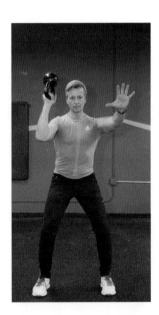
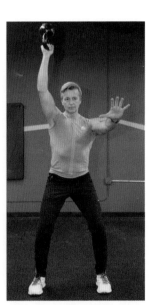

Alternating overhead DB press:
transverse plane.

Upside-down kettlebell lift.

The upside-down kettlebell lift requires tremendous stability of the entire shoulder complex as well as of the wrist and elbow. This is an excellent pattern in which to use irradiation from the grip on the kettlebell handle to aid shoulder stability. Be sure the client maintains scapular control and a neutral wrist position throughout the pattern and uses the contralateral limb to stabilize the thorax and neck. Due to the demanding and unstable nature of this pattern, use a lighter kettlebell to begin with until the client demonstrates an ability to control both the concentric and eccentric phases of the pattern.

Due to the grip, medicine balls add a unique challenge to the overhead press and make this an effective pattern for replicating many activities of daily living, such as lifting children.

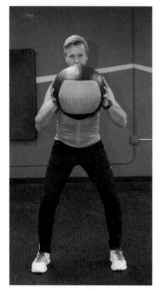
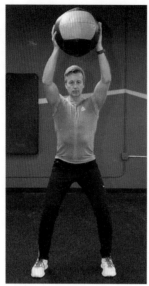
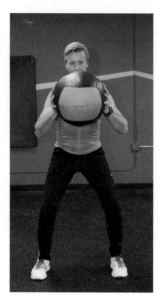
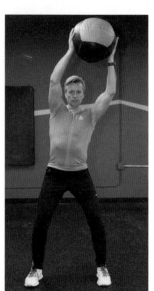

Overhead press with medicine ball: sagittal plane.

Overhead press with medicine ball: frontal plane.

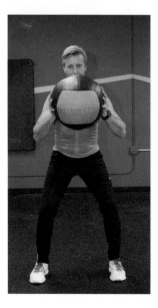
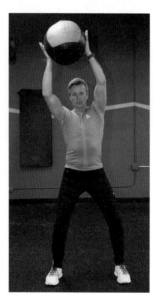
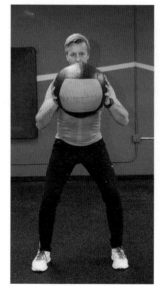
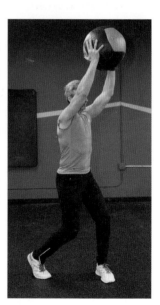

Overhead press with medicine ball: frontal plane.

Overhead press with medicine ball: transverse plane.

HORIZONTAL PULLING PATTERNS

Description: Any pattern where resistance is pulled toward the body (along a horizontal plane) or the body is pulled toward the fixed hands (when the body is in an inclined or horizontal position).

Example: Bent-over row using dumbbells or barbells, seated or standing cable or band row, reclined pull-up using a barbell rack or TRX apparatus.

Another fundamental movement pattern, pulling patterns target the entire extensor chain, posterior scapular stabilizers, and TPC stabilizers. While, in terms of technicality, pulling patterns are relatively easy to perform, many individuals perform them incorrectly. There are three common errors with pulling-type patterns:

1. **Scapular instability:** Clients are cued to pull the scapulae down and back. Recall, the role of the scapular stabilizers is just that – stabilizers. They are not primarily adductors or retractors. **Result:** perpetuation of scapular downward rotation, adduction, and depression.

2. **Glenohumeral instability:** The elbows are pulled far beyond the body, disrupting the ideal GH axis of rotation and driving the humeral head forward in the socket (a and c). **Result:** GH instability.

3. **Spinal instability:** The client is often cued to lift the chest, which often results in thoracolumbar extension (c). This compromise in alignment is compounded by lumbar spine flexion – both in the seated and bent-over row versions – due to most clients' hip flexion deficiency. **Result:** thoracic extension, lumbar flexion, and posterior tilting of the pelvis, leading to TPC instability.

4. **Poor scapular and trunk stability:** In the seated row, he allows his scapulae to over-abduct during the eccentric phase (b) and then over-extends his spine and over-adducts his scapulae during the concentric phases of the pattern (c).

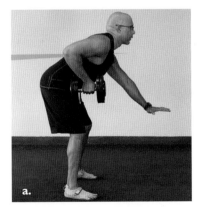 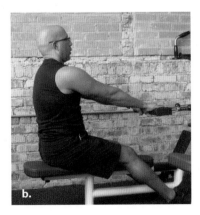 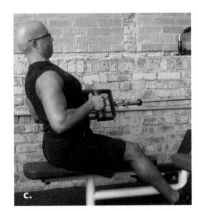

The individual in the image above left is unable to maintain a stable position of either his right scapulothoracic joint or his cervicothoracic junction during the one arm row. Additionally, he pulls his elbow past the body, driving the scapula into an overly adducted position and the humeral head forward relative to the glenoid fossa.

This pattern will overload his cervical spine, leading to movement pattern dysfunctions and early spine degeneration. In the image below left, he is cued to achieve a long spine posture and wrap his scapula around the thorax, thereby improving both the neck and scapula postures.

The client does not maintain scapular or spine stabilization when performing the frontal plane row, which results in anterior humeral glide and lateral neck flexion (image below middle). He is cued to maintain a long spine and scapular stability and to 'pull the arm long', which results in improved alignment and pulling pattern (image below right).

Author's note: The goal of pulling patterns is to pull the shoulders and spine into a neutral or minimally extended position, not to pull into end range shoulder or spine extension.

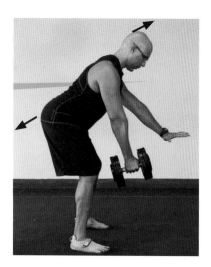 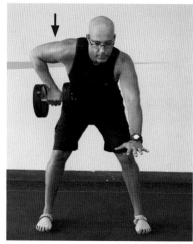 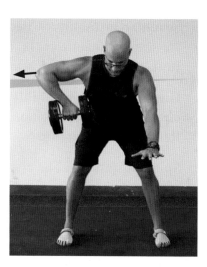

DUMBBELL ROW

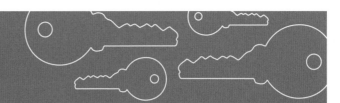

Key To Performance

Dumbbell Row

- The client activates their deep neck flexors, serratus anterior, and trunk stabilizers and maintains a long spine throughout the pattern.
- They bend forward by performing a hip hinge, flexing their hips only as far as their degree of hip flexion. One way to determine this limit is to have the client squat to the deepest point where they can still maintain a neutral spine and then tilt the pelvis forward.
- The client's arms remain straight in this position and the scapulae must be in a neutral position – the scapulae are not allowed to overly abduct, helping the client maintain isometric control of the scapular stabilizers.
- They pull their arms towards the sides, the elbows staying in close, and the scapulae are pulled wide, not back – the motion being similar to a sawing motion. This helps to maintain activation in the serratus anterior, middle trapezius, and lower trapezius.
- The entire GH should rotate along its axis in the glenoid fossa and not be driven forward, which is a frequent occurrence when the client is cued to 'squeeze the shoulder blades together and pull the elbows back.'
- Once they master the supported version, the client progresses to the unsupported, unilateral, rotating, split stance, frontal plane, and single leg support versions.

CLIENT SENSATION: Your client should feel as if they maintain activation and think about pulling their scapulae wide. They should feel significant tension in the extensor chain scapular stabilizers even though they are not directly adducting the scapulae.

Supported DB row: Trainers will often have their clients perform the bent-over row with one arm and knee supported on a bench. This often results in excessive use of the bench for support, negating many of the postural benefits of the unsupported version. If clients require support, they should assume the bent-over position previously described, with one arm supported on a bench or rack. Make sure that the client maintains activation in both the supportive arm as well as in the working arm.

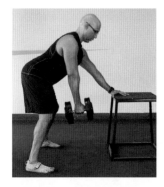
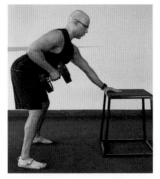
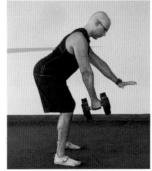
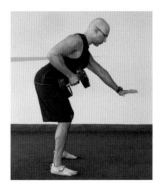

DB row: single arm row; supported (left two images), unsupported (right two images).

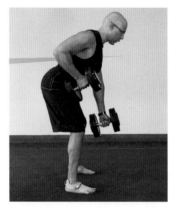 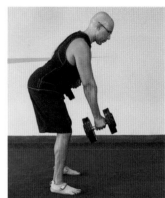

Alternating DB row.

Unilateral DB row with rotation: unilateral patterns introduce a rotary force that needs to be controlled. The client maintains a neutral spine alignment, core activation, and rotates the thorax along a longitudinal axis.

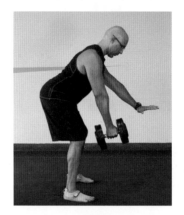 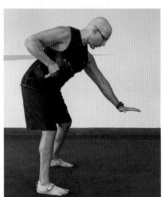

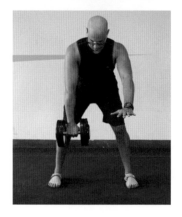 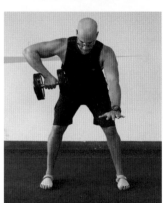

Unilateral DB row: frontal plane.

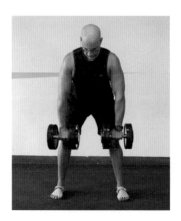 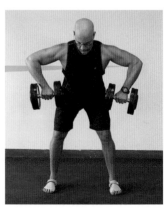

Bilateral DB row: frontal plane.

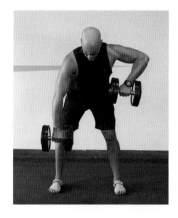 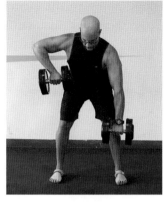

Alternating DB row: frontal plane.

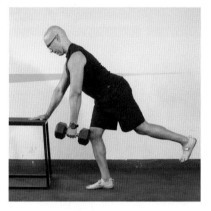 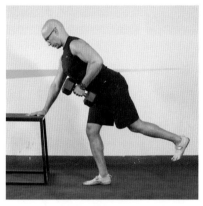

Single leg supported unilateral DB row: ipsilateral support.

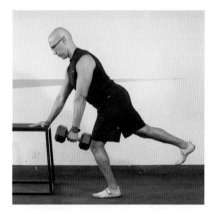 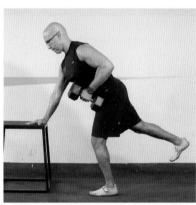

Single leg supported unilateral DB row: contralateral support.

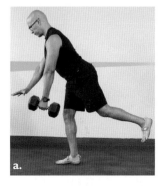 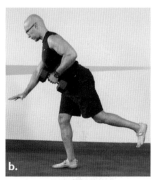 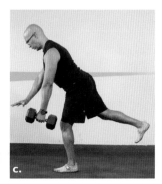 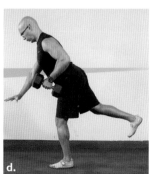

Single leg unilateral DB row: a–b) ipsilateral support, c–d) contralateral support.

All the mechanics described on the previous page apply to the seated cable row versions. Ideal patterning during the alternating seated cable row: the client maintains neutral spine and scapular positions and pulls the scapula wide and the trunk into a long spine posture.

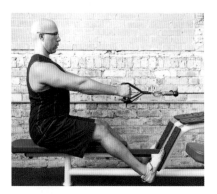 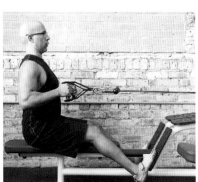

Cable row: bilateral.

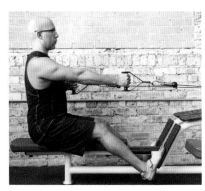 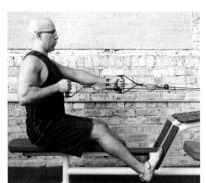

Cable row: alternating.

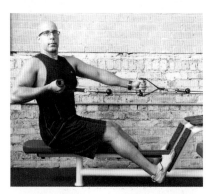 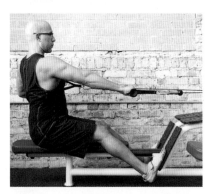

Cable row: rotation.

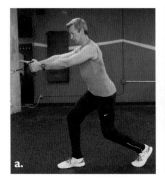 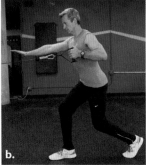 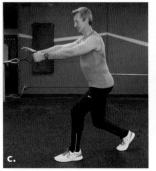 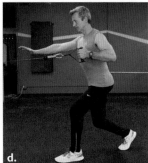

Cable row: (a–b) ipsilateral support, (c–d) contralateral support.

BAND OR CABLE BOW AND ARROW ROW

Band or cable bow and arrow rows are an incredibly effective way to train both acceleration and deceleration of the posterior oblique chain. They offer additional benefits over conventional rowing by including hip motion – external hip rotation with the stepping version and internal hip rotation with the pivot version.

EXERCISE PERFORMANCE

The client initiates the pull through the pelvis, then the trunk, and finishes with the arm. They pull the elbow 'long' as if pulling on a bow-string (white arrow). The level of the elbow always lifts slightly higher than the wrist in low-to-high patterns and slightly lower in high-to-low patterns and becomes an extension of the cable or band. The wrist remains straight and spine remains neutral. The rotation is around the stationary hip, and the hip, knee, and ankle remain aligned. At the end of the pull motion, the client's center of mass should be distributed equally between their feet at the end of the pull (dashed line). They return to the starting position under control.

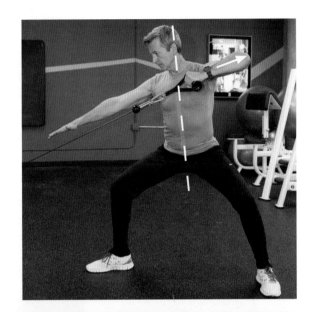

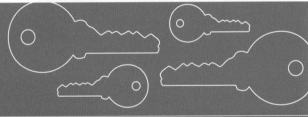

Key To Performance
Band or Cable Pull with Rotation

- The client activates their serratus anterior and trunk stabilizers. They maintain this activation and a long spine throughout the pattern.
- They pull the band or cable, thinking of pulling the arm long along the plane of the body, and the forearm remains in line with the cable, essentially becoming an extension of the cable.

CLIENT SENSATION: Your client should feel as if they maintain activation as they are pulling the cable or band. The movement is initiated and controlled through the hips and thorax rather than the arms.

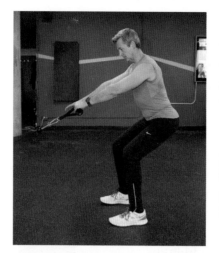 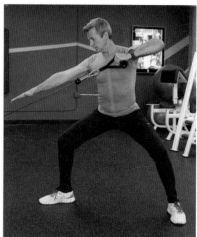

Bow and arrow: low to high.

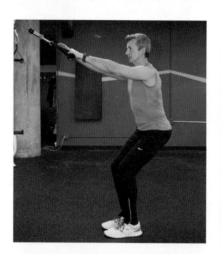 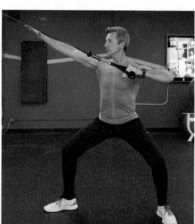

Bow and arrow: high to low.

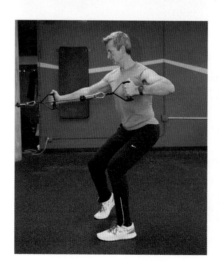 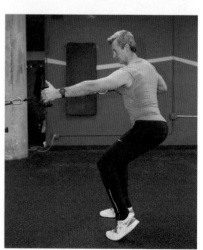

Alternating cable row: with pivot (internal hip rotation).

RECLINED PULL-UP

The reclined pull-up, essentially a reverse motion of the push-up, is a hybrid movement, combining both the benefits of a pull-up and bent-over row. It functions as an initial progression to help a client to understand the nuance of ST control required to properly perform a pull-up. It is a great pattern for both the extensor chain as well as posterior scapular stabilizers, allowing virtually any client, even deconditioned and elderly ones, to derive the benefits of pulling patterns. They can be performed on a barbell rack, a dual cable machine, or a suspension apparatus such as the TRX. Once the client progresses to a point where their body is level with the floor, the pattern is also referred to as an 'inverted row'.

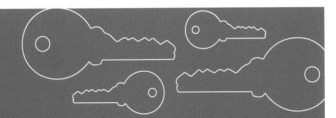

Key To Performance
Reclined Pull-up

- The client activates their serratus anterior and trunk stabilizers. They maintain this activation and a long spine throughout the pattern.

- They grasp the handles and lean back until they are supported.

- They pull themselves up towards the cable and release back to the starting position.

- As the client progresses, their body is lowered to a more horizontal position and then to a point where their legs are elevated on a step or platform.

- They pull themselves up only to the point where they maintain optimal GH rotation or where their upper arms are in line with their torso.

The following guidelines must be adhered to throughout the pattern:

- The spine remains neutral and the core remains activated.

- The ankles remain in dorsiflexion and the wrists remain straight.

- The scapulae remain activated; they adduct slightly as the client pulls up and abduct slightly as the lient lowers themselves, always remaining in a neutral, posteriorly tilted position.

CLIENT SENSATION: Your client should feel as if they maintain activation as they pull their body towards their hands and visualize pulling their shoulders wide and their spine long.

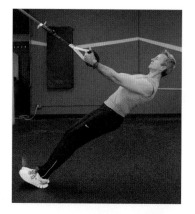
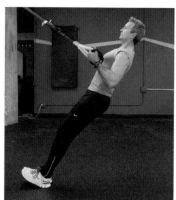

Reclined pull-up: TRX.

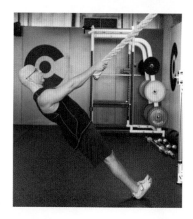
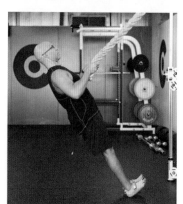

Reclined pull-up: rope.

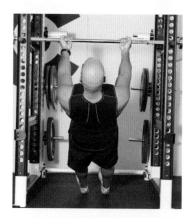
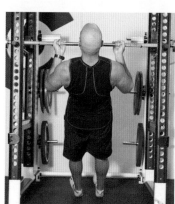

Reclined pull-up: bar.

While the underhand version recruits more the latissimus dorsi and elbow flexors, the overhand grip favors the posterior scapular stabilizers and shoulder complex. The client should pull the elbows wide without over-adduction of the scapula as they pull their body towards the bar.

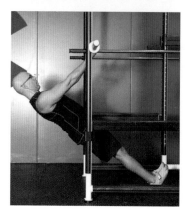
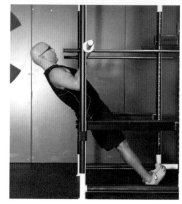

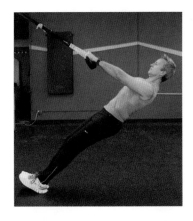 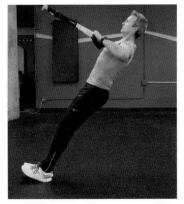

Reclined pull-up: TRX – overhand grip.

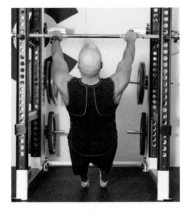 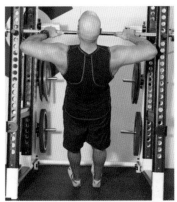

Reclined pull-up: bar – overhand grip, posterior.

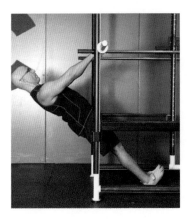 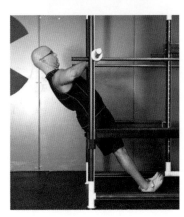

Reclined pull-up: bar – overhand grip, side.

SINGLE ARM ROTATION PATTERNS

The single arm rotation is another hybrid exercise that does not neatly fit into a specific category; however, since the body is pulled toward the fixed arm, it is considered more of a pull pattern. The single arm rotation is a high level pattern that targets the entire shoulder complex while effectively training the rotator cuff in a closed-chain pattern. In other words, the trunk is rotated around a fixed upper extremity, training closed-chain internal rotation, as opposed to the traditional rotator cuff patterns in which the arm is rotated around a fixed trunk. This connection can improve coordination between the wrist/hand, rotator cuff, and scapulothoracic complexes, making this pattern ideal for returning to high level activity. Because of the single arm support and the movement of the free arm, this pattern can also be beneficial after performing pull-ups, to 'free up' the thorax. This pattern can be performed grasping the bar of a Smith machine, a TRX, or similar strap cable apparatus.

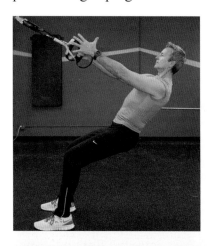 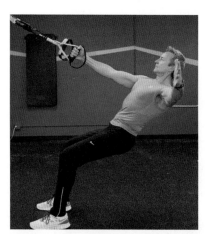

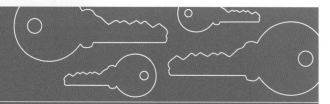

Key To Performance
TRX Single Arm Rotation Patterns

- The client grasps one handle of the TRX, making sure they maintain a strong grip and a straight elbow and wrist.

- They activate the deep neck flexors, serratus anterior, and deep abdominal wall.

- Maintaining a long spine, the client rotates, reaching their arm back while opening the chest.

- They reach back towards the ceiling to return to the starting position.

- The spine must remain long and the scapula must remain stabilized against the thorax throughout the pattern.

Please note: The rotation of the trunk is performed by the glenohumeral internal rotators and scapulothoracic stabilizers – mainly the serratus anterior, pectoralis major, pectoralis minor, subscapularis, latissimus dorsi, teres major, and coracobrachialis.

CLIENT SENSATION: Your client should as if they maintain a long spine and serratus anterior activation and that the work is being done by the stationary arm.

VERTICAL PULLING PATTERNS

Description: Any pattern where the arms pull the resistance along a vertical plane (pull of gravity) or the body is pulled toward the fixed hands along a vertical plane (pull of gravity).

Example: Pull-ups and cable or band pull-downs.

PULL-UP

The pull-up is one of the fundamental patterns and a great movement for training both the trunk and the shoulder complex. In addition to the latissimus dorsi, pull-ups target the posterior deltoid and triceps as well as all the elbow flexors and grip strength, making it a complete functional upper extremity exercise. The challenge with pull-ups is that many clients lack the spine and scapular stability to perform them properly. For these individuals, the reclined pull-up (discussed earlier) is a great alternative, although they are technically not a vertical pull pattern.

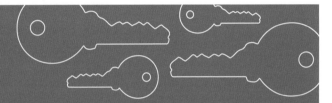

Key To Performance

Pull-up

- The client grasps the handles and sets their scapulae – the scapulae are said to be 'set' when they are pulled down and around the thorax (see image overleaf).
- They pull themselves up towards the bar and release back to the starting position without losing ST control or GH axis of rotation.

The following guidelines must be adhered to throughout the pattern.

- The spine remains neutral and the core remains activated.
- The scapulae remain activated; they adduct slightly as the client pulls up and abduct slightly as they lower themselves, always remaining in a posterior tilted position.
- The client pulls themselves up only to the point where they maintain optimal GH rotation or their upper arms are in line with their torso.
- They maintain a long spine, being careful not to hyperextend through the thoracolumbar junction.

CLIENT SENSATION: Your client should as if they maintain activation and a long spine as they pull their body towards the bar. They visualize pulling their scapula wide and wrapping them around the thorax rather than down and back.

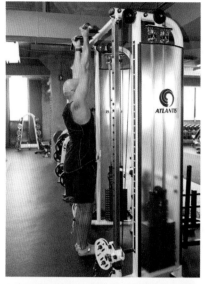
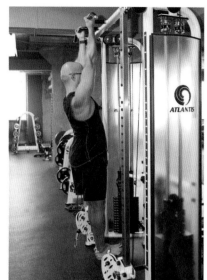

Poor scapular setup (left); proper scapular position (right).

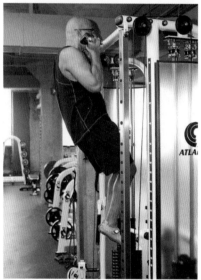
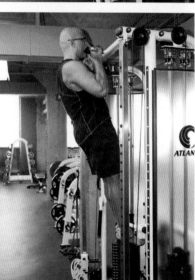

Underhand grip pull-up: poor head and trunk position (left); proper head and trunk position (right).

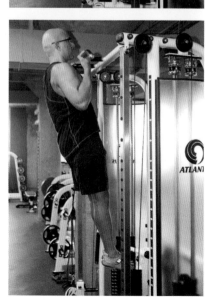

Underhand pull-up.

CABLE PULL-DOWN

Vertical pulls, more commonly referred to as cable pull-downs, challenge the scapular stabilizers in an overhead manner and can be an effective alternative for those clients with decreased range of motion or stability of the shoulder complex. The angle can be changed to accommodate different planes of motions and clients of variable degrees of motion and control. This pattern is relatively easy to learn and develop control, as the starting position places the scapula into upward rotation It is also a great pattern for connecting the latissimus dorsi and scapular stabilizers to the TPC.

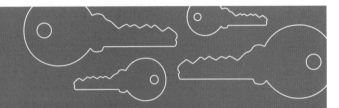

Key To Performance

Cable Pull-Down

- The client activates their serratus anterior and trunk stabilizers. They maintain this activation and a long spine throughout the pattern.

- They pull the cable down, bringing the elbow towards the floor while maintaining a stable scapula – they visualize pulling their scapula wide and around the thorax rather than down and back.

- The client should not pull the scapula down and back or pull the elbow back behind them, as these movements encourage downward rotation of the scapula and anterior humeral glide.

- They should maintain a long spine and be careful not to hyperextend through the thoracolumbar junction.

- These patterns can be performed both seated and standing.

CLIENT SENSATION: Your client should feel as if they maintain activation and a long spine as they pull their body towards their hands. They visualize pulling their shoulders wide, and their elbows should be in front relative to the shoulder joint and point towards the floor at the bottom of the concentric phase of the movement.

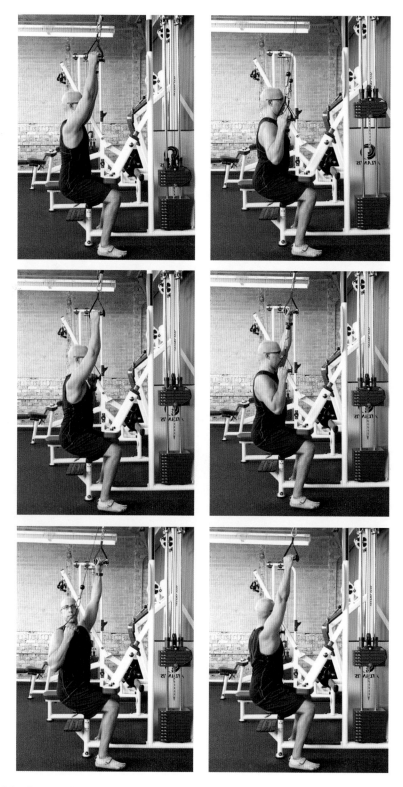

Cable pull-down: ideal scapular and trunk patterning during the alternating cable pull-down pattern – neutral spine posture (above) and with trunk rotation (below). The alternating variations and those with rotation are preferred over the bilateral patterns, as they encourage thoracic motion during the patterns. The client maintains a long spine during all versions.

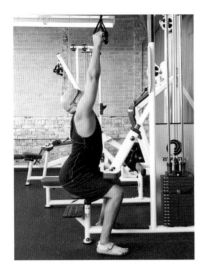 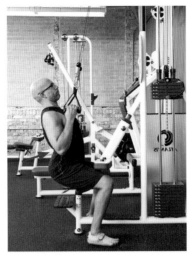

Poor scapular and spine patterning: the client loses scapular control and over-abducts the scapulae during the eccentric phase of the pull-down (image above left), and hyperextends the thoracolumbar junction and over-adducts the scapulae during the concentric phase (image above right).

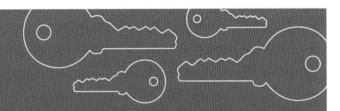

Key To Success

Ratios of Pushing Exercises to Pulling Exercises

There is much debate within the fitness industry regarding the correct ratio of pushing exercises to pulling exercises. The debate should not be about this ratio – it should be all about scapular control. Most general population clients who present with ST dysfunction aren't necessarily 'strong' in pushing motions and 'weak' in pulling motions – they exhibit poor motor control in both pushing and pulling motions. Pushing patterns as well as pulling patterns are required to optimally retrain ST control. Over-reliance on pulling patterns at the expense of pushing patterns does not ensure optimal ST control and in many clients, encourages disruption of normal mechanics. If the scapula is stable and the client engages in a well-rounded conditioning program, there is no debate.

KEY: Focus on improving scapular control, rather than worrying about the number of sets of pushing exercises to pulling exercises. If there is still doubt, err on the side of doing more scapular stabilization exercises (in the corrective exercise section found in chapter 7), as these will improve scapular mechanics and improve function better than any of the higher level fundamental patterns.

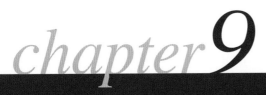

Key Patterns and Movement Progressions for the Hip Complex and Lower Extremity

CHAPTER OBJECTIVES
To identify the key patterns of the hip complex and lower extremity
To develop the specific strategies for progressing the fundamental movement patterns of the hip complex and lower extremity

Progressing lower extremity patterns is necessary for individuals aiming to return to work or return to sport. This chapter will look at the fundamental movement patterns of the hip and lower extremity, including squatting, lunging, stepping, deadlifting, bridging, and reaching.

HIP-DOMINANT VERSUS KNEE-DOMINANT PATTERNS

Lower extremity patterns are generally categorized as hip dominant or knee dominant based upon where the majority of motion occurs and which muscle system is predominately utilized. Hip-dominant patterns are generally patterns where the pelvis is rotating around the femoral heads, and the knees are generally not directly involved in the pattern. The gluteus maximus and hamstring complex – or the posterior chain muscles – eccentrically pulls on the pelvis as the pelvis anteriorly rotates and concentrically pulls to posteriorly rotate the pelvis, so these patterns are sometimes referred to as pulling patterns. Knee-dominant patterns are generally those where the knees are directly involved in the movement of the load and there is much more quadriceps activity. These patterns are sometimes referred to as pushing patterns and include squats, lunges, and step-ups/step-downs.

Hip Dominant	Knee Dominant
Bridges	Squats
Reaches	Lunges
Deadlifts	Step-ups / step-downs

A well-designed conditioning program should stress an equal amount of hip-dominant and knee-dominant patterns. While a delineation is made between these two patterns, every lower extremity pattern should stress hip involvement. The lack of ideal hip and ankle dissociation is a common cause of knee pain in clients during squatting down towards the floor or while descending stairs. For these clients, improving dissociation of the hip and shoulder should be a priority and then followed immediately with a stabilization strategy. Hip-dominant patterns are generally the best patterns to start with for clients with knee problems or where there is pain with loading the knee, as these patterns don't involve direct loading upon the knee. After teaching control of neutral spine and pelvis, clients with back pain generally should be taught knee-dominant patterns first, as control of neutral spine posture during squatting and lunging is the best strategy for sparing the spine through exercise. This latter strategy can then be adapted to the activities of daily life of the client with low back pain.

HIP-DOMINANT PATTERNS

BRIDGES

Bridges are a popular exercise with individuals looking to tone the glutes and are routinely performed in rehabilitation settings for those experiencing low back and hip pain. Bridges are commonly performed to improve hip extension, specifically the function of the gluteus maximus. Commonly, clients and patients, under the guidance of a physical therapist or personal trainer, perform bridges with the instructions to 'squeeze the glutes' or 'push up through the hips.' Performing them in this fashion does increase gluteal activity but also preferentially increases the activation of the superficial fibers of the gluteals, while doing little to improve functional control of the femoroacetabular articulation. This section will look at the bridge pattern, differentiate between the two different types, and provide a strategy for improving hip function using the pattern.

LEVEL I: BRIDGE AND BRIDGE WITH ROTATION

The level I bridge pattern is utilized to improve the function of the core musculature, primarily the abdominals and hamstrings, while subsequently decreasing the tone and increasing the length of the erector spinae. This is an excellent exercise for those requiring decompression/relaxation of the spine (due to increased tonicity through the erectors) and for individuals with hip pain (due to overcompression by the superficial gluteus maximus and deep hip rotators), as well as a coordination movement for the core.

Key To Performance
Bridge

- The client lies supine with the knees bent and the feet flat on the floor.
- The legs are about hip width apart and the hips, knees, ankles, and feet are in a straight line.
- The client is given the cue to begin by activating their core and relax through their hips, spreading through the sit bones (ischial tuberosities) – the hips and gluteals should remain relatively loose and relaxed throughout the movement.
- Next, they perform small range anterior and posterior pelvic tilts while ensuring relaxation of the hip rotators, gluteals, and erector spinae.

- As the performance improves, the individual begins to roll the spine off the floor one segment at a time (spinal flexion), similar to peeling a piece of tape of the floor.

- They lower the spine back onto the floor, reversing the pattern, lowering one segment at a time until the spine and pelvis are in a neutral resting position – Pilates and yoga instructors commonly refer to this as 'imprinting' the spine into the floor.

- The client breathes out as the spine is rotated off the floor and breathes in as the spine is rotated back onto the floor.

- The individual rises off the floor only to the point where they can keep segmentally flexing or 'rolling' through the spine while maintaining core activation and without overactivation of the gluteals and hip rotators.

- The hips, knees, ankles, and feet should remain in a straight line throughout the pattern.

CLIENT SENSATION: The client should feel as if they are relaxing through the hips and spine as they move through the pattern and should feel that it is easier for them to move segmentally through the hips and spine.

LEVEL I: BRIDGE WITH ROTATION

The bridge with rotation is an excellent way to improve rotational flexibility in the hips by dissociating the pelvis from the femurs. Whereas the standing spinal rotation pattern creates rotation in a top-down fashion, the supine version rotates the lumbopelvic-hip complex from the bottom up. Both versions are excellent movements for any individual who demonstrates restriction of hip and spine rotation, but especially for athletes such as golfers and pitchers who need significant dissociation between the pelvis and femoral head.

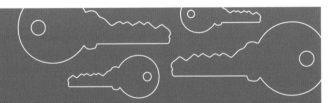

Key To Performance
Bridge with Rotation

- The client breathes in and as they breathe out, rotates their pelvis towards one hip – they breathe in as they rotate the pelvis back to neutral.

- This is repeated in the opposite direction.

- The client's feet should remain flat on the floor and their knees and thighs should remain parallel and stationary throughout the movement – ensure that the rotation is accomplished through the hips and not by moving the lower extremity.

CLIENT SENSATION: The client should feel as if they are relaxing through their hips and rotating around their lower extremities.

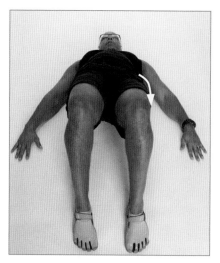 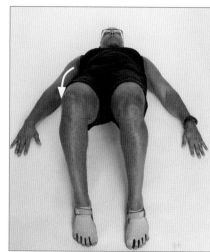

Bridge with rotation, beginning (left image) and (right image).

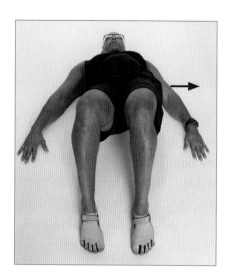

Clients who exhibit poor femoroacetabular dissociation and/or poor TPC stability will often substitute by swaying their pelvis laterally, rather than performing pure hip dissociation.

LEVEL II: HIP EXTENSION BRIDGE

The level I version of the bridge stressed both hip and spinal mobility utilizing the pattern to help a client diminish overall gripping-type stabilization strategies. The level II version is designed to improve hip extension, specifically the function of the posterior hip complex. In fact, the level II bridge pattern is one of the greatest ways to improve hip extension and stabilization function of the gluteal (maximus and medius).

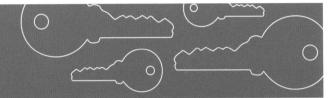

Key To Performance

Hip Extension Bridge

- The client lies on the floor with their legs about hip width apart and their arms resting on the floor.
- They maintain a neutral spine, activate their core, and lift up by activating the hips, not by squeezing through the hips, to both raise and lower the pelvis.
- The client pauses at the top and sits back in the hips as they return to the floor.
- The hips, knees, and feet should remain neutral throughout the pattern – there should be no external rotation or adduction of the hips.
- The movement occurs around the hip – the spine should remain neutral throughout the pattern (dashed line).

CLIENT SENSATION: The client should feel as if they are relaxing through the hips during the eccentric phase and lifting through the hips as they lift up their pelvis.

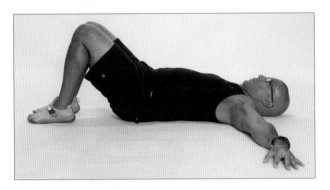

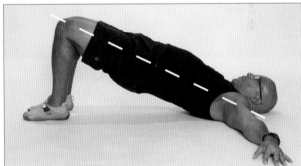

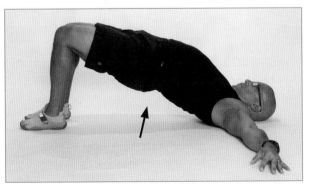

Note the thoracolumbar hyperextension in this client, who is cued to 'squeeze your butt hard'(image left). This destabilizes both the TPC and hip by disconnecting the abdominal wall and by driving the femoral head forward in the acetabulum.

LEVEL III: MARCHING BRIDGE

Along with aiding hip extension, the gluteus maximus shows significant activity during the heel strike phase of gait, suggesting that the gluteus maximus functions to assist unilateral control of the ilium. Marching bridges are an excellent way to train this function of the gluteus maximus and marry the benefits of hip extension, core stabilization, and unilateral loading in a relatively low level position. However, it is important to note that this is not a low level exercise although virtually every trainer and therapist has their clients performing them. Listed below are several keys that increase the effectiveness of this pattern and which must be carefully monitored to ensure maximum benefits are gained from it.

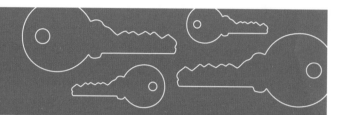

Key To Performance
Marching Bridge

- The client performs a traditional level II bridge as described above.

- They lift up one leg, being sure to maintain a level pelvis, neutral spine, and lower extremity alignment.

- They place the leg back down on the floor and lift the opposite side, making sure to control the pelvic position especially during the transition from leg to leg.

- The client can monitor themselves by placing their hands over their anterior superior iliac spines and assuring that their pelvis remains stationary throughout the pattern.

CLIENT SENSATION: The client should feel as if their pelvis remains neutral with no rotation through the hips, pelvis, or low back.

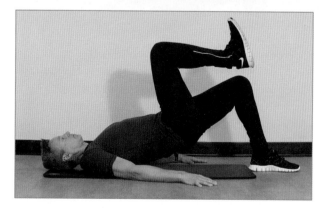
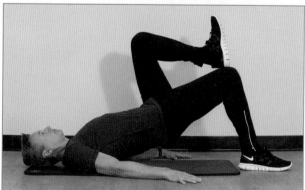

LEVEL IV: SINGLE LEG BRIDGE

Single leg bridges are one of the more challenging exercises for the gluteus maximus and are an excellent pattern for teaching pelvic stability during single leg mechanics prior to progressing the client to the upright posture. To ensure that maximum benefits are achieved from the pattern, the client must adhere to the following guidelines. Throughout the pattern the client must be able to:

- maintain the hip, knee, ankle, and foot in a straight line;
- maintain a level pelvis and a neutral spine posture;
- pivot around the hip joint and contract the posterior hip without driving the femoral head anteriorly in the acetabulum.

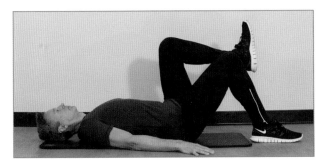 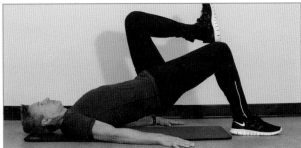

BALL BRIDGE

The ball bridge is a staple exercise for developing triple extension, that is extension of the ankle, knee, and hip. Additional benefits of this pattern include training the extension function of the hamstring, stabilization of the extensor chain, and overall activation of the core. The demands of this pattern make it increasingly important to maintain a neutral spine and pelvic position in order to optimize force production and to minimize the rotational stresses to the spine as well as to the hips and sacroiliac joints.

LEVEL I–II

The pattern begins with the heels on the ball (level I top two images below) and progresses to the toes on the ball (level II bottom two images below). The client should be able to extend through the hips without overextending the lumbar spine and without excessive swaying of the ball.

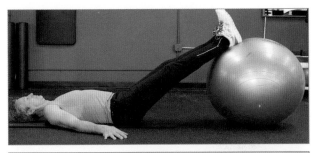 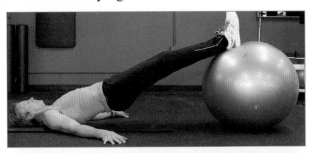

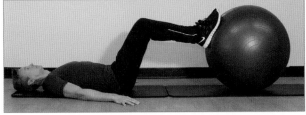 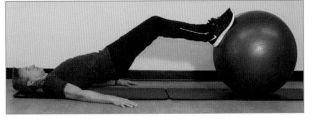

LEVEL III

The bridge with a lift-off combines the benefits of single leg triple extension and stabilization of the lumbopelvic-hip complex. As with the single leg bridge, the client must be able to maintain stabilization of the pelvis and spine as one leg is lifted. There should be no change in spine or pelvic position during the pattern. Begin with the feet on a stable surface, such as a step, before moving the client to a labile surface, such as a stability ball.

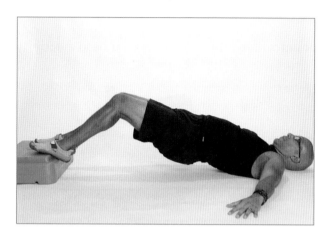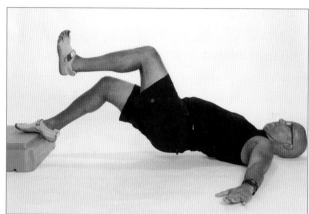

Bridge with single leg lift-off: stable surface.

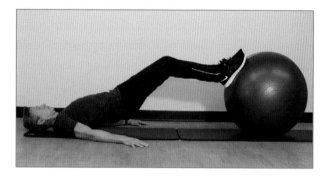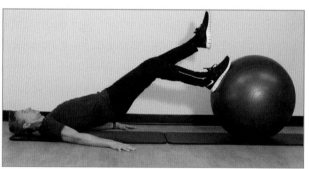

Bridge with single leg lift-off: labile surface.

STABILITY BALL LEG CURL

Since the invention of exercise machines, hamstring training has largely consisted of non-functional variations of seated or lying resisted knee flexion exercises. While knee flexion should only be trained in isolation in cases of true hamstring weakness, such as after a knee injury or surgery, the stability ball leg curl can add a needed knee flexion component to the traditional bridge pattern. In addition to the aforementioned benefits of the bridge pattern, the knee flexion component helps improve the eccentric control of the hamstrings and is a valuable pattern to improve in ACL and PCL rehabilitation. This pattern can be progressed to using a slide board or TRX equipment.

It is important to note that while the ball curl is a common pattern, it is rarely performed properly. The most common movement fault in the leg curl pattern is when trainers cue their clients to keep the hips up and the client substitutes lumbar spine extension for hip extension. These clients will also demonstrate a splayed anterior rib cage posture, demonstrating they have lost control of the TPC and are substituting lumbar extension for hip extension. In the images below it may seem as if the client is not in full hip extension; however, they are holding the position that allows them to maintain a neutral spine, a caudal anterior rib position, and stabilization of the TPC throughout the pattern.

LEVEL I
The client performs a bridge pattern and curls the ball towards the hips; there should be no change in pelvic or spine posture. They essentially lengthen their legs without losing the pelvic or spine position.

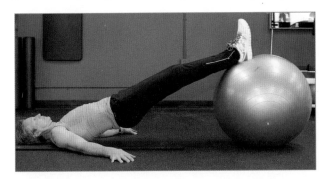 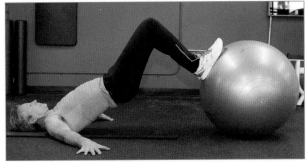

LEVEL II
The single leg curl pattern is the highest level hip extension progression. This pattern requires exceptional core stability and hip control and should only be performed by clients who have progressed through level I of the stability ball leg curl as well as levels I-III of the bridge hip extension patterns. Ensure that the client maintains a level pelvis, neutral spine, and core activation throughout the movement.

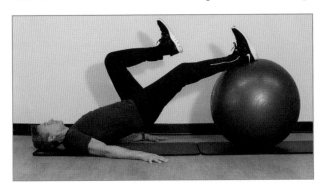 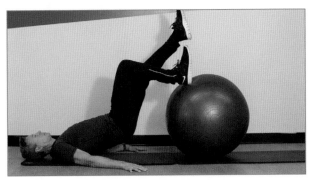

REACHES

As mentioned earlier, hip restriction is one of the greatest contributors to both back and knee injuries, limiting many clients and athletes from ever developing the proper mechanics required to safely perform many movement patterns, including squats, lunges, and deadlifts. The anterior reach is a way to progress the client from the hip hinge to the deadlift while continuing to teach ideal hip mechanics. This pattern is especially effective at cuing the posterior glide of the femoral head within the acetabulum and releasing through the posterior hip capsule. Using proper progressions, reaches can be performed by virtually anyone, including clients requiring improved balance or recovering from lower extremity injuries, or athletes requiring a greater functional challenge.

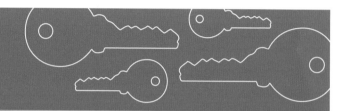

Key To Performance
Reaches

- The client begins the pattern with the feet approximately hip width apart, neutral spine, and core activated. There should be slight flexion in the knees, which is maintained throughout the movement pattern.

- The client begins by flexing the hips while reaching the arms forward at shoulder height. As the arms are reaching forward the hips are driven back. The further the arms reach anteriorly, the further the hips should move posteriorly.

- Ensure that the client maintains their hip hinge, core activation, and a neutral spine throughout the movement. Cue them to keep their hips relaxed and to spread through their ischial tuberosities.

- Once the client can perform 15 repetitions, progress them to the cable version (below), split stance, single leg, stability ball, and overhead versions.

CLIENT SENSATION: The client should feel as if they are able to maintain alignment throughout the pattern and should feel as if their posterior hips are doing most of the work.

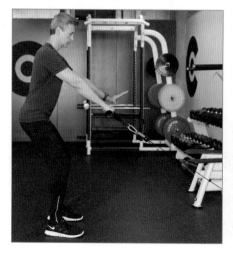
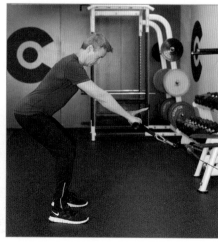

Level I: Bilateral reach with cable resistance.

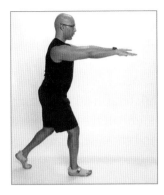 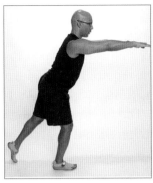 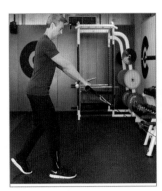 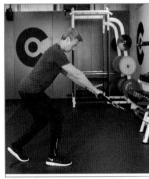

Level II: Split stance reach – unloaded. Level II: Split stance reach – with cable resistance.

LEVEL III: SINGLE LEG REACH

The client initially reaches at shoulder or waist height, and as they gain competence in the pattern, they reach towards the floor (a–d).

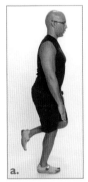 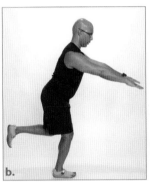 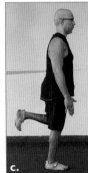 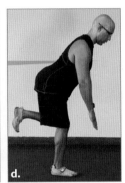 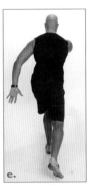 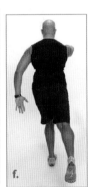

The squared pelvis during the reach: the client is unable to maintain a closed hip position during unilateral stance and externally rotates the hip on their stance leg (e); the client activates their deep, lower gluteus maximus and deep hip rotators to stabilize and 'square' the pelvis (f). If the client is unable to achieve the squared pelvis through verbal or kinesthetic cuing, they must be regressed.

Once the client is able to maintain their stability during the single leg reach, resistance can be added in the form of medicine balls or dumbbells. Using a cable will add increased challenge the posterior chain.

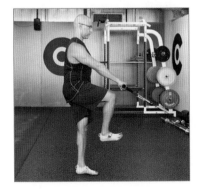 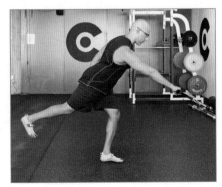

LEVEL IV: OVERHEAD REACH

The overhead reach combines aspects of the anterior reach and the overhead press. It is one of the most functional exercises, incorporating the entire core as well as upper and lower kinetic chains. This is one pattern that every athlete must master, as all sports require some, if not all, aspects of this exercise. Begin the pattern with body weight and reaching the arms overhead. Add a bilateral load (medicine ball), reaching the ball towards the ceiling (arrow). The final progression is a unilateral load with a posterior reach. In all versions, the majority of the motion should be at the hip and shoulder complexes while the spine remains long throughout the patterns.

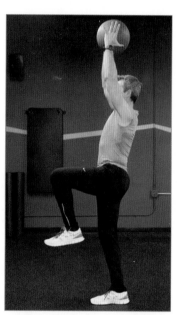

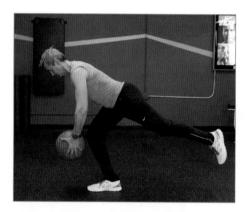

Overhead reach: bilateral – medicine ball.

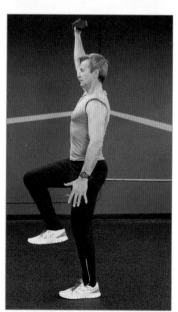

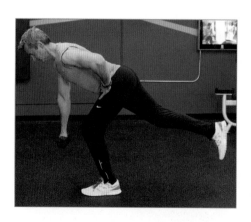

Overhead reach: unilateral with an overhead reach – DB.

WINDMILL

Windmill patterns are essentially hybrid versions of reaches and help improve hip dissociation in single leg support. It is important that the client maintains their TPC as well as femoroacetabular (hip) stability throughout the pattern.

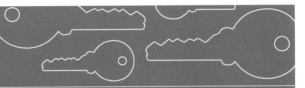

Key To Performance
Windmill

- The client stands in a parallel stance with legs shoulder width apart, maintaining a long spine, core activation, and the arms held out to the sides.
- They rotate towards one side through a vertical axis through the spine.
- The client returns to the starting position and repeats on the other side.

CLIENT SENSATION: The client should feel as if they are rotating through the hips and spine and are able to maintain their posture throughout the pattern.

While any single leg pattern requires rotary stability, the single leg windmill pattern introduces pure transverse plane rotation for the more advanced client and athlete. As with all single leg rotary patterns, it is vital that the motion occurs around a vertical axis and that the pelvis remains 'squared' throughout the pattern. The internal rotation bias helps improve internal rotation mechanics required for sport. The external rotation bias helps train the posterior and external rotation chains necessary for maintaining stability of the lower extremity while in single leg stance.

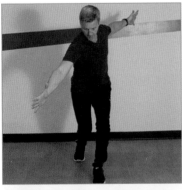 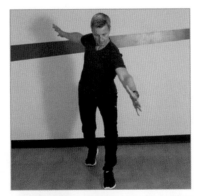

Windmill – split stance: internal rotation (left); external rotation (right).

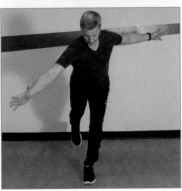 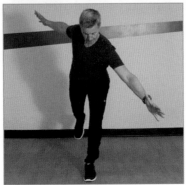

Windmill – unilateral stance: internal rotation (left); external rotation (right).

MECHANICS DURING DEADLIFTS AND SQUATS

Deadlifts and squats are two of the fundamental movement patterns. While the deadlift is a hip-dominant pattern, focusing on development of the posterior chain, the squat is a knee-dominant pattern that equally stresses both the hip and knee complexes. They are both great patterns for improving hip extension as well as improving spine and scapular stability. Unfortunately, the patterning that is taught by many fitness professionals during these patterns can be a major cause of neck, shoulder, and back problems in their clients. There are several causes for concern with these patterns, which will be discussed below.

- **Excessive spine extension and butt gripping:** Clients are often instructed to lift their chest up and pull their shoulder blades down and back during these patterns. This causes overextension of the spine and functionally 'locks' their thoracic spine. Although this may seem like a great strategy for lifting heavy loads, it causes many clients to 'disconnect' or lose anterior abdominal control, limiting the functional stability of the thoracopelvic canister. Over time this leads to poor spinal stabilization, overcompression of the spine, and compensatory hypermobilization of the lumbopelvic region. Additionally, clients are often asked to 'squeeze the glutes' at the top of both lifts, which drives the femoral head anteriorly in the acetabulum, directly leading to compression syndromes of the hip, poor gluteal stabilization strategies, and posterior pelvic rotation.

- **Posterior pelvic rotation and lumbar flexion:** Posterior pelvic rotation and lumbar flexion are common compensations when the client 'runs out of available hip flexion.' In other words, when the client squats or lowers during a deadlift pattern beyond their available range of hip flexion, they will go through obligatory posterior rotation of the pelvis and lumbar flexion (image below right). This problem, exacerbated by thoracic hyperextension as described above, is a leading cause of lumbar disc injuries, overstretching of the facet joints, and sacroiliac joint problems.

- **Excessive neck extension and poor scapular stabilization:** Clients are cued to 'keep the eyes level with the horizon' or even to 'keep the head up' during squat and deadlift patterns. This creates hyperextension of the cervicothoracic junction, which is compounded by using a heavy bar held across the shoulders or holding a heavy weight with the arms during the deadlift. And, during the deadlift, clients often lift weights that are too heavy for their available scapular stability, further stressing the cervicothoracic junction.

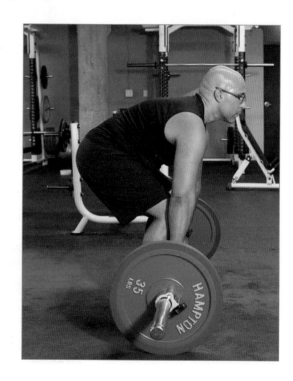

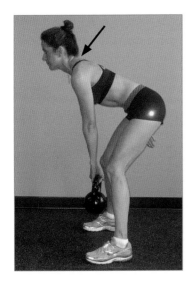 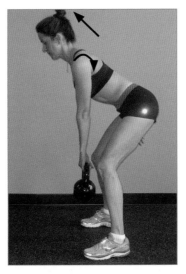

- **Cervicothoracic alignment during the deadlift pattern:** the client hyperextends her neck and overly abducts her scapula during a unilateral deadlift pattern (left image). The client is cued to maintain a long spine and activate her scapular stabilizers, which improves her alignment, reducing stress on her cervicothoracic junction (right image).

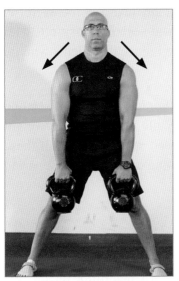 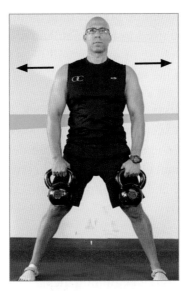

- **Scapular stabilization during the deadlift pattern:** notice the client's scapulae in the image to the left – there is loss of scapular stabilization and resultant downward rotation of the scapulae when the client is cued to 'bring the scapulae down and back.' In the image to the right, the client activates the serratus anterior and lower trapezius and visualizes the shoulders going wide.

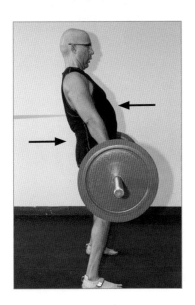 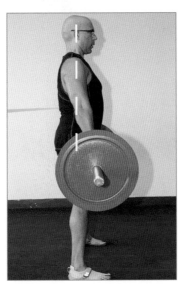

- **Spinal stabilization during the deadlift pattern:** note the loss of anterior stabilization (horizontal left-facing arrow), posterior pelvic rotation, and thoracolumbar hyperextension (horizontal right-facing arrow) when the client is cued to 'lift the chest and squeeze the glutes.' The client achieves the 'long spine' posture (vertical dotted line) and maintains the thoracopelvic canister in the image to the right.

Although these are common cues that are routinely taught during these patterns, and which allow many clients to lift heavier weight, they can drive major dysfunction in clients who exhibit compromised motor control. To gain both the benefits of improving posterior chain function and improving postural control, the following cues must be adhered to during modified deadlift and squatting patterns.

- The spine and pelvis must remain in neutral alignment throughout the pattern. There should be no excessive extension at the top of the motion or loss of alignment in the bottom position. The client must understand how to hip hinge and at what point they reach their end of available range of motion. The end of available range of motion is the point where the client can no longer maintain centrated joints or neutral spine position. As the client lifts, they pull the weight until they are standing in a tall spine posture – they do not pull into thoracolumbar hyperextension.

- The scapulae must remain controlled throughout the pattern. The weight being lifted should not be so heavy as to affect the ability to maintain a neutral scapular position.

- The core must remain activated. There should be no loss of activation at any phase of the exercise. Generally lighter weights will need to be used to help maintain spine and scapular positions with ideal canister stabilization. Additionally, range of motion will need to be reduced in clients who go into a posterior tilt towards the bottom of the motion.

Author's note: Lifting 'purists' will often disagree on the head, neck, and thoracic positions discussed above, arguing that they will lead to poor execution and loss of power. While lifting heavier weight at the expense of injury only matters to the ego-driven lifter, the decreased spinal stress that these modifications offer must be the most important determinant when constructing corrective exercise and training programs for the post-rehabilitative and general population client.

DEADLIFTS

The client must be able to perform a waiter's bow (hip hinge) and a body weight squat with perfect form prior to performing a loaded deadlift. Before beginning the deadlift pattern, determine the client's available range of hip motion statically, through a simple range of motion assessment, and dynamically, through the waiter's bow and body weight squat.

Key To Performance
Deadlift

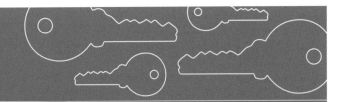

- The client takes a slightly wider than hip width stance, bends their knees to approximately 45 degrees, and performs a hip hinge to grasp the handle of the barbell, dumbbell, or kettlebell.

- Their pelvis and spine, including the head and neck, must remain neutral throughout the pattern – the eyes should look up to activate the extensor reflex.

- The scapular stabilizers must be activated and remain active throughout the pattern – the weight should not be excessive to the point that it pulls the scapulae into downward rotation.

- Once in position, there should be no further motion at the knees, spine, or pelvis – the movement should be pure hip flexion.

- The trainer or therapist should palpate both the lumbar spine, to ensure that it stays neutral, and the lateral abdominal wall, to ensure lateral wall activation throughout the pattern. The client is cued to activate if they lose control and if unable, they are required to stop the pattern.

- The client extends the hips to lift the bar from the floor, but should not hyperextend the hips or thoracolumbar regions.

- Generally, they should breathe in as they descend and breathe out as they lift – this pattern, however, can be altered in the rehabilitation and corrective exercise environments.

- When performing one leg variations, the pelvis must be 'squared' and the spine must remain neutral throughout the pattern (see earlier section for description of the 'squared' pelvis).

CLIENT SENSATION: The client should feel as if their core remains active throughout the pattern and that the gluteal and hamstring complexes are doing the most amount of work.

They should not experience excessive lumbar work as these muscles should be contracting isometrically to stabilize the spine.

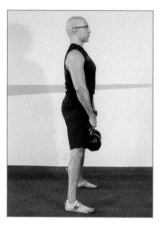 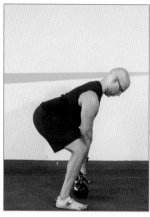 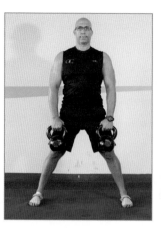 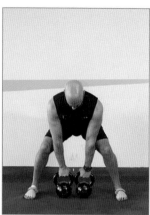

Deadlift pattern: side view (left two images); anterior view (right two images).
Note the maintenance of the long spine throughout the pattern.

Performing the unilateral deadlift pattern introduces a rotary component to the trunk and spine. This pattern can be loaded with a kettlebell or dumbbell. The client must maintain a neutral TPC and rotate through their hips during the pattern.

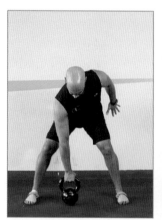 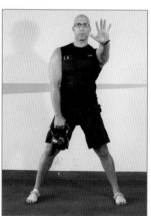 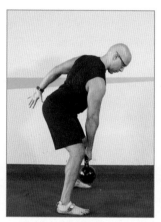 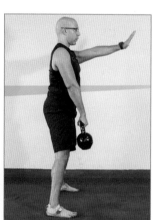

Key To Success
Spinal Stabilization During Deadlift and Squat Patterns

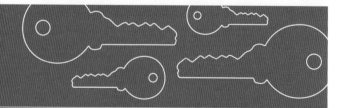

'Maintain the eyes level with the horizon' is a common cue during the deadlift and squat patterns. While this cue is given to maintain activation of the spinal extensors, it directly contributes to overload of the cervicothoracic junction.

KEY: The extensor reflex can be driven by cuing the client to 'look up with the eyes' while maintaining a relative neutral position of the head and neck and upper thoracic spine.

KNEE-DOMINANT PATTERNS

SQUATS

While the squat is considered a knee-dominant pattern, if performed properly it is one of the most effective patterns for loading both the primary movers and stabilizers of the lumbopelvic-hip complex in addition to the trunk. The squat pattern is a must for individuals rehabilitating lumbopelvic-hip injuries and even the elderly can perform the squat pattern by altering the depth and level of stability.

While virtually every trainer, coach, and therapist performs some variation, many misconceptions still exist regarding the proper execution of the squat. For example, there is still the misconception that the knees should not move in front of the toes when squatting, the individual should look up as they squat, and the gluteals should be squeezed as the individuals lifts up during the concentric phase of the squat.

To ensure its effectiveness, several variables need to be taken into consideration when deciding which version of the squat to use with a particular client. Prior exposure to the exercise, level of flexibility, level of motor control, body awareness, and desired outcome of the exercise all play a role in the type of squat and specific cues the trainer, coach, or therapist will decide to use with their client.

This section will evaluate and make suggestions on the most basic version of the squat as this is the safest and easiest to teach most individuals. While this in no way suggests that other versions are not safe or effective, it can often be difficult to teach even the basic versions to some individuals. Although some individuals may choose to perform Olympic, powerlifting-style, or plié-type squats, the majority of the mechanics that are listed below will apply to these other versions as well.

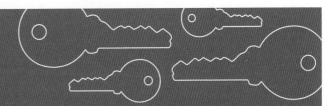

Key To Success
Squatting Mechanics and the Great Knees Over Toes Debate

It is common for trainers and therapists to teach their clients to keep the knees behind the toes during lower extremity patterns such as squats, lunges, and step-ups. The premise is that maintaining the knee behind the toes decreases the pressure on the knee. However, is this really a true interpretation and is this cue really applicable to improving lower extremity mechanics? Fry et al (2003) looked at this notion and did find that a more vertical position of the tibia (less forward position) was effective at reducing knee forces, as compared to participants whose knees were allowed to travel forward unrestricted. However, that is not where the story ends. Increased stress on the hips and low back in the participants whose knees were restricted from moving forward was also noted.

KEY: Restricting the knees from moving forward may be a viable strategy for decreasing knee pressure in clients who have knee pain. However, this strategy will increase the stress on their back and hips, which is often the underlying cause of the client's knee pain to begin with. Therefore, the trainer or therapist is encouraged to evaluate the hip and knee mechanics and use the 'knee behind the toes' cue judiciously for clients who are experiencing knee pain.

Key To Performance
Squat

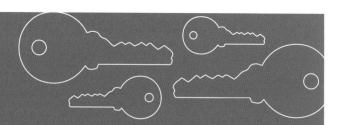

- The client sets up in a parallel stance position with neutral spine posture and their feet approximately shoulder width or slightly wider apart. The hands are held in front of body.

- The head, trunk, and pelvis should be in neutral position to begin and remain relatively stationary throughout the motion.

- The head and eyes should remain level with the horizon – the client should not look up as this encourages cervicothoracic extension.

- Core activation should be maintained throughout the motion.

- The client's trunk and pelvis should fall equidistant between the feet as they descend into the squat.

- Their knees should track in the same plane as the feet (knees should track approximately between digits 1–3 of the foot).

- The knees should not deviate medially (adduction) or laterally (abduction) at any point throughout the motion.

- The tibia (lower leg) and feet should remain neutral throughout the movement.

- The client should be able to maintain the foot tripod throughout the pattern.

- They squat until their thighs are approximately parallel or slightly below. The depth of squat is dependent on the client's ability to maintain neutral alignment – as soon as they are unable to maintain any of the aforementioned keys, they are stopped from descending any lower.

- They lift up from the hips, being sure not to overactivate the glutes at the top of the motion.

CLIENT SENSATION: The client should feel as if they are able to maintain alignment throughout the pattern.

Note: During all lower extremity patterns that involve squatting, deadlifting, and reaching – the hips should shift posteriorly to initiate the movement. Be sure to watch your clients that initiate these types of patterns by bending their knees and cue them to prioritize hip movement.

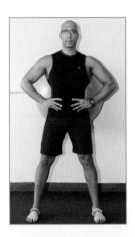
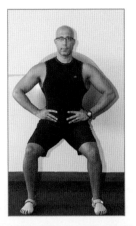

LEVEL I: BALL SQUAT

The ball squat is a great alternative for those individuals who are just learning the squat mechanics, cannot perform a free standing squat because of instability or pain, or have not yet progressed sufficiently to perform the unsupported squat pattern.

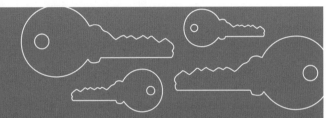

Key To Performance
Ball Squat

- The client sets up in a parallel stance, neutral spine posture with their feet approximately shoulder width or slightly wider apart. The ball is placed just above their sacrum and their hands are held in front of the body or at the sides.

- The head, trunk, and pelvis should be in neutral position to begin and remain relatively stationary throughout the motion.

- The head and eyes should remain level with the horizon – the client should not look up as this encourages cervicothoracic extension.

- Core activation should be maintained throughout the motion.

- The client's trunk and pelvis should fall equidistant between their feet as they descend into the squat.

- The knees should track in the same plane as the feet (knees should track approximately between digits 1–3 of the foot).

- The knees should not deviate medially (adduction) or laterally (abduction) at any point throughout the motion.

- The tibia (lower leg) and feet should remain neutral throughout the movement.

- The client should be able to maintain the foot tripod throughout the pattern.

- They squat until their thighs are approximately parallel or slightly below. The depth of squat is dependent on the client's ability to maintain neutral alignment – as soon as they are unable to maintain any of the aforementioned keys, they are stopped from descending any lower.

- They lift up from the hips, being sure not to overactivate the gluteals at the top of the motion.

CLIENT SENSATION: The client should feel as if they are able to maintain alignment throughout the pattern.

Key To Success
Determining the Depth of the Squat

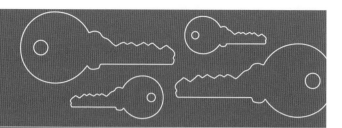

Recently, it has become rather trendy in the training industry to have clients perform deep squats – that is, to have a client's butt approximate their ankles in the descent phase of the pattern. There seem to be two driving factors for this recent phenomenon:

1. Gray Cook utilizes the deep squat as part of his functional movement assessment so individuals took that to mean that their clients should deep squat. However, Gray Cook never said that this should be a pattern for training clients, but rather that it should not be used unless the clients have earned the right through proper stability and mobility.

2. Trainers often point to the study that demonstrates that an increased depth of squatting shows better EMG activity, as compared to shallower depth squatting (Caterisano et al 2002).

However, what these studies often don't consider is whether or not the client can, or more precisely should, be performing deep squatting. In other words, it is true that the greater the range of motion of a particular exercise (in this case the squat), the greater the activation of the prime movers (i.e. the gluteus maximus for the squat). However, the question that needs to be asked is whether or not the client possesses the hip range of motion to squat properly without creating posterior rotation of the pelvis, or has adequate ankle dorsiflexion to prevent compensatory valgus and/or internal rotation at the knee during the squat pattern. So, while the deep squat is great for activating the gluteus maximus in the client with ideal range of motion and stabilization patterns, it can be detrimental to the joints of the low back, pelvis, and/or knees in the client who does not possess those same capabilities.

KEY: The client should be instructed to squat to the depth where they can maintain ideal alignment and centration of all the joints of the spine, pelvis, and lower kinetic chain.

ALTERNATIVE SQUAT PATTERNS

Supporting the arms on a stable surface or TRX can help a client develop competency and confidence in performing the squat pattern. This also allows for easier maintenance of the TPC during the movement. The client squats as deep as they are able while maintaining lower extremity joint centration and TPC stability. During either pattern, the client can hold isometrically at the bottom of their range and take 3–5 deep breaths. This helps to coordinate hip loading and diaphragmatic breathing, which has a functional carry-over to activities of daily living.

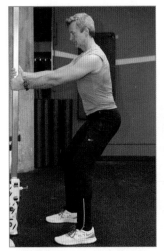 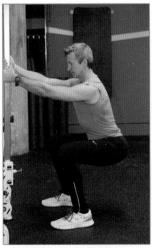 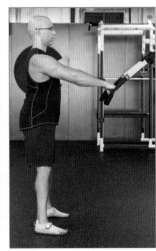 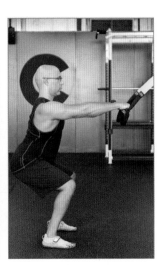

Supported squat.   TRX supported squat.

Once the client understands how to maintain their form through supported squats, they are progressed to unsupported versions. The client can place one hand upon his chest and one hand upon his abdomen to help cue proper maintenance of the TPC during the squat pattern.

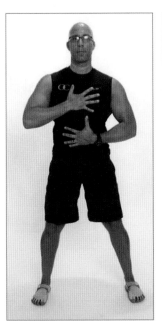 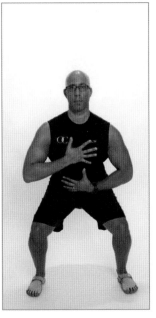 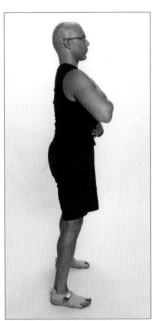 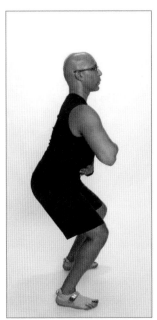

TPC control during squat (anterior-left); (side-right).

LEVEL II: LOADING THE SQUAT PATTERN

Once the client can achieve a perfect squat pattern, the pattern can be loaded with dumbbells, cable machines, or medicine balls. The placement of the barbell on the upper thoracic spine tends to fixate the thoracic spine, so barbell squats are not performed by those individuals with poor TPC stability. Additionally, keeping the hands in front or at the sides of the body helps unload the spine from the deleterious effects of heavy barbell squats when training the general population client.

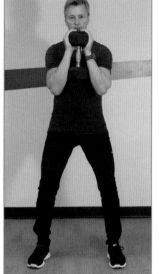 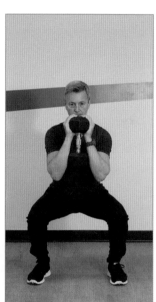

Goblet squats and dumbbell squats are safer squat patterns than the behind-the-neck barbell versions and allow the individual to maintain their TPC (Goblet squat, right).

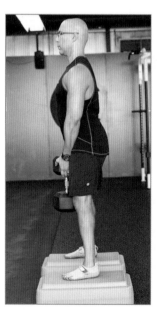 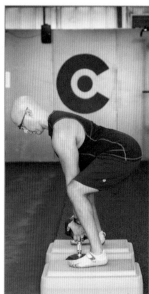 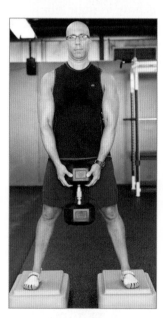 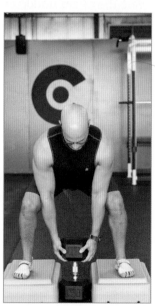

DB squat, side view (left); anterior view (right). The DB squat pattern as demonstrated above is very similar to the deadlift pattern described on page 278. The biggest difference is there is more knee flexion in the squat version. To make it more like a traditional squat pattern, the client should position their trunk in a more upright position.

LEVEL III: OVERHEAD SQUAT

Given the demands on the core musculature and scapular stabilizers, the overhead squat pattern should only be performed with clients who demonstrate perfect squat mechanics. Additionally, the overhead version requires significant flexibility of the shoulder and hip complexes to enable the spine and pelvis to remain in a neutral position, so these positions should be closely monitored during the pattern.

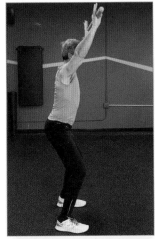
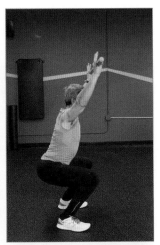

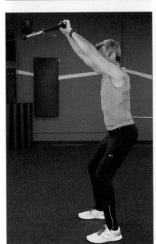
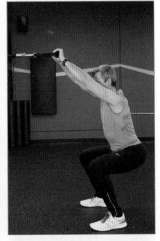

The overhead squat against resistance requires even greater shoulder and core stability as well as upper extremity flexibility. This requires that the client is able to upwardly rotate and posteriorly tilt the scapula while maintaining the upper arms in a locked, overhead position. It is important that the client only squat to the point where they can maintain a neutral alignment of their spine, pelvis, and lower and upper extremities throughout any of the overhead squat patterns.

Be sure that the client can maintain a neutral spine and scapular position throughout the pattern.

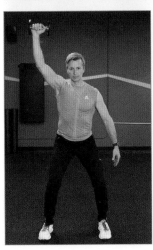
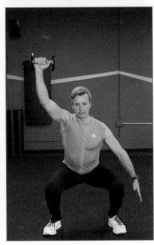

Because the asymmetrical overhead squat is one of the most demanding integrative patterns, it should only be performed by those individuals demonstrating complete core, scapular, and lower extremity stability.

LEVEL IV: SINGLE LEG SQUAT

For clients who have progressed to a more advanced level, there is no exercise that has better functional carry-over to real life and sport than the single leg squat (SLS). The SLS can directly improve every aspect of the lower extremity, from the feet through to the pelvis. Additionally, the SLS increases the load on the lower extremity without the additional spinal loads that accompany more traditional barbell squats. And the SLS can be the litmus test for return to sport for clients or athletes – if they cannot perform a perfect SLS squat, they are not ready to return to their sport. There are several keys to performing a single leg squat, which will be described below.

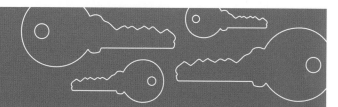

Key To Performance
Single Leg Squat

- The client stands on one leg with the foot, knee, and hip aligned.
- The head, trunk, and pelvis must remain in a neutral position and remain relatively stationary throughout the motion.
- The head and eyes should remain level with the horizon – the client should not look up as this encourages cervicothoracic extension.
- Core activation should be maintained throughout the motion.
- The knees should track in the same plane as the feet (knees should track approximately between digits 1–3 of the foot).
- The knees should not deviate medially (adduction) or laterally (abduction) at any point throughout the motion.
- The tibia (lower leg) and feet should remain neutral throughout the movement.
- The client should be able to maintain the foot tripod throughout the pattern.
- They squat until their thighs are approximately parallel or slightly below. The depth of squat is dependent on the client's ability to maintain neutral alignment – as soon as they are unable to maintain any of the aforementioned keys, they are stopped from descending any lower.
- They lift up from the hips, being sure not to overactivate the glutes at the top of the motion.
- The pattern can be progressed by introducing arm and leg motion, simulating a running gait. Begin in split stance to single leg, progressing to maintaining the SLS for the entire exercise.
- If the client is unable to maintain spine or lower extremity alignment, or demonstrates excessive instability through the lower extremity, pelvis, or trunk, they must be regressed to the split squat or supported version.

CLIENT SENSATION: The client should feel as if they are able to maintain alignment throughout the pattern. They should feel as if their posterior hip is doing most of the work.

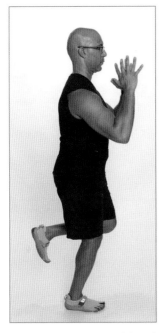 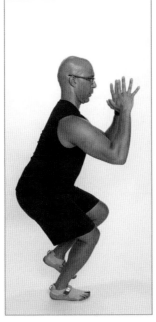 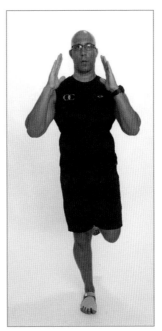 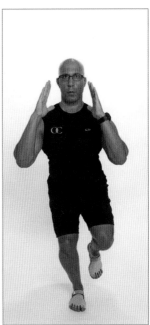

Single leg squat (side view).   Single leg squat (anterior view).

SPLIT SQUAT

Split squat patterns are a progression of the basic squat pattern and are another effective way to train the lumbopelvic-hip complex, as rarely in life are movements performed with the legs in a parallel position. The ball split squat is a great way to perform the pattern with clients who are just learning the movement, rehabilitating an injury, or have stability issues.

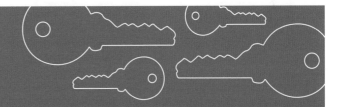

Key To Performance
Split Squat

- The client sets up in a split stance position with their lumbar spine against a stability ball.

- The feet are approximately a comfortable hip width apart and the hands are held in front of the body.

- The head, trunk, and pelvis should be in neutral position to begin and remain relatively stationary throughout the motion. Core activation should be maintained throughout the pattern.

- The head and eyes should remain level with the horizon – the client should not look up, as this encourages thoracolumbar extension.

- The client should begin the movement by sitting back in their lead hip and lowering the body.

- The knees should track in the same plane as the feet (knees should track approximately between digits 1–3 of the foot).

- The knees should not deviate medially (adduction) or laterally (abduction) at any point throughout the motion.

- The client's feet should remain neutral throughout the movement and they should be able to maintain the foot tripod throughout the pattern.

- They squat until their thighs are approximately parallel to the floor. The depth of squat is dependent on the client's ability to maintain neutral alignment – as soon as they are unable to maintain any of the aforementioned keys, they are stopped from descending any lower.

- They lift up from the hips, being sure not to overactivate the glutes at the top of the motion.

- Once the pattern has been learned, it can be loaded with medicine balls, kettlebells, or dumbbells.

- This pattern can be progressed to the unsupported, elevated, and single leg stance.

CLIENT SENSATION: The client should feel as if they are able to maintain alignment throughout the pattern and should feel as if the hips are doing most of the work.

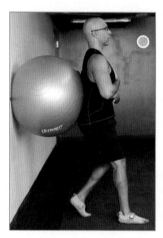 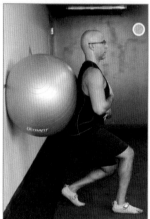 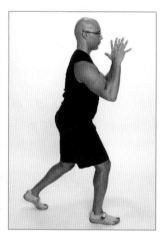 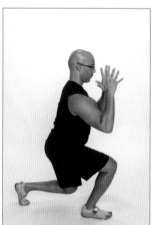

Level I: Split squat against a ball.

Level II: Split squat without support.

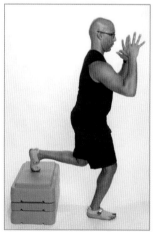 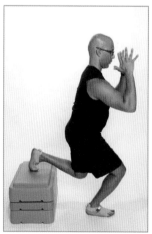 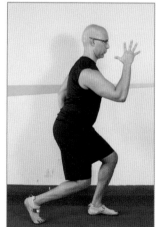 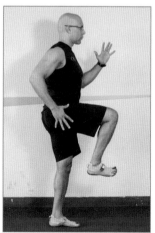

Level III: Split squat with elevated rear leg.

Level IV: Split squat to single leg stance.

LUNGES

Lunges are among the most functional exercises that can be performed for both the core and lower kinetic chain. Proper lunge mechanics are necessary, whether for picking up a child or a bag of groceries, or for performing a lateral maneuver while engaging in a sporting activity. What makes lunges extremely effective is that they emphasize loading of the hips, knees, and ankles and can be performed in several planes of motion. Frontal and transverse patterns improve athletic movements in activities such as reaching in tennis, cutting to the side in basketball, or the pivot and go movement that a defensive back may perform in football.

Proper progressions begin with maintaining a neutral spine position throughout the loading (eccentric) and unloading (concentric) phases of the movement. The focus on the pattern is movement through the hips while maintaining a neutral, stable spine position, which helps to limit spinal loading and lower extremity instability.

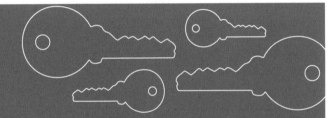

Key To Performance
Reaching Lunge

- The client starts in an upright, neutral spine posture with their core activated.
- They take a step forward, reaching the arms towards the floor.
- They pivot around the forward hip, maintaining a neutral spine posture.
- Using the front hip, the client pushes themselves back to the starting position.
- There should be no excessive motion in the spine as they push themselves back to the start.
- The head, trunk, and pelvis should be in neutral position to begin and remain relatively stationary throughout the motion.
- Progress the client to the frontal and transverse patterns.

CLIENT SENSATION: The client should feel as if they are able to maintain alignment throughout the pattern and should feel as if their front hip and leg are doing most of the work.

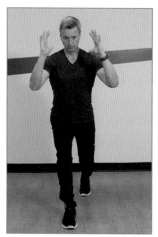 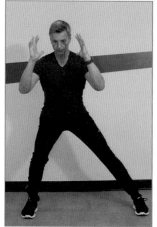 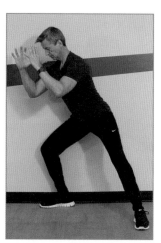

Lunge: sagittal plane, frontal plane, transverse plane (anterior view).

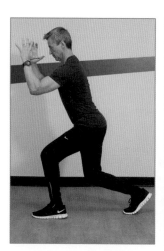 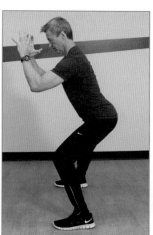 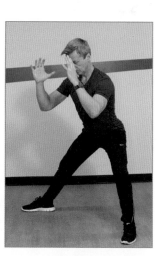

Lunge: sagittal plane, frontal plane, transverse plane (side view).

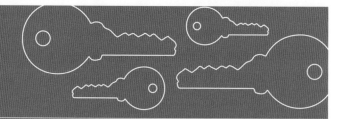

Key To Success
Lunge Patterns

Lunge patterns are an excellent way to train the entire extensor chain while improving overall balance and flexibility of the lower extremity. By modifying the length and depth, nearly anyone can benefit from performing lunges. Decreasing the length, depth, and speed will be appropriate for older clients or for those with low back or hip instabilities, whereas increasing the length, depth, speed, and external loads will benefit more athletic individuals.

After mastering the movement with body weight, lunges can be loaded with dumbbells, weight vests, medicine balls, or resistive bands to increase the demand on the entire extensor chain. Be sure the client maintains neutral spine and scapular positions throughout the patterns. Likewise, there should be no changes in lower extremity positioning between the body weight and loaded versions.

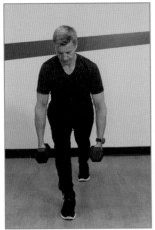 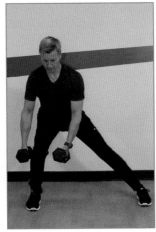 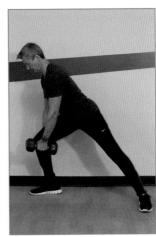

Lunge:
sagittal plane (left),
frontal plane (middle),
transverse plane (right).

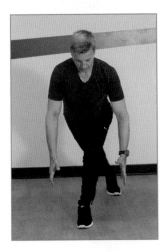

The cross-over lunge with reach adds additional challenges to the hip complex, making it an ideal return-to-sport or higher level progression. The key is to ensure that the rotation comes from the hip and not the knee – the hip, knee, and ankle should remain in a straight line throughout the pattern.

LUNGE WITH ROTATION

The lunge with rotation is utilized to improve internal hip rotation and deceleration mechanics of the forward hip. The client begins with neutral spine and core activation and then proceeds by taking a step forward while rotating the pelvis towards the forward leg. They stabilize and then push through the hip and thigh to return to the starting position. The rotation comes from the hip with minimal rotation from the spine. Although both are necessary parts of normal biomechanics, there should be minimal rotation at the knee and pronation through the ankle during the motion. The client places their arms on the pelvis so that they can monitor its movement around the stationary lower limb. Their head faces straight forward so rotation occurs through their spine, making this a great way to train dissociation of the head from the trunk.

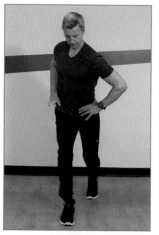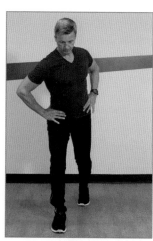

Stepping lunge with rotation: internal rotation (above left); external rotation (above right).

Additionally, the lunge with rotation is an excellent way to train stabilization mechanics in the lower extremity while subsequently training trunk rotation. The client begins by holding the arms in front of the body, parallel to the floor. They step into a lunge position, simultaneously rotating towards the forward leg, inducing internal hip rotation. They then step back to the starting position and repeat. Performing the same pattern while rotating away from the forward leg is used to train deceleration of an external rotation force of the forward leg. Rotation should occur through the forward hip and spine, and the client must maintain alignment of the ankle, knee, hip, and pelvis. If the client has difficulty maintaining balance or stability, shorten the length of the stance and/or the amount of trunk rotation.

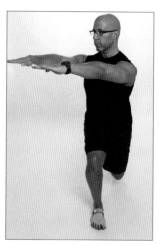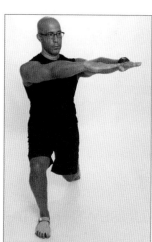

Stepping lunge with rotation: internal rotation bias (left); external rotation bias (right).

SLIDE BOARD AND STABILITY BALL LUNGE PATTERNS

The basic sagittal and frontal plane lunge can be performed on a slide board or stability ball, thereby adding an additional challenge to the pattern. The client begins by flexing the forward hip while the opposite foot is slid along the board. The range of motion during any of the slide board or ball lunges is determined by the client's ability to maintain neutral spine and pelvis; the available range of hip flexion of the forward leg; the available length in the rectus femoris and hip flexors in the rear leg (sagittal plane version); and the available length of the hip adductors in the sliding leg (frontal plane version).

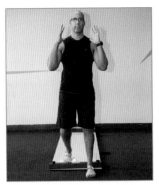 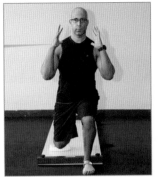 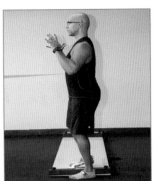 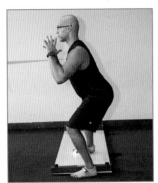

Sagittal and frontal plane slide board lunge, anterior (left); side (right).

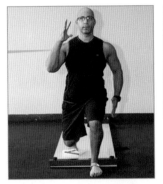 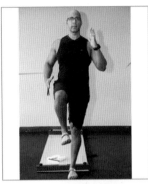 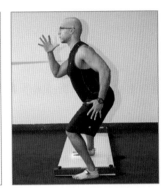 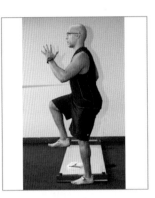

Sagittal and frontal plane slide board lunge to single leg stance, anterior (left); side (right).

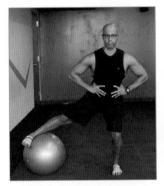 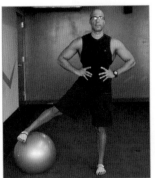 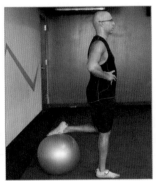 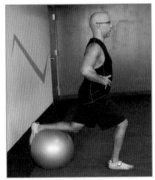

Sagittal and frontal plane ball lunge, anterior (left); side (right).

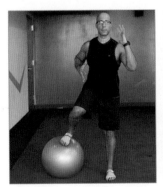 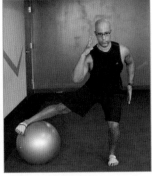 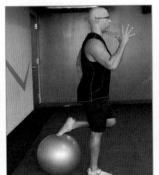 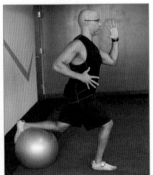

Sagittal and frontal plane slide board lunge with arm drivers, anterior (left); side (right).

STEP-UPS

Whether walking down a flight of stairs or stepping onto a curb, stairs are a necessary task of modern life. Unfortunately, stairs present a real challenge for many clients with knee pain. The step-up pattern is a great way to improve a client's mechanics so they can successfully handle stairs or step up and down off a raised surface. Additionally, step-ups are an excellent way to train the entire extensor chain (gluteus maximus, hamstrings, and gastrocnemius/soleus complex) while ensuring proper mechanics through the ankle, knee, and hip complexes. Nearly every client, regardless of their ability, can perform step-ups if they are progressed appropriately. The challenge with the step-up is in clients with decreased ankle or hip mobility and poor instructions in its execution. Clients lacking hip and/or ankle range of motion generally make it up with increased knee motion, generally by shearing through the knee. The other mistake clients generally make is to turn the step-up into a knee-dominant motion by extending the knees rather than lifting through the hips and bringing the body up over the foot. The key to improving the step-up pattern lies in improving dissociation at the ankle and/or hip and then improving mechanics. Equally important is using a step height that is appropriate for the client's hip range of motion that allows them to square the pelvis to make this a hip-dominant pattern (see below).

Squaring the pelvis during the step-up pattern: the client cannot maintain a squared pelvis because the step is too high for his available range of hip flexion (left); this creates unleveling of the pelvis. If he is unable to start in a neutral pelvic position, he will compensate through his spine or lower extremity as he steps up. Notice that he is able to level his pelvis once the steps are lowered to his available range of motion (right).

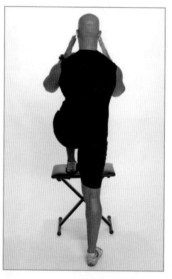
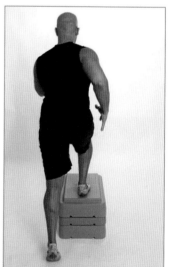

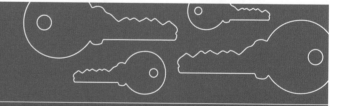

Key To Performance
Step-ups

- The client begins with one leg on the step – their pelvis is level, their spine is in alignment, and they maintain alignment through the foot, knee, and hip.

- The majority of their weight should be on the front leg (approximately 75%) with less on the back leg (25%). The client plantar flexes the ankle of the back leg, keeping the hip, knee, and foot of the back leg in alignment.

- The client steps up onto the step, lifting through the medial stabilization chain, and then steps back down, eccentrically controlling the descent through the medial stabilization chain. The weight is maintained on the forward leg even as they step back down – they step back and place the toes back on the floor, maintaining the majority of the weight on the forward leg.

- A level pelvis and neutral spine should be maintained throughout the pattern.

- Progress to the unilateral pattern once the client can perform twenty repetitions of the basic version.

CLIENT SENSATION: The client should feel as if they are lifting through the forward hip and maintains the majority of the weight on the forward leg in both the step-up (concentric) and step-down (eccentric) phases.

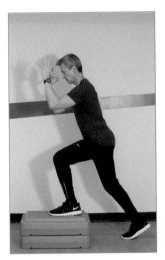 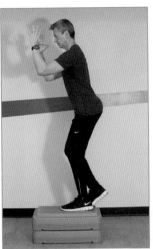 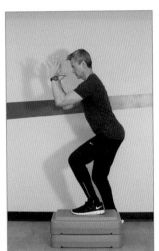 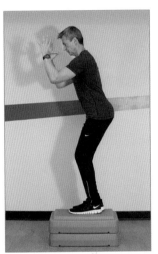

Step-up: sagittal (left); frontal (right).

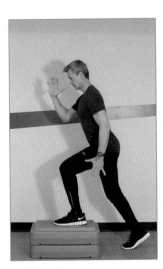 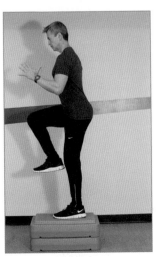 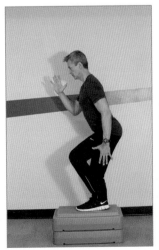 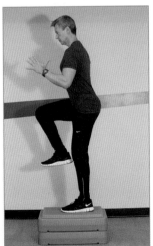

Step-up to single leg stance: sagittal (left); frontal (right).

FARMER'S WALKS, SLED PUSHES, AND SLED DRAGS

Farmer's walks and pushing and pulling sleds are some of the most effective functional patterns for improving trunk and hip stability and developing overall functional strength, while limiting the potentially high spinal loads that result when performing traditional barbell squats and deadlifts. Although these are relatively high level functional patterns, clients who have developed optimal stability and strength can be progressed safely into them. Unilateral farmer's walks are great patterns for developing rotary stability of the thoracopelvic canister (TPC). As with all patterns, the client should be able to maintain a long spine, ideal scapular alignment, and TPC stabilization throughout the patterns.

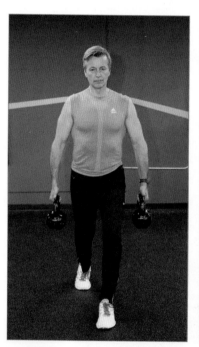 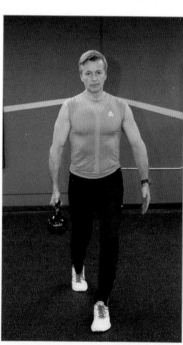

Farmer's walk: bilateral pattern (left); unilateral pattern (right).

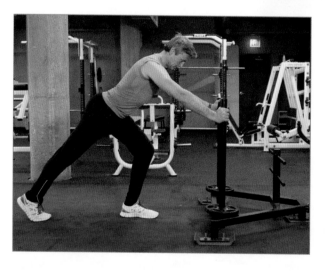 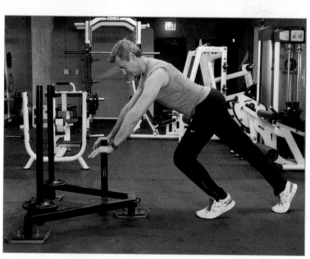

Sled push: high grip; low grip.

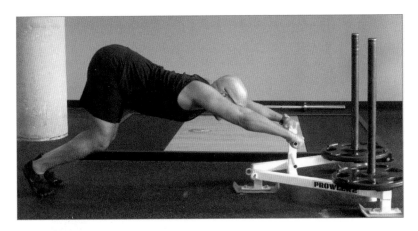

The client in the image above flexes through his lumbar spine and hyperextends through his thoracic spine. This is a common position in clients with stiffness in the thorax and hips and hypermobility of the lumbar spine. Additionally, he over-elevates his scapula and hyperextends at the cervicothoracic junction which overloads both the shoulder and neck region.

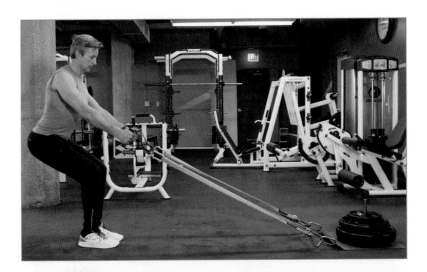

Sled drags. The sled drag pattern is very effective at improving knee stability in those clients that have developed relatively good control of their lower extremities. The client maintains a neutral spine and scapulothoracic control throughout the pattern. He steps backwards being sure to step through the ankle and foot and then extending the knee. He maintains alignment of the hip, knee, and ankle-foot throughout the pattern.

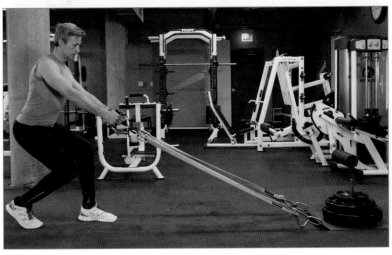

PROPRIOCEPTIVE NEUROMUSCULAR FACILITATION FLEXION AND EXTENSION PATTERNS

Proprioceptive neuromuscular facilitation (PNF) flexion and extension patterns are functional progressions of pushing and pulling patterns. They are among the most functional core exercises as they coordinate movements between the entire upper and lower kinetic chain. The extension patterns condition the entire extensor chain and posterior rotator cuff, while the flexion pattern does likewise for the entire flexor chain and anterior rotator cuff. Either of these patterns can be made more challenging by increasing the load or increasing the speed of execution. Be sure that the individual can perform and control both the shoulder and hip complexes individually prior to incorporating them into the following patterns.

PNF FLEXION PATTERNS

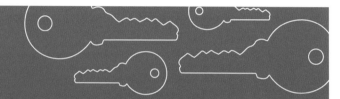

Key To Performance
PNF Flexion Patterns

- The client begins in a neutral spine and pelvic position with slight hip flexion and core activation.

- The cable or bands are set in the high position.

- The client initiates the pattern by rotating through their trunk and lead leg while simultaneously flexing and adducting their shoulder.

- They slowly return to the beginning position and repeat on the other side.

CLIENT SENSATION: The client should feel as if they are able to maintain alignment throughout the pattern and should feel that the trunk and pelvis are driving the motion.

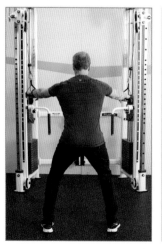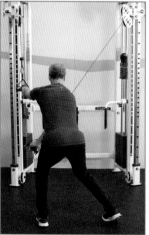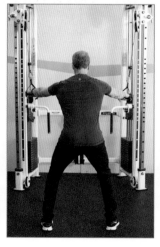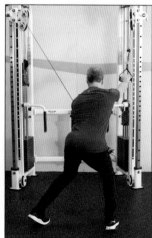

PNF flexion patterns: training the anterior oblique chain.

PNF EXTENSION PATTERNS

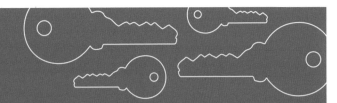

Key To Performance
PNF Extension Patterns

- The client begins in a neutral spine and pelvic position with slight hip flexion and core activation.

- The cable or bands are set in the low position.

- The client initiates the pattern by rotating through their trunk and lead leg while simultaneously extending through their shoulder.

- They slowly return to the beginning position and repeat on the other side.

CLIENT SENSATION: The client should feel as if they are able to maintain alignment throughout the pattern and should feel that the trunk and pelvis are driving the motion.

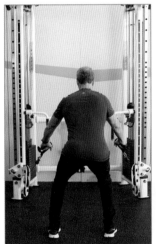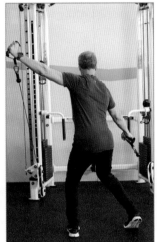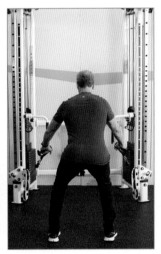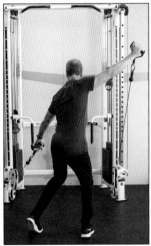

PNF extension patterns: training the posterior oblique chain.

chapter *10*

Contraindicated Exercises

CHAPTER OBJECTIVES
To identify contraindicated patterns for clients with shoulder or hip dysfunction

While it is inaccurate to categorize an exercise as either 'good' or 'bad' (they would be better classified as 'appropriate' or 'non-appropriate'), there are several exercises that are contraindicated for patients and clients who experience some of the more common movement dysfunctions that have been discussed in this book.

CONTRAINDICATED PATTERNS FOR THE CLIENT WITH SHOULDER DYSFUNCTION

For clients with a painful and/or unstable shoulder joint, there are several contraindicated exercises including upright rows, dips, anterior and lateral dumbbell raises, and the barbell bench press. One problem with these exercises is that clients with an unstable scapulothoracic articulation will tend to overload the cervical and upper thoracic spine as well as the glenohumeral joint as they perform these patterns. These clients will be better served to work through the corrective exercise patterns discussed earlier in the book and then perform less challenging patterns working up to these patterns should they want or need to perform them for sport or for aesthetic purposes. Additional causes of concern with these exercises is listed below.

UPRIGHT ROW AND SHRUGS

The upright row (image right) is a poor exercise pattern for the painful and unstable shoulder because it places the glenohumeral (GH) joint into abduction and internal rotation, the exact position that creates impingement of the rotator cuff and subacromial bursa. Often clients substitute for inefficient ST stabilization or GH internal rotation by elevating the scapulae and protracting the head as they raise the bar. The additional problem with this pattern is that the trunk is fixed and the arms are mobilized, which perpetuates rigidity of the thorax and hypermobility of the ST articulation.

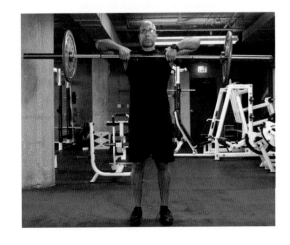

Although popularized by bodybuilders in their pursuit of overdeveloped 'traps', loaded shrugs (image right) are contraindicated for anyone except those participating in contact sports, such as American football, rugby, wrestling, and mixed martial arts. There is absolutely no benefit to this pattern and it will effectively overload the cervical spine, drive forward head posture, and drive scapulothoracic instability. Forward head shear is a common movement fault when performing the shoulder shrug pattern.

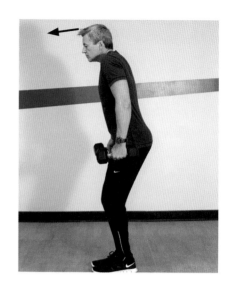

DIPS

Dips, both the traditional bar dip (image below left) and the bench versions (image below right), are particularly hard on the shoulder because the majority of the motion is derived from driving the head of the humerus forward in the glenoid fossa. Most clients with a painful or unstable shoulder are unable to support much additional resistance, let alone their entire body weight on an unstable GH or ST joint. This exercise can directly lead to or perpetuate anterior humeral glide syndrome, scapular elevation, and a forward head posture. Notice the forward head and shoulder position in the bar and bench dips.

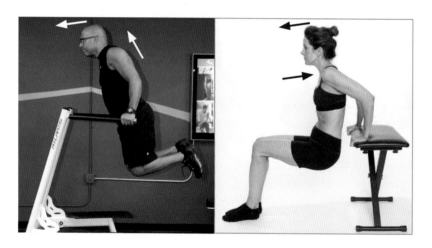

DUMBBELL ANTERIOR AND LATERAL RAISE

Although a common exercise, DB anterior and lateral raises are two of the most damaging exercises for the client with an unstable neck and shoulder. Not only does this exercise increase compressive loads on the cervical spine, but it also contributes to scapular instability. During the DB anterior and lateral raise, the neck becomes the anchor for the moving arms and the long lever arm only increases the stress on the neck. The eccentric load is extremely challenging to

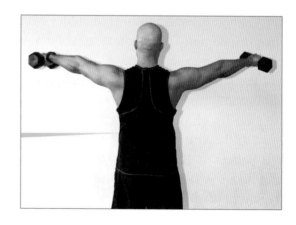

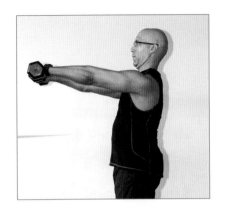

control even for those clients without neck and scapular issues. During the anterior raise (image left), clients will compensate for the weight and long lever arm by hyperextending through both the cervicothoracic and thoracolumbar junctions, adding to de-stabilization of the thoracopelvic canister.

BARBELL BENCH PRESS

The barbell bench press also presents a challenge for an unstable shoulder because, in addition to the thorax, the ST joint is fixed, while the GH joint is mobilized under usually large loads. This overloads the rotator cuff muscles and joint capsule due to the large loads that are used. Additionally, most clients perform the bench press with excessive arching of their back, essentially 'disconnecting' their thoracopelvic stabilizers and increasing activity in the pectoralis major and minor, further perpetuating the anterior scapular tilt and anterior

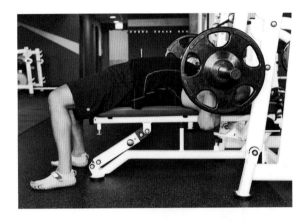

humeral positions. As noted above with upright rowing, the thorax becomes the fixed point and the scapulothoracic and glenohumeral articulations become the mobile points during this movement, which is a problem for the client and patient with the unstable shoulder or hypomobile thorax.

As an additional side note, any exercise performed behind the neck – such as behind the neck pull-downs, pull-ups, and overhead presses – need to be eliminated from the client's program. There is a huge risk of injuries to the neck and shoulders and absolutely no benefits of performing exercises in this manner. Stick with safer versions of these exercises.

CONTRAINDICATED PATTERNS FOR THE CLIENT WITH HIP DYSFUNCTION

 As with the shoulder complex, there are several contraindicated exercises for the hip complex. These include the leg lift, deep squat, bench step-over, leg press, and leg machine exercises.

LEG LIFT

Although not considered a pure hip exercise, the leg lift – along with its related versions, the inclined leg lift and the leg throw (where the trainer or therapist throws the legs down after the client raises them) – is a poor exercise choice for clients who lack optimal thoracopelvic stability and hip mobility. These patterns are extremely high level and place some of the highest compression forces

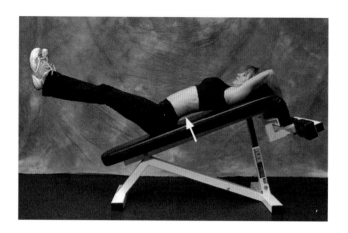

on the spine in relation to other abdominal exercises. Clients with poor hip dissociation preferentially move more from their lumbar spine to begin with and this pattern only perpetuates the dysfunction (arrow). This pattern also leads to loss of the thoracopelvic canister (TPC) control in clients with poor stability strategies, leading to overactivity of the superficial hip flexors.

DEEP SQUAT

While the deep squat may be a good evaluation tool for assessing hip and ankle range of motion, as well as the client's ability to stabilize their TPC, it is not a pattern that promotes improved biomechanics for the majority of individuals with hip and TPC dysfunction. Performing deep squats in clients without proper hip flexibility will directly lead to instabilities of the lumbar spine and/or sacroiliac joints as they try to compensate for the loss of range of motion in these areas. Very few clients possess the

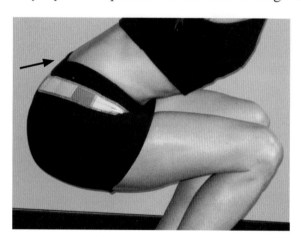

necessary hip flexion range of motion to make this an acceptable part of their corrective exercise or conditioning program. As she descends deeper into the squat, she will compensate by moving into posterior pelvic tilting and lumbar spine flexion. The client must be able to maintain a neutral spine and pelvis throughout the pattern and must stop the descent of the squat once they are no longer able to maintain control of their TPC. Notice the posterior tilt of the pelvis and lumbar spine flexion in this client as she squats to 'parallel'.

BENCH STEP-OVER

While it is not a bad exercise per se, the way most individuals perform this pattern is sure to make their physical therapists and chiropractic physicians grimace. It is intended to work the gluteals, but most clients perform the bench step-over pattern on a bench that is far too high for their available hip range of motion and stability. Therefore, they de-centrate their entire lower extremity and TPC to perform this pattern. (Notice the de-centration and over-stretching of the knee in this individual as he is about to load it by stepping over the bench.)What types of movement cause the highest number of menisci and anterior cruciate ligament injuries in the knee? – movements in which the menisci and cruciate ligaments are

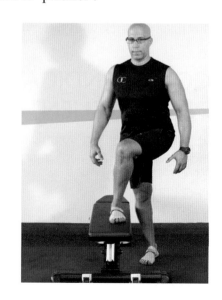

loaded and then repetitively compressed and overstretched. The way that most clients perform the bench step-over almost inevitably guarantees that they will have to visit their orthopedic surgeon in a few years.

LEG PRESS

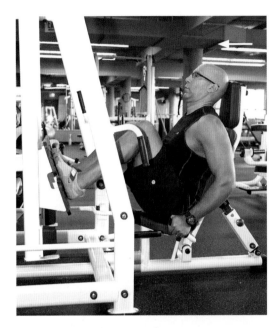

Leg presses are a poor exercise choice for individuals with limited hip flexibility and lumbar instability, or those who have chronic knee pain. Most clients lack the available range of hip flexion and are therefore unable to maintain a neutral spine and pelvic position as the weight is lowered and their knees are brought towards their chest. They compensate by posteriorly rotating through the pelvis and flexing their lumbar spine. This puts a tremendous load on the lumbar spine and perpetuates the dysfunctional pattern. This is also a problem with the more vertical versions of the leg press; however, the greater challenge with these versions is the increase in shear forces through the knee in clients with degenerative knee conditions. Recall, most clients with knee problems require improved hip function, which isn't adequately addressed with leg presses. Another problem with most versions of the leg press is that most individuals will lock their scapulothoracic articulation by holding onto the handles, and subsequently drive increased cervicothoracic extension (arrow in image above).

LEG MACHINE EXERCISES

An entire chapter could be dedicated to the pros and cons of leg machines, which include the seated leg extension (image left), the seated leg curl (image right), and abductor/abductor machines. While they are extremely effective at isolating the muscles of the legs and may have a role in the early phases

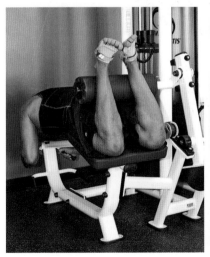
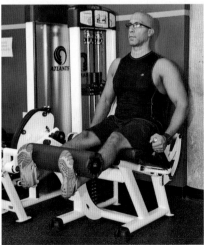

of rehabilitation or as part of a corrective exercise strategy, their overall effectiveness in improving long-term function is questionable. First of all, there is rarely, if ever, a time when there is more resistance placed on the leg beneath the knee than above it (unless a child or opponent is hanging on a client's lower leg). In other words, during daily activities and in sport, the load is usually above the hip. Second, because the client is seated, these machines fail to coordinate activity between the regions of the kinetic chain and may disrupt normal kinematic sequencing of the lower kinetic chain. Third, because the foot is off the ground the feedback loop from the foot to the nervous system is negated even though the lower extremity is still being loaded. Although there have been studies demonstrating short-term improvements in strength and performance with the use of machines, no studies are available to substantiate the long-term use of these machines over other lower body exercises. While there is no doubt that machines improve strength and muscle mass, which can have a functional benefit in the real world, their practical application remains somewhat limited in corrective exercise and improving fundamental movements.

SUMMARY

The goal of this chapter is not to suggest that the exercises highlighted are not good or can never be performed by healthy individuals. Rather, the purpose is to point out several problems with common exercises that are performed in the rehabilitation and gym settings. It means that clinicians, coaches, and trainers need to take a closer look at the exercise recommendations and determine the risk versus reward for their clients and patients on a case-by-case scenario.

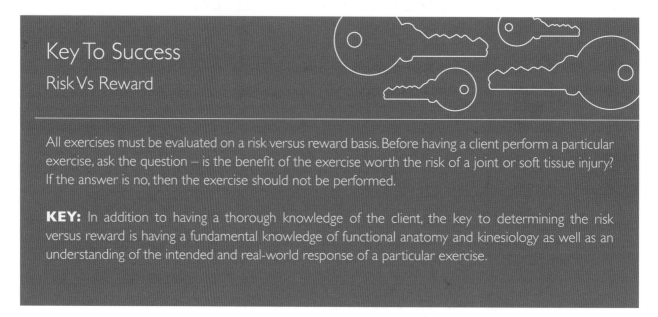

Key To Success
Risk Vs Reward

All exercises must be evaluated on a risk versus reward basis. Before having a client perform a particular exercise, ask the question – is the benefit of the exercise worth the risk of a joint or soft tissue injury? If the answer is no, then the exercise should not be performed.

KEY: In addition to having a thorough knowledge of the client, the key to determining the risk versus reward is having a fundamental knowledge of functional anatomy and kinesiology as well as an understanding of the intended and real-world response of a particular exercise.

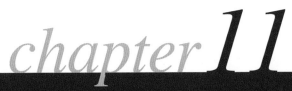

Conclusion

CHAPTER OBJECTIVES
To summarize the key principles of improving function
and developing optimal movement patterns presented in this book

"If we could give every individual the right amount of nourishment and exercise, not too little and not too much, we would have found the safest way to health." (Hippocrates)

PRINCIPLES OF FUNCTIONAL MOVEMENT

The fundamental philosophy of this book is based upon the three basic principles of movement that are frequently overlooked in the rehabilitative, corrective exercise, and conditioning industries. At first glance, these principles may seem to be too simplistic to warrant consideration when seeking a solution to the multiple levels of dysfunction that are seen in the majority of clients. However, once the impact that these small corrections can have on the nervous and neuromusculofascial system is recognized and understood, one begins to realize that an exercise program that overlooks these simple principles could be considered negligent, even harmful. It is even possible to consider the likelihood that many of the most common exercise prescriptions and corrective cues can actually exacerbate rather than correct dysfunctional movement patterns.

The key to this book is in the principles of human movement and to recognize they are universal laws that apply to all clients regardless of their functional goals. They are not just techniques, strategies, or methods that serve to reach a temporary goal such as accelerating weight loss or improving athletic performance. However, these principles will help the client achieve their individual functional goal, whether it be losing weight, improving their golf swing, or simply getting through their activities of daily living with greater ease and less discomfort by creating a framework in which to base all other aspects of the fitness program. The three principles are: 1) respiratory patterns must be normalized; 2) there must be centration of the joints; and 3) the client must be able to integrate respiration and maintain centration during the fundamental movement patterns of lunging, squatting, pushing, pulling, rotation, and gait.

1. RESPIRATION

The importance of functional breathing cannot be overstated. When working to create stabilization of the core, if the integration of respiration is overlooked, the body will choose breathing over stabilization, and stability of the trunk and spine will suffer with every breath the client takes.

The diaphragm attaches to the inside of the rib cage from the xiphoid process all the way around the rib cage to insert into the thoracolumbar junction. When fully relaxed, the central tendon of the diaphragm sits high in the chest cavity. As it contracts, the diaphragm flattens down to the level of the lower ribs. For the diaphragm to flatten, the abdominal muscles must eccentrically lengthen to allow the abdominal contents to be moved down and out (as addressed with the diaphragmatic breathing technique). The aspect most often overlooked is that the lower ribs must move anteriorly and posteriorly as well as laterally to accommodate and assist in increasing the circumference of the diaphragm. And finally, upon the exhalation, the anterior ribs must drop back down to the start position, so that the diaphragm is optimally aligned for the next breath cycle.

This method of breathing additionally provides all the benefits of diaphragmatic breathing: increased oxygenation of the cells, activation of the parasympathetic nervous system, and improved lymphatic function due to the 'milking' effect on the entire lymphatic system. However, functional breathing has the added benefit of improving thoracic mobility while enhancing stability of the spine and trunk.

Many clients are rigid in their thorax due to several factors, including overcorrection of postural faults, exercises that fixate the ribs and thoracic spine, poor breathing patterns, surgeries, and repetitive or cumulative traumas as a result of their activities of daily living. Poor thoracic mobility leads to a breakdown at the more mobile regions, including the lumbopelvic complex, due to the alterations in the transference of forces through the kinetic chain. This also causes compensatory movements through areas that are better designed to provide stability, including the lumbopelvic region, knees, and scapulae.

Perhaps most important, when this type of breathing is integrated with activation of the local system muscles (primarily transversus abdominis, multifidii, psoas major, and the pelvic floor), a powerful stabilization strategy known as the 'intra-abdominal pressure mechanism' is activated. The co-contraction of the local system muscles creates a tightening of the thoracolumbar fascia, which attaches these structures together. As the diaphragm contracts during functional breathing, it is aligned parallel to the pelvic floor, producing a stable 'canister' support of the trunk, spine, and pelvis. From this position, it powerfully increases the pressure inside the canister created by the diaphragm, pelvic floor, transversus abdominis and multifidi, which functions to elongate and decompress the spine while enabling pure rotational movement. The muscles push out into the fascial system of the TPC which creates a solid foundation for the extremities to work from without having to overuse the extremities to aid TPC stabilization. Hydraulic amplifier occurs when the multifidii and lumbar erector spinae contract into the thoracolumbar fascia and contraction of the transversus abdominus which draws the thoracolumbar fascia taut and thereby produces a stiffening effect on the thoracopelvic canister. This provides the trunk, spine, and pelvis the ability to simultaneously stabilize and decompress the spine, which is key to providing long-term health of the overall musculo-skeletal-fascial system.

2. CENTRATION

The goal for optimal movement in the human body is to optimally centrate or align the joint surfaces and to able to lengthen through the articulations, which provides the base for pure axial rotation. An important concept overlooked in many core stabilization strategies is joint centration and the local stabilization system of individual joints. The local system muscles attach close to the axis of rotation and are not direction specific, meaning that the position of the joints has no bearing on the effectiveness of their contractions. This enables these muscles to function efficiently in stabilizing joint motion. Joint centration is compromised when the larger global muscle system overpowers the local system, disrupting the optimal axis of rotation. While the global system muscles are extremely effective at producing global stabilization, their attachments, which tend to be further from the axis of rotation than the local stabilizers, cannot provide adequate intersegmental stabilization and tend to overcompress the joints when this stabilization strategy becomes chronic, as is common in individuals who have chronic pain.

The second component of joint centration is that the joints should move independently of each other under neuromuscular control. Referred to as 'dissociation', this essentially means that the right area is moving at the right time with the right amount of control. For example, a client should be able to initiate hip flexion without moving into a posterior pelvic tilt, and produce shoulder flexion without having to over-elevate the scapulae.

When a joint is stabilized and is able to dissociate appropriately from adjoining joint articulations, it allows for equal co-contraction of the surrounding musculature and the ability to lengthen through the joint structures, thereby producing efficient, coordinated, and fluid movements of each articulation within that portion of the kinetic chain.

3. INTEGRATION

Once the first two principles have been addressed, meaning that the client can breathe and stabilize appropriately, as well as efficiently stabilize and dissociate at the appropriate segments of the kinetic chain, these principles must be integrated into functional movement patterns. This optimal pattern of coordination between respiration, stabilization, and dissociation is the key to producing smooth, efficient movement. These optimal movement patterns have been lost in many of our clients through development (recall Vojta mentioned that one-third of children do not develop optimal neuromotor patterns), as well as modern conveniences such as baby activity centers (Johnny Jump Ups and similar apparatus), shoes and orthotic support, walking on flat surfaces, seated occupations, and modern conveniences such as computers, elevators, and cars. All of these factors drive and perpetuate dysfunction, creating many of the muscle imbalance syndromes so prevalent in modern society. To give these clients the best chance for success and keep up with their ever-changing environment that conspires to keep them sedentary and void of natural developmental activity, it is the job of the fitness professional, physical therapist, and movement specialist to help these individuals integrate these lost movement patterns back into their daily lives. When this goal is accomplished, the client has the best chance for success and the opportunity to live an active and full life.

FINAL WORD

While these concepts drive the fundamental ideas of corrective exercise and functional conditioning that have been presented in this book, there is one last component that is equally important in determining the effectiveness of this approach. At the end of the day, despite all the best efforts and intentions, it is likely more important who the therapist or trainer is as a person, and the extent that they are willing to be that person and give of themselves to serve their client, that will be the greatest determinant of their client's success. As the renowned poet Ralph Waldo Emerson so eloquently summed it up:

"The purpose of life is not to be happy. It is to be useful, to be honorable, to be compassionate, to have it make some difference that you have lived and lived well."

CASE STUDIES

Three case studies will be presented in this section. The goal is not to provide in-depth analysis of each client or of the exact corrective exercise and progressive training program that was utilized with each individual. They are presented to demonstrate a guideline to how the principles presented in this book can be used to re-establish function in the general population client and help restore them to a high level of function.

I. CLIENT WITH A ROTATOR CUFF TEAR AND THORACIC PAIN

A middle-aged female presented with left shoulder pain and an MRI diagnosis of a supraspinatus tear. She also reported thoracic pain on the same side of the shoulder tear. These symptoms have been present for the past three months and she has not responded favorably to conservative physical therapy or deep myofascial release. Her work included long hours on the computer and her discomfort limited how long she could work. She has been unable to exercise due to the intensity of her symptoms. Surgeries included left foot surgery approximately five years previously and bilateral breast augmentation.

PRIMARY FINDINGS

The client presented with stiffness of her left thorax and a forward, internally rotated left shoulder complex. She had poor respiratory patterns, demonstrating poor use of her left side diaphragm and overutilization of her accessory muscles of respiration. She had limited dorsiflexion in her left ankle and overall limited shoulder range of motion. During left single leg stance, she demonstrated a left lateral trunk shift and toe gripping.

PRIMARY TREATMENT

Initial treatment was focused on releasing soft-tissue restrictions and mobilizing her left thorax. Diaphragmatic breathing and core activation was instituted to restore balance to her system as well as improve thoracopelvic stabilization on her left side, and she was instructed to practice this at home. She was instructed to discontinue deep tissue massage in place of indirect myofascial techniques to help further calm down her nervous system and provide a more gentle form of myofascial release. After the initial few weeks of treatment, she was progressed to functional patterns of mini-squats, seated trunk rotation focusing on maintaining axial rotation, and wall supported plank isometric positions to restore scapular control. Over the next few weeks, her patterns were progressed to the point where she was able to perform each of the fundamental movement patterns with optimal neuromotor control. After eight weeks of treatment, she was released to work with a fitness professional to continue to progress her movement patterns.

2. CLIENT WITH MEDIAL KNEE PAIN

A 30-year-old male triathlete presented with right medial knee pain, which was present for approximately three weeks of the final two months of triathlon training. The pain was localized to the medial region of the knee and he did not experience the pain when biking or swimming. He reported a knee injury approximately ten years previously, although he did not recall any significant residual effects of the injury. He had tried conservative treatment, including massage and physical therapy, with no significant relief.

PRIMARY FINDINGS

The client presented with a thoracic lordosis and right internal hip rotation on postural evaluation. He primarily breathed utilizing an accessory dominant pattern. He demonstrated toe gripping and increased internal rotation of the hip during right single leg. There was bilateral gluteus medius inhibition on muscle testing.

PRIMARY TREATMENT

Initially the client was taken off running, although he was allowed to continue swimming and biking. Treatment included mobilization and soft-tissue techniques to the client's thorax. He was instructed in proper diaphragmatic breathing and core activation. In the initial phases he was instructed in isolated closed clam and supported squat patterns and progressed to the split squat and crab walk patterns. After two weeks he was progressed to split squat to single leg stance, with focus on maintaining a long spine, a squared pelvis, and the foot tripod. He was worked back into a run-walk routine to transition him back into running. This client progressed well and was able to complete his triathlon.

3. CLIENT WITH BILATERAL PLANTAR FASCIITIS

A 53-year-old female presented with bilateral plantar fasciitis. She failed to respond to conservative physical therapy treatment, which included soft-tissue work as well as ultrasound and exercise. Cortisone injections and orthotics provided only minimal relief. Significant history included one caesarian section and one vaginal birth. She had also undergone a hysterectomy several years prior to the onset of foot pain. The foot discomfort made walking unbearable and she was unable to exercise due to the pain. Her job required her to stand for several hours per day.

PRIMARY FINDINGS

The client presented with a thoracic extension (lordosis), posterior pelvic rotation, thoracolumbar hyperextension, and gripping through both her thoracic extensors and external obliques. Her thorax was rigid upon rocking and there was minimal lateral and posterior diaphragmatic excursion during respiration. There was palpable tenderness at the insertion of the plantar fascia and hypertonicity along the medial aspect of both feet. There was bilateral inhibition of her quadratus lumborum and gluteus medius as well as of the intrinsic muscles of her feet.

PRIMARY TREATMENT

Given her extensive surgical history and lack of response to both conservative as well as surgical approaches, this client's approach included specific soft-tissue release of her abdomen, mobilization of her thorax, and visualization techniques including diaphragmatic breathing to quiet the overactivity of the global muscles of the trunk. She was instructed to practice these visualizations and diaphragmatic breathing routinely throughout her day. The trunk was targeted because she had received extensive therapeutic intervention to her feet and ankles for the previous 18 months, with very minimal benefit. After two weeks she had a 50% decrease in foot tenderness and was able to stand for longer periods of time throughout the day with less pain. Specific soft-tissue techniques were instituted to activate inhibited foot muscles. She was instructed in the foot tripod and to hold this isometric position while standing for three repetitions of ten-second holds, five times per day. Her pain continued to decrease over the next few weeks and she was able to eventually return to short distances of pain-free walking before she was discharged from care.

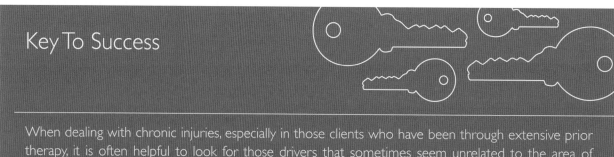

Key To Success

When dealing with chronic injuries, especially in those clients who have been through extensive prior therapy, it is often helpful to look for those drivers that sometimes seem unrelated to the area of complaint. In chronic pain and dysfunction, rarely is the area of complaint the driving factor — if it was, the client would have generally been rehabilitated as a result of their previous therapeutic interventions.

KEY: Perform a thorough history and evaluation on the client, making sure that special attention is paid to situations and regions that may not seem related, including prior surgeries (abdominal), traumas (acute as well as broken bones), and exercises (such as if they were a gymnast, dancer, etc. in their younger years). These are often the key to discovering the factors driving their current issues and are often overlooked.

KEY TERMINOLOGY

ABBREVIATIONS

AC – acromioclavicular joint

GH – glenohumeral joint

FA – femoroacetabular joint

FMT – functional muscle test

LPH – lumbo-pelvic-hip complex

MMT – manual muscle test

NMS – neuromusculoskeletal system

SIJ – sacro-iliac joint

SC – sternoclavicular joint

ST – scapulo-thoracic articulation

TL – thoracolumbar

TPC – thoracopelvic canister

ACTIVATION

Techniques to stimulate the proprioceptive system to increase the strength or response of the muscle system. Techniques for activation include visualization, isometric contractions, palpation (of musclofascial attachments, ligaments, skin, or joint capsule), and breathing.

ARTHROGENIC INHIBITION

Muscle inhibition caused by overstretching, overcompression, swelling, and/or internal derangement of a joint.

AUTOGENIC INHIBITION

A protective reflex regulated by the golgi tendon organs that causes muscle inhibition in response to excessive increases in muscle tension.

AXIS OF ROTATION

The imaginary central point or line through a joint around which the joint rotates. This axis is determined by the shape of the joints as well as the soft tissue structures (joint capsule and ligaments) that surround the articulation. Maintaining an ideal axis of rotation is dependent on ideal muscle synergy, optimal motor control, and the subsequent control of joint centration.

BRACING STRATEGY

Co-contraction of the muscles around a joint to improve gross stabilization. For example, co-contraction of the abdominals and erector spinae around the trunk and spine for improved stabilization. This strategy may become detrimental if maintained for long periods of time and/or it is the individual's only stabilization strategy.

CENTRAL NERVOUS SYSTEM

The part of the nervous system that includes the brain and spinal cord.

CENTRATION

Maintaining optimum congruency between articular surfaces while ensuring an optimal axis of rotation. Relies upon the ability to elicit the optimal neuromotor control to both stabilize and dissociate joint structures.

CO-ACTIVATION

A contraction of the muscles surrounding the joint to maintain an optimum axis of rotation and joint centration.

CONCENTRIC CONTRACTION

A muscle contraction in which the attachments of the muscle are getting closer together in order to move or accelerate a resistance.

CORRECTIVE EXERCISE

Exercise designed to specifically address postural alterations, faulty stabilization, and/or dysfunctional movement patterns, with the primary objective being enhanced efficiency of the neuromusculoskeletal system and with less detrimental stresses placed upon the joint and soft tissue structures.

DISSOCIATION

The ability to move one bone of a joint articulation independent of another under optimal motor control.

DRIVERS

Drivers are situations, conditions, or strategies that create a specific reaction in the body. For example, abdominal surgery is a strong driver of low back dysfunction because it can lead to inhibition of the local system and up-regulation of the global system of the lumbopelvic-hip complex. Other drivers that contribute to movement dysfunction include poor performance of exercise patterns, learned behaviors, poor cuing, fatigue, emotional stress, and poor nutrition.

ECCENTRIC CONTRACTION

A muscle contraction in which the muscle attachments are getting further apart in order to decelerate a movement.

FACILITATION

The hastening or enhancement of a reflexive reaction. Facilitation of a movement and/or activity can be enhanced by the use of palpations and reflexive stretching, as well as tactile, verbal cues, and/or visualization cues.

FEEDBACK

Sensory responses detected by various proprioceptors of the proprioceptive system in the periphery and relayed to the central nervous system regarding the direction, speed, amplitude, and force of movement or resistance in a particular body region.

FEED-FORWARD MECHANISM

Anticipatory pre-contraction of certain muscles (generally the one-joint muscles) milliseconds before a prime movement occurs in order to stabilize the joint structures. For example, research has demonstrated the transversus abdominis and pelvic floor pre-activate prior to the initiation of limb motion in individuals without pain or trauma.

FLEXION INTOLERANCE

The inability to tolerate flexion positions. An affected individual will tend to lose range of motion and/or strength due to articular and/or soft tissue stresses. This individual requires improved stabilization strategies and education as to proper ergonomics and exercise.

FOOT TRIPOD

The position of foot stability where the pressures on the foot are balanced and supported on the plantar surfaces of the first metatarsophalangeal, fifth metatarsophalangeal, and calcaneus.

FORCE COUPLE

Two or more muscles that pull relatively equally and oppositely, creating rotation. For example, contraction of the upper trapezius and lower trapezius creates upward rotation of the scapula.

FUNDAMENTAL MOVEMENT PATTERNS

The movement patterns that form the basis of all functional movement. These include squatting, lunging, pushing, pulling, rotation, breathing, and gait.

HILTON'S LAW

A nerve that innervates a specific joint also innervates the muscles and skin associated with that joint. This is the benefit of using kinesthetic feedback such as tapping, scratching, and kinesiotape.

HYPERMOBILITY

A joint that moves too freely secondary to loss of passive restraint of the joint capsule, ligaments and/or insufficient motor control.

HYPOMOBILITY

A joint that does not possess adequate mobility due to capsular or myofascial contracture as well as scar tissue or adhesions.

INHIBITION

The desensitization or lack of optimal neurological input into the contractile units (myofascial) of the body that is different from pure muscle weakness. In an inhibited muscle, there is sufficient neurophysiological support of the myofascial structures, whereas weakness often results secondary to the lack of ideal physiological support. Inhibited muscles that test weak will often test strong directly after an activation strategy such as origin-insertion palpation, isometric position, joint centration, or other type of kinesthetic (tactile) facilitation.

INTEGRATION

Coordination of fundamental movement patterns with optimal centration and ideal sequencing of stabilization, dissociation, and breathing.

ISOMETRIC CONTRACTION

A muscle contraction where there is no net change in the length of the muscle. These types of contractions are used to stabilize a joint or body position as well as aid the transition between eccentric and concentric contractions.

KINETIC CHAIN

The conjoined osseous, articular, myofascial, and neural structures that are interrelated and function together to produce an action within the body. For example, all the structures of the foot, ankle, knee, hip, and pelvis make up the lower kinetic chain, while the structures of the thorax, scapula, humerus, elbow, wrist, and hand comprise the upper kinetic chain.

LAW OF FACILITATION

When an impulse moves repeatedly through a certain neural pathway, it tends to move along this pathway with greater ease, meeting less resistance with each successive passing. Isometric positions, tactile or kinesthetic palpation, or kinesiotape are effective ways of facilitating muscle contraction.

LAW OF IRRADIATION

Irradiation is the spreading of excitement throughout the nervous system. Facilitation of a muscle along a kinetic chain or centration of one joint can improve functional muscle activation or centration along the entire kinetic chain. For example, centration of the ankle joint can help centrate the knee, the hip, and the pelvis. Similarly, activation of the scapular stabilizers can facilitate activation along the stabilizers of the entire upper arm.

LAW OF SUCCESSIVE INDUCTION

Contraction of an agonist followed by the contraction of its functional antagonist will result in a stronger contraction of the agonist. For example, contraction of the gluteus maximus followed by a contraction of the psoas major will result in a stronger contraction of the gluteus maximus on subsequent attempts.

LONG SPINE

Neutral alignment of the spine over top the pelvis where there is maximum length and stabilization at each region. The individual visualizes a string pulling cephalically (up) on the posterior aspect of the occiput and a string pulling caudally (down) upon the coccyx.

PERIPHERAL NERVOUS SYSTEM
The part of the nervous system that includes the cranial and spinal nerves.

PROPRIOCEPTION
The awareness of the parts of the body detected through the various proprioceptors and processed by the central nervous system. Improving proprioception is an important concept in motor control as injury, atrophy of one-joint stabilizers, and joint infusion have all been shown to decrease proprioceptive awareness of both joint position awareness and muscle activation.

RECIPROCAL INHIBITION
A normal muscle inhibition of the antagonist secondary to the contraction of the agonist. For example, contraction of the hip flexors inhibits the hip extensors.

REFLEXIVE INHIBITION
Muscle inhibition secondary to joint injury, which often results in the selective atrophy of the muscles most responsible for joint stabilization.

REVERSE MUSCLE FUNCTION
The distal attachment of a muscle pulling the proximal portion of the muscle towards itself. For example, the metatarsal attachment of the tibialis anterior pulling the tibia forward over the foot to aid ankle dorsiflexion during the gait cycle.

SQUARED PELVIS
The position where the pelvis is in a relatively neutral alignment and centrated between the two hip articulations when standing on two legs or upon the one hip when standing on one leg.

STABILIZATION
The ability to hold and maintain a joint position with the correct amount of tension and motor control for the task at hand.

SYNDROME
A syndrome is a group of signs and symptoms that together are indicative of a characteristic pathology or neuromusculofascial dysfunction. Syndromes are often the combined result of poor stabilization and movement strategies.

SYNERGIST DOMINANCE
In the presence of muscle or joint inhibition, the synergists assume the role of the primary stabilizers or movers. For example, inhibition of the gluteus maximus causes the hamstrings to become the prime movers of hip extension.

REFERENCES

Arnason, A., Sigurdsson, S.B., Gudmundsson, A., Holme, I., Engebretsen, L., Bahr, R.: 2004. Risk factors for injuries in football; *American Journal of Sports Medicine*; 32(1 Suppl): 5S–16S.

Askling, C., Tengvar, M., Sarrtok, T., Thorstensson, A.: 2000. Sports related hamstring strains-two cases with different etiologies and injury sites; *Scandinavian Journal of Medicine & Science in Sports*; 10(5): 304–307.

Baechle, T.R., Earle, R.W.: 2000. *Essentials of Strength Training and Conditioning*. Human Kinetics, Champaign, IL.

Bandy, W.D., Sanders, B.: 2001. *Therapeutic Exercise: Techniques for Intervention*. Lippincott Williams & Wilkins, Baltimore, MD.

Barker, K.L., Shamley, D.R., Jackson, D.: 2000. Changes in the cross-sectional area of multifidus and psoas in patients with unilateral back pain: the relationship to pain and disability: *Clinical Journal of Sport Medicine*; 10(4): 239–244.

Batmanghelidj, F.: 1995. *Your Body's Many Cries for Water: You Are Not Sick, You Are Thirsty! Don't Treat Thirst With Medications*. Global Health Solutions, Falls Church, VA.

Beardall, A.G.: 1982. *Clinical Kinesiology Instruction Manual*. A.G. Beardall, D.C., Lake Oswego, OR.

Beardall, A.G.: Beardall C.A.: 2006. *Clinical Kinesiology Vol I: Low Back and Abdomen*. Woodburn, OR.

Beardall, A.G.: Beardall C.A.: 2006. *Clinical Kinesiology Vol II: Pelvis and Thigh*. Woodburn, OR.

Beardall, A.G.: Beardall C.A.: 2006. *Clinicial Kinesiology Vol III: TMJ, Hyoid, and Other Cervical Muscles and Cranial Manipulation*. Woodburn, OR.

Beardall, A.G.: 1983. *Clinical Kinesiology Vol IV: Muscles of the Upper Extremities, Shoulder, Forearm, and Hand*. Lake Oswego, OR.

Beardall, A.G.: 1985. Clinical Kinesiology Vol V: *Muscles of the Lower Extremities, Calf, and Foot*. Lake Oswego, OR.

Beckman, S.M., Buchanan, T.S.: 1995. Ankle inversion injury and hypermobility: effect on hip and ankle muscle electromyography onset latency; *Archives of Physical Medicine and Rehabilitation*; 76(12): 1138–1143.

Binningsley, D.: 2003. Tear of the acetabular labrum in an elite athlete; *British Journal of Sports Medicine*; 37: 84–88.

Biondino C.R.: 1999. Anterior cruciate ligament injuries in female athletes. *Conn Med.* 63(11):657–660.

Bogduk, N.: 2005. *Clinical Anatomy of the Lumbar Spine and Sacrum. 4th ed.* Elsevier Churchill Livingstone, Philadelphia, PA.

Borich, M.R., Bright, J.M., Lorello, D.J., Cieminski, C.J., Buisman, T., Ludewig, P.M.: 2006. Scapular angular positioning at end range internal rotation in cases of glenohumeral internal rotation deficit; *Journal of Orthopaedic & Sports Physical Therapy*; 36(12): 926–934.

Boyle, M.: 2010. *Advances in Functional Training: Training Techniques for Coaches, Personal Trainers and Athletes*. On Target Publications, Aptos, CA.

Buhler, C.: 2004. *The Evaluation and Treatment of Low Back & Abdomen*. Course handouts, Kaysville, UT.

Burstein, A.H.: 1989. "The spine engine: a unified theory of the spine?" *Journal of Bone & Joint Surgery*; 71: 1580.

Caterisano, A., Moss, R.F., Pellinger, T.K., Woodruff, K., Lewis, V.C., Booth, W., Khadra, T.: 2002. The effect of back squat depth on the EMG activity of 4 superficial hip and thigh muscles; *Journal of Strength & Conditioning Research*; 16(3): 428–32.

Caulfield, B., Garrett, M.: 2004. Changes in ground reaction force during jump landing in subjects with functional instability of the ankle joint; *Clinical Biomechanics (Bristol Avon)*; 19(6): 617–21.

Cech, D., Martin, S.: 1995. *Functional Movement Development Across the Life Span*. W.B. Saunders, Philadelphia, PA.

Chek, P.: 2000. *Movement That Matters: a Practical Approach to Developing Optimal Functional Movement Skills*. C.H.E.K. Institute, Encinitas, CA.

Chek, P.: 2004. *How to Eat, Move and Be Healthy!: Your Personalized 4-step Guide to Looking and Feeling Great From the Inside Out*. C.H.E.K. Institute, San Diego, CA.

Cholewicki, J., Silfies, S.P., Shah, R.A., Greene, H.S., Reeves, N.P., Alvi, K., Goldberg, B.: 2005. Delayed trunk muscle reflex responses increase the risk of low back injuries; *Spine*; 30(23): 2614–2620.

Cohen, R.: 2010. *Introduction to Reflex Locomotion According to Vojta*. Course handouts. Philadelphia, PA.

Cole Lukasiewicz, A., McClure, P., Michener, L. Praff, N., Senneff, MD, B.: 1999. Comparison of 3-dimensional scapular position and orientation between subjects with and without shoulder impingement; *Journal of Orthopaedic & Sports Physical Therapy*; 29(10): 574–586.

Comerford, M.J., Mottram, S.L., Gibbons, S.G.T.: 2008. *Motor Control & Functional Stability Retraining for Sacro-Iliac Joint and Pelvic Stability Dysfunction*. Northeast Seminars, East Hampstead, NH.

Comerford, M.J., Mottram, S.L.: 2005. *Diagnosis & Musculoskeletal Management of Shoulder Impingements and Instabilities*. Northeast Seminars, East Hampstead, NH.

Comerford, M.J.: *Core Stability: Priorities in Rehabilitation of the Athlete*; www.Sportex.Net; 15–22.

Comerford, M.J.: *Screening to Identify Injury and Performance Risk: Movement Control Testing – The Missing Piece of the Puzzle*; Www.Sportex.Net; 21-26.

Cook, G.: 2003. *Athletic Body in Balance*. Human Kinetics, Champaign, IL.

Cowling, E.J., Steele, J.R., McNair, P.J.: 2003. Effect of verbal instructions on muscle activity and risk of injury to the anterior cruciate ligament during landing; *British Journal of Sports Medicine*; 37(2): 126–30.

Cowling, E.J., Steele, J.R.: 2001. Is lower limb muscle synchrony during landing affected by gender? Implications for variations in ACL injury rates; *Journal of Electromyography and Kinesiology*; 11(4): 263–8.

Cowling, E.J., Steele, J.R.: 2001. The effect of upper-limb motion on lower-limb muscle synchrony. Implications for anterior cruciate ligament injury; *Journal of Bone & Joint Surgery*; 83A(1): 35–41.

Coyle, D.: 2009. *The Talent Code*. Bantam Bell, New York, NY.

Croce, R.V., Russell, P.J., Swartz, E.E., Decoster, L.C.: 2004. Knee muscular response strategies differ by developmental level but not gender during jump landing; *Electromyography Clinical Neurophysiology*; 44(6): 339–348.

Cuthbert, S.C., Goodheart, Jr., G.J.: 2007. On the reliability and validity of manual muscle testing: a literature review; *Chiropractic & Osteopathy*; 15(4).

Cuthbert, S.C.: 2009. What are you doing about muscle weakness: Part I? *Dynamic Chiropractic*; 27(10).

Cuthbert, S.C.: 2009. What are you doing about muscle weakness: Part II: cervical spine? *Dynamic Chiropractic*; 27(14).

Cuthbert, S.C.: 2009. What are you doing about muscle weakness: Part III: lumbar spine? *Dynamic Chiropractic*; 27(18).

Dadebo, B., White, J., George, K.P.: 2004. A survey of flexibility training protocols and hamstring strains in professional football clubs in England; *British Journal of Sports Medicine*; 38(4): 388–394.

Dangaria, T.R. & Naesh, O.: 1998. Changes in cross-sectional area of psoas major muscle in unilateral sciatica caused by herniation. *Spine*; 15:928–931.

Dash, M., Telles, S.: 2001. Improvement in hand grip strength in normal volunteers and rheumatoid arthritis patients following yoga training; *Indian Journal of Physiology & Pharmacology*; 45(3): 355–360.

Decker, M.J., Hintermeister, R.A., Faber, MD, K.J. Hawkins, MD, R.J.: 1999. Serratus Anterior Muscle Activity During Selected Rehabilitation Exercises; *The American Journal of Sports Medicine*; 27(6): 784–791.

Decker, M.J., Tokish, MD, J.M., Ellis, H.B., Torry, M.R., Hawkins, MD, R.J.: 2003. Subscapularis muscle activity during selected rehabilitation exercises; *The American Journal of Sports Medicine*; 31: 126–134.

de Marche Baldon, R., Helissa Nakagawa, T., Batista Muniz, T., Ferreira Amorim, C., Dias Maciel, C., Viadanna Serra~ o, F.: 2009. Eccentric hip muscle function in females with and without patellofemoral pain syndrome; *Journal of Athletic Training*; 44(5): 490–496.

Eliasz, J., Mikuliszyn, R.S., Deren, M.: 2004. Measurement of force exerted on footplates by centrifuge subjects; *Aviation, Space and Environmental Medicine*; 75(6): 551–553.

Ellison, J.B., Rose, S.J., Sahrmann, S.A.: 1990. Patterns of hip rotation range of motion: a comparison between healthy subjects and patients with low back pain; *Physical Therapy*; 70(9): 537–541.

Fagenbaum, R., Darling, W.G.: 2003. Jump landing strategies in male and female college athletes and the implications of such strategies for anterior cruciate ligament injury; *American Journal of Sports Medicine*; 31(2): 233–240.

Fagerson, T.L.: 1998. *The Hip Handbook*. Butterworth-Heinemann, Woburn, MA.

Farrokhi, S., Pollard, C.D., Souza, R.B., Chen, Y.J., Reischl, S., Powers, C.M.: 2008.Trunk position influences the kinematics, kinetics, and muscle activity of the lead lower extremity during the forward lunge exercise; *Journal of Orthopaedic & Sports Physical Therapy*; 38(7): 403-409.

Forda, K.R., Manson, N.A., Evansa, B.K., Myera, G.D., Gwinnb, R.C., Heidtb, R.S., Hewetta, T.E.: 2006. Comparison of in-shoe foot loading patterns on natural grass and synthetic turf; *Journal of Science and Medicine in Sport*; 42: 1–8.

Franklin, E.N.: 2004. *Conditioning for Dance: Training for Peak Performance in All Dance Forms*. Human Kinetics, Champaign, IL.

Franklin, E.N.: 1996. *Dynamic Alignment Through Imagery*. Human Kinetics, Champaign, IL.

Frost, R.: 2002. *Applied Kinesiology: a Training Manual and Reference Book of Basic Principles and Practice.* North Atlantic, Berkeley, CA.

Fry, A.C., Smith, J.C., Schilling, B.K.: 2003. Effect of knee position on hip and knee torques during the barbell squat; *Journal of Strength & Conditioning Research;* 17(4): 629–33.

Gabbe, B.J., Finch, C.F., Bennell, K.L., Wajsweiner, H.: 2005. Risk factors for hamstring injuries in community level Australian football; *British Journal of Sports Medicine;* 39(2): 106–110.

Gibbons, S.: 2005. *Assessment & Rehabilitation of the Stability Function of the Psoas Major & the Deep Sacral Gluteus Maximus Muscles.* Kinetic Control, Ludlow, UK.

Gibbons, S.G.T., Comerford, M.J., Emerson, P.L.: 2002. Rehabilitation of the stability function of psoas major; *Orthopaedic Division Review;* January / February: 9–16.

Gibbons, S.G.T., Comerford, M.J.: 2001. Strength versus stability: part 1: concepts and terms; *Orthopaedic Division Review;* March / April: 21–27.

Gibbons, S.G.T., Comerford, M.J.: 2001. Strength versus stability: part 2: limitations and benefits; *Orthopaedic Division Review;* March / April: 28–33.

Gibbons, S.G.T., Mottram, S.L., Comerford, M.J., Phty, B.: 2001. Stability and movement dysfunction related to the elbow & forearm; *Orthopaedic Division Review;* Sept/Oct, 2001.

Gladwell, M.: 2005. *Blink.* Time Warner Book Group. New York, USA.

Gracovetsky, S.: 2008. *The Spinal Engine.* Serge Gracovetsky, PhD, St. Lambert, Q.C., Canada.

Grandjean, A.C., Reimers, K.J., Haven MC, Curtis G.L.: 2003. The effect on hydration of two diets, one with and one without plain water; *Journal of the American College of Nutrition;* 22(2): 165–173.

Grandjean, A.C., Reimers, K.J., Bannick, K.E., Haven, M.C. 2000. The effect of caffeinated, non-caffeinated, caloric and non-caloric beverages on hydration. *Journal of the American College of Nutrition;* 19(5):591–600.

Grimaldi, A, Richardson, C, Stantonb, W, Durbridgec, G, Donnellyd, W, & Hidesab, J.: 2009. The association between degenerative hip joint pathology and size of the gluteus medius, gluteus minimus and piriformis muscles. *Manual Therapy*, 14(6); p.605–610.

Groh, M.M., Herrera, J.: 2009. A comprehensive review of hip labral tears; *Current Reviews in Musculoskeletal Medicine;* 2:105–117.

Guyton, A.C.: 1991. *Textbook of Medical Physiology. 8th ed.* W.B. Saunders, Philadelphia, PA.

Hagins, M., Pietrek, MD, M., Sheikhzadeh, A., Nordin, M., Axen, K.: 2004. The effects of breath control on intra-abdominal pressure during lifting tasks; *Spine*; 29(4): 464–469.

Hannaford, C.: 1995. *Smart Moves: Why Learning Is Not All in Your Head.* Great Ocean, Alexander, NC.

Harris-Hayes, M., Sahrmann, S.A., Van Dillen, L.R.:2009. Relationship between the hip and low back pain in athletes who participate in rotation-related sports; *Journal of Sport Rehabilitation;* 18(1): 60–75.

Health, United States, 2008: *With Special Feature on the Health of Young Adults.* National Center for Health Statistics, Hyattsville, MD, 2009.

Hodges, P.W., Heijnen, I., Gandevia, S.C.: 2001. Postural activity of the diaphragm is reduced in humans when respiratory demand increases; *Journal of Physiology;* 537(3): 999–1008.

Hoskins, W., Pollard, H.: 2005. The management of hamstring injury – part 1: issues in diagnosis; *Manual Therapy;* 10(2): 96–107.

Hoskins, W., Pollard, H.: 2005. The management of hamstring Injury – part 2: issues in diagnosis; *Manual Therapy;* 10(3):180–190.

Hulme, J.A.: 2008. *Beyond Kegels: Bladder Health and the Pelvic Muscle Force Field.* The Prometheus Group; Chicago, IL.

Hungerford, B.: 2007. *Functional Load Transfer Through the Pelvic Girdle: An Overview of the Research Applicable to the Stork (One Leg Standing) Test.* 6th World Congress of Low Back & Pelvic Pain, Barcelona, Spain.

Kendall, F.P., McCreary, E.K., Provance, P.G., Rodgers, M.M., Romani, W.A.: 2005. *Muscles: Testing and Function With Posture and Pain.* 5th ed. Lippincott Williams & Wilkins, Baltimore, MD.

Khan, K.M., Cook, J.K.: 2004. Overuse tendon injuries: where does the pain come from? *Spine;* 29(22): E515–E519.

Kibler, MD, W.B, Ludewig, P.M., McClure, P., Uhl, T.L., Sciascia, A.: 2009. Scapular Summit 2009; *Journal of Orthopaedic & Sports Physical Therapy;* 39(11): A1–A13.

Kolar, P., Holubcova, Z., Frank, C., Liebenson, C., Kobesova, A.: 2009. *Exercise & the Athlete: Reflexive, Rudimentary & Fundamental Strategies.* International Society of Clinical Rehabilitation Specialists – course handouts, Chicago, IL.

Kolar, P., Kobesova, A., Holubcova, Z.: 2009. *Dynamic Neuromuscular Stabilization: A Developmental Kinesiology Approach.* Rehabilitation Institute of Chicago – course handouts, Chicago, IL.

Kujala, U.M., Orava, S., Jarvinen, M.: 1997. Hamstring injuries. Current trends in treatment and prevention; *Sports Medicine.* 23(6): 397–404.

Langevin, H.: 2002. Relationship of Acupuncture Points and Meridians to Connective Tissue Planes; The *Anatomical Record;* 269: 257–265.

Leaf, D.: 1995. *Applied Kinesiology Flowchart Manual.* David W. Leaf, Plymouth MA.

Lee, D.: 2003. *The Thorax: An Integrated Approach. 2nd ed.* Diane G. Lee Physiotherapist Corp, White Rock, BC.

Lee, D.: 2004. *The Pelvic Girdle: An Approach to the Examination and Treatment of the Lumbopelvic-Hip Region. 3rd ed.* Churchill Livingstone, Edinburgh.

Lee, L.: 2008. *Discover the Sports Pelvis: The Role of the Pelvis in Recurrent Groin, Knee, and Hamstring Pain & Injury.* The Mid-Atlantic Physical Therapy Associates course handouts, LLP.

Lee, L.: 2008. Is it time for a closer look at the thorax? *InTouch;* 1: 13-16.

Leetun, D.T., Ireland, M.L., Willson, J.D., Ballantyne, B.T., Davis, I.M.: 2004. Core stability measures as risk factors for lower extremity injury in athletes; *Medicine & Science in Sports & Exercise;* 36(6): 926–934.

Lephart, S.M., Ferris, C.M., Riemann, B.L., Myers, J.B., Fu, F.H.: 2002. Gender differences in strength and lower extremity kinematics during landing; *Clinical Orthopaedics and Related Research;* (401): 162–169.

Levine, S., Nguyen, T., Kaiser, L.R., Rubinstein, N.A., Maislin, G., Gregory, C., Rome, L.C., Dudley, G.A., Sieck, G.C., Shrager, J.B..: 2003. Human diaphragm remodeling associated with chronic obstructive pulmonary disease: clinical implications; *American Journal of Respiratory Critical Care Medicine;* 168(6):706–713.

Lewis, C.L., Sahrmann, S.A., Moran, D.W.: 2007. Anterior hip joint force increases with hip extension, decreased gluteal force, or decreased iliopsoas force; *J Biomech;* 40(16): 3725–3731.

Lewis, J.S., Wright, C., Green, A.: 2005. Subacromial impingement syndrome: the effect of changing posture on shoulder range of movement; *Journal of Orthopaedic & Sports Physical Therapy;* 35(2): 72–87.

Lewit, K.: 1994. The functional approach; *The Journal of Orthopaedic Medicine;* 16(3): 73–74.

Lewit, K.: 2008. Lessons for the future; *International Musculoskeletal Medicine;* 30(3): 133–140.

Liebenson, C.: 2007. *Rehabilitation of the Spine: a Practitioner's Manual. 2nd ed.* Lippincott Williams & Wilkins, Philadelphia, PA.

Lindsay, M.: 2008. *Fascia – Clinical Applications for Health and Human Performance.* Cengage Learning. Clifton Park, NY.

Lombard, W.P., & Abbott, F.M.: 1907. The mechanical effects produced by the contraction of individual muscles of the thigh of the frog. *American Journal of Physiology,* 20, 1–60.

Lubeck, D.P.: 2003. The costs of musculoskeletal disease: health needs assessment and health economics; *Best Practice & Research Clinical Rheumatology;* 17(3): 529–539.

Lum, L.C.: 1987. Hyperventilation syndromes in medicine and psychiatry: a review; *Journal of the Royal Society of Medicine;* 80: 229–231.

Lunden, J.B., Braman, J.P., Laprade, R.F., Ludewig, P.M.: 2010. Shoulder kinematics during the wall push-up plus exercise; *Journal of Shoulder and Elbow Surgery*; 19(2):216–23.

Magarey, M.E., Jones, M.A.: 1995. Dynamic evaluation and early management of altered motor control around the shoulder complex. *Applied Kinesiology Flowchart Manual – 3rd Edition,* David Leaf, Plymouth, MA – self published.

Malliaropoulos, N., Papalexandris, S., Papalada, A., Papacostas, E.: 2004. The role of stretching in rehabilitation of hamstring injuries: 80 athletes follow-up; *Medicine & Science in Sports & Exercise;* 36(5): 756–759.

Massery, M. The patient with multi-system impairments affecting breathing mechanics and motor control. In: Frownfelter D, Dean E, eds. *Cardiovascular and Pulmonary Physical Therapy Evidence and Practice, ed. 4.* St. Louis, MO.: Mosby & Elsevier Health Sciences; 2006:Chapter 39:695–717.

Massery, M.: 2009. *If You Can't Breathe, You Can't Function – Integrating the Pulmonary, Neuromuscular, and Musculoskeletal Systems in Pediatric Populations.* Pathways Center – course handouts, Glenview IL.

McClure, P.W., Michener, L.A., Karduna, A.R.: 2006. Shoulder function and 3-dimensional scapular kinematics in people with and without shoulder impingement syndrome; *Physical Therapy;* 86(8): 1075-1090.

McGill, S.: 2004. *Ultimate Back Fitness and Performance.* Wabuno, Waterloo, Ont.

McGill, S.: 2007 *Low Back Disorders: Evidence-based Prevention and Rehabilitation. 2nd ed.* Human Kinetics, Champaign, IL.

McGuine, T.A., Greene, J.J., Best, T., Leverson, G.: 2003. Balance as a predictor of ankle injuries in high school basketball players; *Manual Therapy;* 8(4): 195–206.

Meyerowitz, S.: 2001. *Water – The Ultimate Cure.* Sproutman Publications, Great Barrington, MA.

Michaud, T.C.: 1997. *Foot Orthoses and Other Forms of Conservative Foot Care.* T.C. Michaud, Newton, MA.

Mitchell, L.C.J., Ford, K.R., Minning, S., Myer, G.D., Mangine, R.E., Hewett, T.E.: 2008. Medial foot loading on ankle and knee biomechanics; *North American Journal of Sports Physical Therapy;* 3(3): 133–40.

Moeller, J., Lamb, M.M.: 1997. Anterior cruciate ligament injuries in female athletes: why are women more susceptible? *The Physician and Sports Medicine;* 25(4).

Muscolino, J.E.: 2006. *Kinesiology: the Skeletal System and Muscle Function.* Mosby Elsevier, St. Louis, MO.

Myer, G.D., Chu, D.A., Brent, J.L., Hewett, T.E.: 2008. Trunk and hip control neuromuscular training for the prevention of knee joint injury; *Clinics in Sports Medicine;* 27(3): 425–448.

Myer, G.D., Paterno, M.V., Ford, K.R., Hewett, T.E.: 2008. Neuromuscular training techniques to target deficits before return to sport after anterior cruciate ligament reconstruction; *Journal of Strength and Conditioning Research;* 22(3) 1–28.

Myer, G.D., Paterno, M.V., Ford, K.R., Quatman, C.E., Hewett, T.E.: 2006. Rehabilitation after anterior cruciate ligament reconstruction: criteria-based progression through the return-to-sport phase; *Journal of Orthopaedic & Sports Physical Therapy*; 36(6): 385–402.

Myers, J.B., Ju, Y., Hwang, J., McMahon, MD, P.J., Rodosky, MD, M.W., Lephart, S.M.: 2004. Reflexive muscle activation alterations in ahoulders with anterior glenohumeral instability; *The American Journal of Sports Medicine;* 32(4): 1013–1021.

Myers, J.B., Pasquale, M.R., Laudner, K.G., Sell, T.C., Bradley, J.P., Lephart, S.M.: 2005. On-the-field resistance-tubing exercises for throwers: an electromyographic analysis; *Journal of Athletic Training;* 40(1): 15–22.

Myers, T.W.: 2009. *Anatomy Trains: Myofascial Meridians for Manual and Movement Therapists. 2nd ed.* Elsevier, Edinburgh.

Nadler, S.F., Malanga, G.A., Bartoli, L.A., Feinberg, J.H., Prybicien, M., Deprince, M.: 2002. Hip muscle imbalance and low back pain in athletes: influence or core strengthening; *Medicine & Science in Sports & Exercise;* 34(1): 9–16.

Nadler, S.F., Malanga, G.A., Feinberg, J.H., Rubanni, M., Moley, P., Foye, P.: 2002. Functional performance deficits in athletes with previous lower extremity injury: *Clinical Journal of Sports Medicine;* 12(2): 73–78.

Nelson-Wong, E., Flynn, T., Callaghan, J.P.: 2009. Development of active hip abduction as a screening test for identifying occupational low back pain; *Journal of Orthopaedic & Sports Physical Therapy;* 39(9): 649-657.

O'Dell: 2006. *A Comprehensive Approach to Shoulder Training and Injury Resistance.* Explosively fit Strength Training, Nine Mile Falls, WA.

Page, P., Frank, C.C., Lardner, R.: 2010. *Chapter 10 - Restoration of Muscle Balance. Assessment and Treatment of Muscle Imbalance: the Janda Approach.* Human Kinetics, Champaign, IL. pp. 145.

Petersen, J, Holmich, P. Evidence based prevention of hamstring injuries in sports; *British Journal of Sports Medicine;* 39(6): 319–323.

Richardson, C., Hides, J., Hodges, P.W.: 2004. *Therapeutic Exercise for Lumbopelvic Stabilization: a Motor Control Approach for the Treatment and Prevention of Low Back Pain. 2ND ed. u.a.:* Churchill Livingstone, Edinburgh.

Roussel, N., Nijs, J., Truijen, S., Vervecken, L., Mottram, S., Stassijns, G.: 2009. Altered breathing patterns during lumbopelvic motor control tests in chronic low back pain: a case study; *European Spine Journal;* 18(7): 1066_1073.

Sahrmann, S.: 2002. *Diagnosis and Treatment of Movement Impairment Syndromes.* Mosby, St. Louis, MO.

Salci, Y., Kentel, B.B., Heycan, C., Akin, S., Korkusuz, F.: 2004. Comparison of landing maneuvers between male and female college volleyball players; *Clinical Biomechanics (Bristol, Avon);* 19(6): 622_628.

Schleip, R., Klingler, W., and Lehmann-Horn, F.: 2004. *Active Contraction of the Thoracolumbar Fascia - Indications of a New Factor in Low Back Pain Research With Implications for Manual Therapy, 5th Interdisciplinary World Congress on Low Back & Pelvic Pain.* Downloaded June 1, 2010: www.fasciaresearch. de/MelbourneReport.pdf.

Schleip, R., Klingler, W., and Lehmann-Horn, F.: 2004. Active fascial contractility: fascia may be able to contract in a smooth muscle-like manner and thereby influence musculoskeletal dynamics. *Medical Hypotheses;* 65: 273–277.

Schleip, R., Klingler, W., and Lehmann-Horn, F.: 2007. *Fascia Is Able to Contract in a Smooth Muscle-like Manner and Thereby Influence Musculoskeletal Mechanics.* 5th World Congress of Biomechanics; MEDIMOND International Proceedings; Munich, Germany. Downloaded June 1, 2010: www.fasciaresearch.com

Schleip, R., Klingler, W.,: 2005. Active fascial contractility: fascia is able to contract and relax in a smooth muscle-like manner and thereby influence biomechanical behavior. Department of Applied Physiology, Ulm University, Ulm, Germany. Downloaded June 1, 2010: www.fasciaresearch.de/2005PosterFreiburg.pdf.

Schleip, R., Naylor, I., Ursu, D., Melzer, W., Zorn, A., Wilke, H-J., Lehmann-Horn, F., Klingler, W.: 2006. Passive muscle stiffness may be influenced by active contractility of intramuscular connective tissue; *Medical Hypotheses;* 66: 66–71.

Schmidt, R.A., Wrisberg. C.A.: 2008. *Motor Learning and Performance: a Situation-based Learning Approach. 4th ed.* Human Kinetics, Champaign, IL.

Scott, M., Comerford, M.J., Mottram, S.L.: 2006. Transversus training – a waste of time in the gym; *Fitpro Network;* 30-32.

Sharkey, J.: 2008. *The Concise Book of Neuromuscular Therapy: a Trigger Point Manual.* Lotus Pub., Chichester, England.

Sher, J.S., Uribe, J.W., Posada, A., Murphy, B.J., Zlatkin, M.B.: 1995. Abnormal findings on magnetic resonance images of asymptomatic shoulders; *Journal of Bone and Joint Surgery:* 77: 10–15.

Sherry, M.A., Best, T.M.: 2004. A comparison of 2 rehabilitation programs in the treatment of acute hamstring strains; *Journal of Orthopaedic & Sports Physical Therapy;* 34(3): 116–125.

Shier, D., Butler, J., Lewis, R.: 2007. Hole's Human Anatomy & Physiology. 11th ed. McGraw-Hill, Dubuque, IA.

Shultz, S.J., Carcia, C.R., Perrin, D.H.: 2004. Knee joint laxity affects muscle activation patterns in the healthy knee; *Journal of Electromyography and Kinesiology;* 14(4): 475–483.

Smith, M., Coppieters, M., Hodges, P.: 2005. Effect of experimentally induced low back pain on postural sway with breathing; *Experimental Brain Research;* 166(1): 109–117.

Smith, M., Russell, A., Hodges, P.: 2006. Disorders of breathing and incontinence have a stronger association with back pain than obesity and physical activity; *Australian Journal of Physiotherapy;* 52(1): 11–16.

Stedman, TL. 1990. *Stedman's Medical Dictionary – 25th Edition*. Williams and Wilkins, Baltimore MD.

Strachan, D.P.: 1991. Ventilatory function as a predictor of fatal stroke; *BMJ;* 302(6768): 84–87.

Swartz, E.E., Decoster, L.C., Russell, P.J., Croce, R.V.: 2005. Effects of developmental stage and sex on lower extremity kinematics and vertical ground reaction forces during landing; *Journal of Athletic Training;* 40(1): 9–14.

Taleb, N. 2007. *The Black Swan: The Impact of the Highly Improbable*. Random House, New York, NY.

Taunton, J.E., Ryan, M.B., Clement, D.B., McKenzie, D.C., Lloyd-Smith, D.R., Zumbo, B.D.: 2002. A retrospective case-control analysis of 2002 running injuries; *British Journal of Sports Medicine;* 36: 95–101.

Thie, J.F., Thie., M.: 2005. *Touch for Health: the Complete Edition : a Practical Guide to Natural Health With Acupressure Touch and Massage*. DeVorss, Camarillo, CA.

Umphred, D. A.: 2007. *Neurological Rehabilitation*. 5th ed. Mosby Elsevier, St. Louis, MO.

Valtin, H. 2002. "Drink at least eight glasses of water a day." Really? Is there scientific evidence for "8x8"? *American Journal Regulatory, Integrative and Comparitive Physiology;* 283: R993–R1004.

Van Dillen, L.R., Bloom, N.J., Gombatto, S.P., Susco, T.M.: 2008. Hip rotation range of motion in people with and without low back pain who participate in rotation-related sports. *Phys Ther Sport;* 9(2): 72–81.

Verall, G.M., Slavotinek J.P., Barnes, P.G.: 2005. The effect of sports specific training on reducing the incidence of hamstring injuries in professional Australian Rules football players; *Br. J Sports Med;* 39(6): 363–368.

Verrall, G.M., Slavotinek, J.P., Barnes, P.G., Fon, G.T., Spriggins, A.J.: 2001. Clinical risk factors for hamstring muscle strain injury: a prospective study with correlation of injury by magnetic resonance imaging; *British Journal of Sports Medicine;* 35: 435–440.

Verrall, G.M., Slavotinek, J.P., Barnes, P.G., Fon, G.T.: 2003. Diagnostic and prognostic value of clinical findings in 83 athletes with posterior thigh injury: comparison of clinical findings with magnetic resonance imaging documentation of hamstring muscle strains; *American Journal of Sports Medicine;* 31(6): 969–973.

Walther, D.S.: 2000. *Applied Kinesiology: Synopsis. 2nd ed*. Systems DC, Pueblo, CO.

Ward, M.Glasoe, W.M., Yack, H.J., Saltzman, C.L.: 1999. Anatomy and biomechanics of the first ray physical therapy; *Physical Therapy;* 79 (9): 854–859.

Woods, C., Hawkins, R.D., Maltby, S., Hulse, M., Thomas, A., Hodson, A.: 2004. The Football Association Medical Research Programme: an audit of injuries in professional football—analysis of hamstring injuries; *British Journal of Sports Medicine;* 38: 36–41.

Xu, M.D., J.Kochanek, K.D., Murphy, S.L.; Tejada-Vera, B.: 2010. *Deaths: Final Data for 2007;* National Vital Statistics Report; 58(19).

Zanulak, B.T., Ponce, P.L., Straub, S.J., Medvecky, M.J., Avedisian, L., Hewett, T.E.: 2005. Gender comparison of hip muscle activity during single-leg landing; *Journal of Orthopaedic & Sports Physical Therapy;* 35(5): 292–299.

Zazulak, B.T., Hewett, T.E., Reeves, N.P., Goldberg, MD, B., Cholewicki, J.: 2007. Deficits in neuromuscular control of the trunk predict knee injury risk: a prospective biomechanical-epidemiologic study; *The American Journal of Sports Medicine;* 35(7): 1123-1130.

INDEX

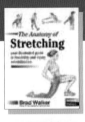
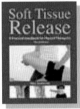
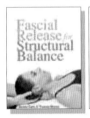 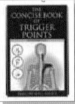 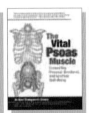 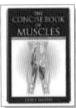

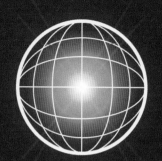

Institute for Integrative Health & Fitness Education

EDUCATE. EMPOWER. EXCEL.

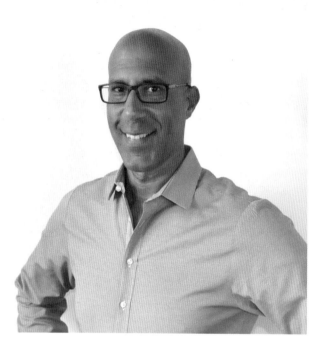

Dr. Evan Osar is an internationally recognized speaker, author, and expert on assessment, corrective exercise, and movement. Audiences around the world have heard Dr. Osar's dynamic presentations. He is known for helping make complicated topics such as assessment and corrective exercise easy to apply. He has developed the industry's most advanced training certifications: Integrative Corrective Exercise Instructor™ and Integrative Movement Specialist™. With his wife Jenice Mattek, Dr. Osar created the Institute for Integrative Health and Fitness Education™, an on-line educational resource for the health and fitness professional that specializes in posture and movement.

To book Dr. Osar to lead a workshop or keynote your event , contact:
helpdesk@fitnesseducationseminars.com

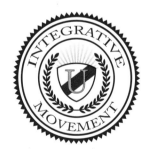
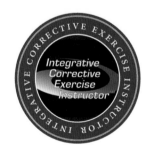
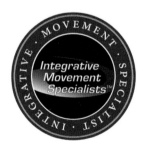

www.IIHFE.com